The Special Care Patient

Guest Editor

BURTON S. WASSERMAN, DMD, DABSCD

DENTAL CLINICS OF NORTH AMERICA

www.dental.theclinics.com

April 2009 • Volume 53 • Number 2

SAUNDERS an imprint of ELSEVIER, Inc.

W.B. SAUNDERS COMPANY
A Division of Elsevier Inc.

1600 John F. Kennedy Boulevard • Suite 1800 • Philadelphia, Pennsylvania 19103-2899

http://www.dental.theclinics.com

DENTAL CLINICS OF NORTH AMERICA Volume 53, Number 2
April 2009 ISSN 0011-8532, ISBN-13: 978-1-4377-0467-9, ISBN-10: 1-4377-0467-0

Editor: John Vassallo; j.vassallo@elsevier.com
Developmental Editor: Theresa Collier

Dental Clinics of North America (ISSN 0011-8532) is published quarterly by Elsevier Inc., 360 Park Avenue South, New York, NY 10010-1710. Months of issue are January, April, July, and October. Business and Editorial Offices: 1600 John F. Kennedy Boulevard, Suite 1800, Philadelphia, PA 19103-2899. Customer Service Office: 11830 Westline Industrial Drive, St. Louis, MO 63146. Periodicals postage paid at New York, NY and additional mailing offices. Subscription prices are $207.00 per year (domestic individuals), $347.00 per year (domestic institutions), $100.00 per year (domestic students/residents), $246.00 per year (Canadian individuals), $437.00 per year (Canadian institutions), $297.00 per year (international individuals), $437.00 per year (international institutions), and $150.00 per year (international and Canadian students/residents. International air speed delivery is included in all *Clinics* subscription prices. All prices are subject to change without notice. **POSTMASTER:** Send address changes to *Dental Clinics of North America*, 11830 Westline Industrial Drive, St. Louis, MO 63146. **Customer Service (orders, claims, online, change of address): Elsevier Periodicals Customer Service, 11830 Westline Industrial Drive, St. Louis, MO 63146. Tel: 1-800-654-2452 (U.S. and Canada). Fax: 314-523-5170. E-mail: journalscustomerservice-usa@elsevier.com (for print support); journalsonlinesupport-usa@elsevier.com (for online support).**

Reprints. For copies of 100 or more, of articles in this publication, please contact the Commercial Reprints Department, Elsevier Inc., 360 Park Avenue South, New York, NY 10010-1710. Tel.: 212-633-3812; Fax: 212-462-1935; E-mail: reprints@elsevier.com.

The Dental Clinics of North America is covered in *MEDLINE/PubMed (Index Medicus), Current Contents/Clinical Medicine, ISI/BIOMED* and *Clinahl.*

Printed and bound by CPI Group (UK) Ltd, Croydon, CR0 4YY
Transferred to Digital Print 2011

Contributors

GUEST EDITOR

BURTON S. WASSERMAN, DMD, DABSCD
Founding Chairman and Program Director, Dental and Oral Medicine, New York Hospital Queens, Flushing; Chairman, Dental Medicine, Wyckoff Heights Medical Center, Brooklyn; Chairman, Committee for Network Dental Services, New York Presbyterian Healthcare System, New York City; Clinical Professor of Dentistry, Columbia University, College of Dental Medicine; Clinical Professor of Surgery, Weill Medical College of Cornell University, New York City; Assistant Professor of Community Dentistry, SUNY Stony Brook, School of Dental Medicine, Stony Brook; Private Practice, Flushing, New York

AUTHORS

DEBRA CINOTTI, DDS
Clinical Associate Professor, Department of General Dentistry; and Program Coordinator, Dental Care for the Developmentally Disabled Program; and Associate Dean for Admissions and Student Affairs, School of Dental Medicine, Stony Brook University, Stony Brook, New York

JOHN M. COKE, DDS
Professor, Department of Diagnostic Sciences; and Director of Hospital Dentistry; and Director of General Dental Residency, University of Alabama-Birmingham School of Dentistry, Birmingham, Alabama

MARTIN J. DAVIS, DDS
Associate Dean, Student and Alumni Affairs, Columbia University College of Dental Medicine and Professor of Pediatric Dentistry, Columbia University College of Dental Medicine, New York

NANCY J. DOUGHERTY, DMD, MPH
Associate Clinical Professor, Department of Pediatric Dentistry, New York University College of Dentistry, New York; Clinical Assistant Professor, Departments of Dentistry and Pediatrics, Albert Einstein College of Medicine; Director, Postgraduate Program in Pediatric Dentistry, Department of Dentistry, North Bronx Healthcare Network, Jacobi Medical Center, Bronx, New York

MICHAEL D. EDWARDS, DMD
Clinical Associate Professor, Department of Comprehensive Dentistry, University of Alabama-Birmingham School of Dentistry, Birmingham, Alabama

JUNE FALAGARIO-WASSERMAN, MA, LMHC
Coordinator, Child and Adolescent Services; and Clinical Supervisor, Advanced Center for Psychotherapy, Jamaica Hospital and Medical Center, Jamaica Estates, New York

FRED S. FERGUSON, DDS
Distinguished Teaching Professor; and Professor of Pediatric Dentistry; and Acting Chair; and Director, Dental Care for the Developmentally Disabled Program, Department of Children's Dentistry, School of Dental Medicine, Stony Brook University, Stony Brook, New York

PAUL GLASSMAN, DDS, MA, MBA
Professor of Dental Practice, and Director of Community Oral Health, University of the Pacific Arthur A. Dugoni School of Dentistry, San Francisco, California

KELLY P. HALLIGAN, DDS, RCSEd-SND
Assistant Professor, Department of Restorative Dentistry, The University of Texas Health Science Center at San Antonio Dental School, San Antonio, Texas

TIMOTHY J. HALLIGAN, DMD
Colonel and 59th Dental Group Commander, Lackland Air Force Base, San Antonio, Texas

ROBERT G. HENRY, DMD, MPH
Acting Chief, Department of Dental Services, Veterans Affairs Medical Center; Clinical Associate Professor, University of Kentucky College of Dentistry; Research Associate, Sanders-Brown Center on Aging, Lexington, Kentucky

ARTHUR H. JESKE, DMD, PhD
Professor and Dean for Strategic Planning, The University of Texas at Houston Health Science Center Dental Branch, Houston, Texas

SHEILA H. KOH, DDS
Associate Professor and Director of the Special Patient Clinic, The University of Texas at Houston Health Science Center Dental Branch, Houston, Texas

SHANTANU LAL, DDS
Division of Pediatric Dentistry, Columbia University College of Dental Medicine, New York, New York

BURTON L. NUSSBAUM, DDS, RCS Ed
Adjunct Professor of Pediatric Dentistry, University of Pennsylvania School of Dental Medicine, The Children's Hospital of Philadelphia; Special Needs Dentist, Thomas Jefferson University Medical School and Hospital, Philadelphia, Pennsylvania; Dentistry for Special People, Cherry Hill, New Jersey

STEVEN P. PERLMAN, DDS, MScD
Global Clinical Director, Special Olympics, Special Smiles; Associate Clinical Professor of Pediatric Dentistry, The Boston University School of Dental Medicine, Boston, Massachusetts

RICK RADER, MD
Director, Morton J Kent Habilitation Center, Orange Grove Center; Adjunct Professor of Human Development, University of Tennessee, Chattanooga, Tennessee

KAREN A. RAPOSA, RDH, MBA
Senior Manager of Professional Relations, Colgate Oral Pharmaceuticals, Inc., New York

MIRIAM R. ROBBINS, DDS, MS
Clinical Associate Professor and Associate Chair, Department of Oral and Maxillofacial Pathology, Radiology and Medicine, New York University College of Dentistry, New York, New York

MAUREEN ROMER, DDS, MPA
Associate Professor and Director of Special Care Dentistry, Arizona School of Dentistry and Oral Health, A.T. Still University, Mesa, Arizona

MARK SLOVIN, DDS
Director, Dental Phobia Program; and Assistant Clinical Professor, Department of General Dentistry, Stony Brook University School of Dental Medicine, Stony Brook, New York

BARBARA J. SMITH, PhD, RDH, MPH
Manager, Geriatric and Special Needs Populations, Council on Access, Prevention, & Interprofessional Relations, American Dental Association, Chicago, Illinois

BENJAMIN H. SOLOMOWITZ, DMD
Director of Residency Education, and Dentist Anesthesiologist, Department of Dentistry, Interfaith Medical Center; General Dentistry and Dental Anesthesiology, Brooklyn, New York

PAUL SUBAR, DDS
Assistant Professor of Dental Practice, University of the Pacific Arthur A. Dugoni School of Dentistry, San Francisco, California

S. THIKKURISSY, DDS, MS
Assistant Professor, Pediatric Dentistry, The Ohio State University College of Dentistry, Nationwide Children's Hospital, Columbus, Ohio

MARY L. VOYTUS, DDS
Director, Dental Residency Program; and Director of Medical Education, Division of Dentistry, Department of Medical Education, Mountainside Hospital, Montclair, New Jersey

H. BARRY WALDMAN, DDS, MPH, PhD
Distinguished Teaching Professor, Department of General Dentistry, School of Dental Medicine, Stony Brook University, Stony Brook, New York

ALLEN WONG, DDS, FACD
Assistant Professor, Department of Dental Practice, University of the Pacific Arthur A. Dugoni School of Dentistry, San Francisco, California

Contents

Dedication xiii

Burton S. Wasserman

Preface xv

Burton S. Wasserman

Issues in Access to Oral Health Care for Special Care Patients 169

Martin J. Davis

Access to oral health care for persons with special health care needs is quite limited. Psychologic, economic, and physical barriers exist that prevent these patients, who may have complex medical histories and physical or psychologic disabilities, from accessing appropriate continuing dental care. There are ways to surmount each of these barriers, typically with both positive and negative aspects that must be considered. Education of the health care professionals, the patients, government officials, third-party payers, and colleagues in all aspects of health care, is needed. The ultimate answer is education of and cooperation by all concerned, including the patients and caretakers.

Health Related Issues for Individuals with Special Health Care Needs 183

H. Barry Waldman, Rick Rader, and Steven P. Perlman

More than 50 million individuals in the United States with developmental disabilities, complex medical problems, significant physical limitations, and a vast array of other conditions considered under the rubric of "disabilities" live in our communities, many as a result of deinstitutionalization and mainstreaming. Children and adults with special health care needs have become a much more integral and visible component of everyday life. This process represents an ongoing change in perceptions about individuals with disabilities and subsequent reform of policies concerning the rights and the principles of care for people with special needs. The reform was built upon an increased role for the family and community health practitioners in providing needed care.

Planning Dental Treatment for People with Special Needs 195

Paul Glassman and Paul Subar

People with disabilities and other special needs present unique challenges for oral health professionals in planning and carrying out dental treatment. This article presents a schema for planning dental treatment that encourages the oral health provider to fully consider multiple medical, social, psychologic and dental findings when preparing treatment recommendations for a patient with special needs. If these factors are fully integrated, the resulting treatment recommendations provide the best chance of helping the individual achieve and maintain a lifetime of oral health.

Special Needs of Anxious and Phobic Dental Patients **207**

Mark Slovin and June Falagario-Wasserman

Dentally anxious and phobic individuals are an underserved special needs population because of their avoidance of treatment. Dentists and their auxiliary staff, with an understanding of the etiologies leading to this potentially serious health obstacle, can enhance the patient's overall quality of life. Techniques are available for dentists to evaluate and treat this critical phenomenon. Through proper information, education, and staff sensitivity, these individuals can be rehabilitated and enjoy improved oral and systemic health.

Minimal and Moderate Oral Sedation in the Adult Special Needs Patient **221**

John M. Coke and Michael D. Edwards

Oral minimal/moderate sedation can be an effective tool to aid in the dental management of adult special needs patients. Specific sedative drugs must be chosen by the dentist that can be used safely and effectively on these patients. This article focuses on a select number of these drugs, specific medical and pharmacologic challenges presented by adult special needs patients, and techniques to safely administer oral minimal and moderate sedation.

Treatment of Mentally Disabled Patients with Intravenous Sedation in a Dental Clinic Outpatient Setting **231**

Benjamin H. Solomowitz

Treating the special care patient is challenging for the treating dentist and dentist anesthesiologist. The goal is to have a patient free of disease and pain restored with aesthetic and functional use of his/her oral cavity. The challenge is to incorporate the patient's medical, physical, behavioral, financial, and oral hygiene considerations into this goal. This article describes clinical techniques used to treat special care patients under intravenous sedation in an outpatient dental clinic setting. The discussion includes how to make a preoperative dental diagnosis, how to start an intravenous line painlessly, intravenous medications used in outpatient sedation, clinical tips for dentistry with special care patients, and postoperative evaluation.

Evaluation, Scheduling, and Management of Dental Care Under General Anesthesia for Special Needs Patients **243**

Mary L. Voytus

Dental care in the operating room requires expertise to be efficient, effective, and comprehensive. By gathering appropriate information preoperatively, intraoperatively, and postoperatively, the dentist can assume the leadership role that is required for effective dental care. Standardizing procedures, while including the training of residents, can meet the dental goals for comprehensive dental management.

Treatment Planning Considerations for Adult Oral Rehabilitation Cases in the Operating Room **255**

Allen Wong

Treatment planning for adult oral rehabilitation starts before cases are scheduled and continues after the discharge phase. Practitioners providing dental care must be competent in all phases of dentistry and comfortable in the operating room setting. Dental caries risk assessment and medical risk assessment are important in developing comprehensive and predictable treatment plans. Oral rehabilitation in the operating room for patients who have special needs is a growing concern. Coordinating medical procedures with oral rehabilitation procedures while patients are under general anesthetic is an efficient use of sedation. A systematic approach for treatment plan consideration is explored for oral rehabilitation cases using general anesthesia or monitored anesthesia care.

Managing Older Patients Who Have Neurologic Disease: Alzheimer Disease and Cerebrovascular Accident **269**

Robert G. Henry and Barbara J. Smith

Neurologic diseases represent some of the most common disabling and costly conditions in older age. Alzheimer disease and cerebrovascular accidents (strokes) are two of the most common neurologic conditions, and represent the leading causes of nursing home placement. Dental professionals will be caring for older patients who have age-associated neurologic diseases, including Alzheimer disease and stroke because of the increased longevity of the United States population coupled with improved survivorship of these conditions as a result of advanced medical diagnosis and treatment. Understanding the clinical manifestations of these two common, but distinctly different, neurologic conditions will enable dental professionals to provide safe and rational dental care.

Dental Management of Special Needs Patients Who Have Epilepsy **295**

Miriam R. Robbins

Patients who have developmental disabilities and epilepsy can be safely treated in a general dental practice. A thorough medical history should be taken and updated at every visit. A good oral examination to uncover any dental problems and possible side effects from antiepileptic drugs is necessary. Stability of the seizure disorder must be taken into account when planning dental treatment. Specific considerations for epileptic patients include the treatment of oral soft tissue side effects of medications and damage to the hard and soft tissue of the orofacial region secondary to seizure trauma. Most patients who have epilepsy can and should receive functionally and esthetically adequate dental care.

etiologies for SIB. This complication necessitates a team approach that includes medical and behavioral specialists.

Oral Health Burden in Children with Systemic Diseases **351**

S. Thikkurissy and Shantanu Lal

Children who have systemic diseases face a burden of disease distinctly greater than their healthy counterparts. Neglect or delay of addressing this burden can lead not only to significant morbidity for the child, but also to family dysfunction. This article addresses issues salient to the understanding of oral health burden in children and families living with systemic disease. Topics include the parent as caregiver, children who have cerebral palsy, juvenile arthritis, developmental delay, and organ diseases.

Behavioral Management for Patients with Intellectual and Developmental Disorders **359**

Karen A. Raposa

Intellectual and developmental disorders can severely impair a patient's ability to communicate and socialize. Individuals with such disorders tend to have unusual ways of learning, paying attention, and reacting to different sensations. Symptoms can range from very mild to very severe. To properly treat these patients and, if necessary, refer them for appropriate medical care, dental professionals must be able to recognize the signs and symptoms of each patient's specific disability. This article gives details about behavior associated with intellectual and developmental disorders and describes specific techniques for care that may be used routinely at home and carried into the dental setting.

Home Oral Health Practice: The Foundation for Desensitization and Dental Care for Special Needs **375**

Fred S. Ferguson and Debra Cinotti

As oral health is increasingly recognized as a foundation for health and wellness, caregivers for special needs patients are an essential component of the oral health team and must become knowledgeable and competent in home oral health practice. Education and training for caregivers should become a standard of care early in the first year of life for any child with developmental delay or any person, regardless of age, who experiences an illness or event that compromises their ability to provide self oral health care. Given the implication of poor oral health to general health and health care costs, home oral health practice is a significant factor in dental care, general health, quality of life, and controlling health care costs.

Index **389**

FORTHCOMING ISSUES

July 2009

Oral Health Care Access

Gary A. Colangelo, DDS, MGA
Guest Editor

October 2009

Trauma and Emergency Care

Gerald A. Ferretti, DDS, MS, MPH
and Sami Chogle, BDS, DMD, MSD
Guest Editors

January 2010

Treatment of Periodontics

Frank A. Scannapieco, DMD, PhD
Guest Editor

RECENT ISSUES

January 2009

Evidence-based Dentistry

Mark V. Thomas, DMD *Guest Editor*

October 2008

Contemporary Dental and Maxillofacial Imaging

Steven L. Thomas, DDS, MS and
Christos Angelopoulos, DDS, MS
Guest Editors

July 2008

Handbook of Dental Practice

Harry Dym, DDS and Orrett E. Ogle, DDS
Guest Editors

RELATED INTEREST

Pediatric Clinics of North America October 2008 (Vol. 55, No. 5)
Developmental Disabilities, Part I
Donald E. Greydanus, MD, Dilip R. Patel, MD, and Helen D. Pratt, PhD,
Guest Editors

Pediatric Clinics of North America December 2008 (Vol. 55, No. 6)
Developmental Disabilities, Part II
Donald E. Greydanus, MD, Dilip R. Patel, MD, and Helen D. Pratt, PhD,
Guest Editors

Dedication

I am honored to dedicate this book to all the special needs dental patients who often are challenged in finding willing and well-trained providers to deliver optimal dental and oral health care.

Burton S. Wasserman, DMD, DABSCD
55-14 Main Street
Flushing, NY 11355, USA

E-mail address:
bswasser@nyp.org (B.S. Wasserman)

Dent Clin N Am 53 (2009) xiii
doi:10.1016/j.cden.2008.12.019

dental.theclinics.com

Preface

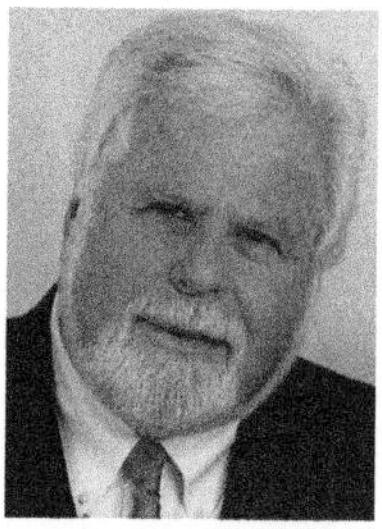

Burton S. Wasserman, DMD, DABSCD
Guest Editor

During the past decade, dental treatment for special needs patients has received national attention. These patients face unique challenges in accessing oral health care. Special needs patients traditionally have been treated by pediatric dentists, and general dentists often are not trained adequately or do not have the necessary physical facilities to provide optimal care. As the patients reach adulthood, it becomes increasingly difficult to continue treatment with a pediatric dentist or to find a general dentist who is willing and appropriately trained to deal with complex behavioral management issues.

Dental schools have become aware of this national dental problem and have made inroads to incorporate special needs training in their respective core curricula. Schools like S.U.N.Y. Stony Brook School of Dental Medicine have partnered with hospital general practice residency programs (New York Hospital Queens) to include special needs training in a postgraduate setting.

A combination of current trends, increased interest, and lack of comprehensive education to our profession has stimulated the idea that a text devoted to the special needs dental patient was long overdue.

Mr. John Vassallo, the Editor of *Dental Clinics of North America*, spearheaded the initiative to develop a "world class" text that would clearly define the aspects and issues that face the special needs dental patient.

I was humbled to accept the guest editorship of this very important issue. Our primary goal was to make a very readable and informative issue that would touch all the relevant elements of special care dentistry, including access, definition, disease entities, treatment options, and national trends.We assembled the best practitioners in special care dentistry to develop articles in their particular areas of expertise. Of course, the outcome of this outstanding edition of *Dental Clinics of North America* is dedicated to the oral health care of all special needs patients.

Dent Clin N Am 53 (2009) xv–xvi
doi:10.1016/j.cden.2008.12.012

I thank my wife, June Wasserman, my children, grandchildren, and my entire family as well as my hospital support staff and private practice staff for their love and patience during the preparation of this important project.

Burton S. Wasserman, DMD, DABSCD
55-14 Main Street
Flushing, New York 11355, USA

E-mail address:
bswasser@nyp.org (B.S. Wasserman)

Issues in Access to Oral Health Care for Special Care Patients

Martin J. Davis, DDS

KEYWORDS

- Oral health • Special health care needs • Access
- Barriers to care • Third part insurers
- Dental health coordinators • Continuing education
- Underestimating oral health care needs

THE SCOPE OF THE ACCESS ISSUE

Access to health care is a widely examined, emotion-laden issue. Not only life and death reflect access to adequate health care, but so do presidential elections and the rise and fall of major businesses. Dental care access is a complex subset of the debate. In a recent *New York Times* article entitled, "Boom Times for U.S. Dentists, But Not for Americans' Teeth," it was noted that access to health care, oral health care in particular, presents a well-documented challenge worldwide and specifically in the United States. The article contrasted the substantial incomes of United States dentists with data reflecting the limited or complete lack of access of individuals in lower socioeconomic status.[1] The article referenced the now well-known death of 12-year-old Deamonte Driver in Maryland as a result of his Medicaid status and, consequently, limited access to oral health care. His mother could not identify a dentist who would accept him as a patient. His dental caries produced infection, and eventually a brain abscess took his life. He died after two brain operations and an estimated quarter million dollars in medical care.[2]

The American Dental Association (ADA) and multiple oral health organizations continually report on the limitations of access, generally agreeing that 30% of Americans have limited or no access to oral health care. The ADA president, Dr. Mark Feldman, responded to the *New York Times* article in the ADA News on September 17, 2007, by stating, "We can't expect to meet this need by charity work alone. Legislators need to act to provide funds for needed care." Feldman further noted, "All of us must work harder to improve the oral health of the millions of Americans who don't have adequate access to dental care."[3] Pointedly demonstrating the acute nature of the oral health care access problem, Dr. Bernard J. Machen, President of the University of Florida and a pediatric dentist, noted that three-fourths of dentists provide charitable care, and yet only 30% of Medicaid children receive any dental care at all.[4]

Columbia University, College of Dental Medicine, 630 West 168th Street, NY 10032, USA
E-mail address: mjd2@columbia.edu

Dent Clin N Am 53 (2009) 169–181
doi:10.1016/j.cden.2008.12.003
dental.theclinics.com

Nowhere is the unmet need more critically visible than for persons with special health care needs (PSHCN), most of whom are concomitantly economically disadvantaged. It is estimated that one in six Americans has some disability.[5] "Special care dentistry is the delivery of dental care tailored to the individual needs of patients who have disabling medical conditions beyond routine conditions or mental or psychologic limitations that require consideration beyond routine approaches ... approximately 12% of the population is considered to have severe disabilities."[6] In simple numbers "more than fifty million U.S. residents have a developmental, physical, or intellectual disability that hinders them in functioning on their own or contributing fully to work, education, family, and community life. About 17% of U.S. children under 18 years have a developmental disability."[7] Honeycutt and colleagues further noted in 2004 the following incidences per two thousand United States births:

12,500 children with cerebral palsy
5,000 children with hearing loss
4,400 children with vision impairment
5,000 children with heart malformations
5,500 children with other circulatory/respiratory anomalies
800 children with spina bifida/meningocele
3,300 children with cleft lip/palate
8,600 children with a variety of musculo-skeletal/integumental anomalies

The numbers listed represent 1 year in the United States alone. In 2005, Steinberg noted, "One of the neediest yet most under-served groups of dental patients in the United States today is the special needs population. This is a rather diverse group of children and adults, including those with disabilities—whether medical related, mental, or psychologic—and those with physically handicapping conditions that require more than our routine approach to care."[8] In the 2004 National Survey of Children with Special Care Needs, it was noted that the most needed health service reported, but not received, was dental care. The survey estimated that possibly as many as 75% of children with special health care needs are unable to access oral health care in any given year.

Are there other factors that exacerbate the access issue or increase demand for care? Is there data that the individual dental disease rate for PSHCN is generally higher? It is challenging to document the same, given the many subset populations included in the definition of PSHCN. In 2000, the United States Surgeon General issued a report, "Oral Health in America," which noted the access disparities for oral health care, especially for PSHCN, with the added commentary that this group generally is at significantly measurably higher levels of systemic disease incidence and are at a higher risk for developing oral disease than is the general population.[9] In a similar report, the U.S. Department of Health and Human Services Health Resource Services Administration in 2001 noted, "Disabled persons exhibit poor oral hygiene, more severe periodontal disease, more decayed tooth surfaces, and greater treatment needs than persons without disabilities."[10]

PSYCHOLOGIC BARRIERS

Given the restricted access to care for PSHCN, and yet the general willingness of most dentists—be they general practitioners or specialists—to do charitable works, what are the causes of access problems? What are the specific barriers to oral health care? They are numerous and they are challenging. The most often cited barrier is the economic one; practitioners frequently state that providing care to a special needs patient is poorly reimbursed. This article will address that legitimate concern subsequently. Perhaps more central to the issue is the dearth of individual dentists who are prepared or comfortable providing such care. A clear case can be made that lack of education regarding the PSHCN is the greatest barrier. For an oral health care professional with no knowledge of or experience providing care to PSHCN, there is certainly an emotional or even more complex psychologic initial threshold that must be crossed. Just as for a dental student or a dental hygiene student who is preparing to care for their first ever patient, there are emotional aspects that have direct bearing on willingness to see the patient. In dental college the student has limited choices in attaining the prescribed lengthy list of competencies. The final degree and the ability to practice, as documented through licensure, are the motivating goals on which their careers depend. Resultantly, students are highly motivated to overcome their anxieties regarding their adequate knowledge and the ability to identify disease and provide needed services for that first patient, and to deliver care with excellence, both expeditiously and comfortably.

Similar "first patient" anxiety issues emerge later when that same professional, now with clinical experience, is first asked to care for a PSHCN. Given the broad list of conditions that constitute PSHCN, practitioner anxiety and frequently resultant reluctance is understandable, especially if the practitioner is not well prepared educationally. As noted, special health care needs include not only physical disabilities, but also psychologic and complex medical conditions. Hematologic disorders, metabolic disorders, and general medical fragility in a patient can create a practitioner who is fraught with concern over understanding and properly addressing the myriad conditions and contingencies present. Finally, it is not unusual for a patient with disabilities or other special health care needs to present with a constellation of medical problems concomitant to the main condition. Understanding all ramifications of such complex histories requires a broad-based education in the subject. Caring for that very first PSHCN is tantamount to a leap of faith in oneself as a practitioner, and obviously it best occurs in a carefully guided setting. Competent backup and the ability to carefully analyze the complexities and outcomes of the treatment support the growth of the novice's confidence to proceed.

Dentistry is, by frequent public survey, one of the most respected and trusted of the learned professions. Much of this respect comes from the care, pride, and sense of accomplishment derived from practice by the caregiver, which in turn reinforces those attitudes. Contemporary dentistry, like many other professions, entertains much discussion about maintaining its historically stringent ethics and standards. A value historically held closely by dentistry is the personal satisfaction derived from accomplishing complex procedures at an exceptional level to improve the health of the patient. Exceeding expectations and standards is a value at the head of the list of things taught in colleges of dental education. The typical student bemoans the extraordinary precision and 100% accuracy expected for every procedure, many of which have multiple sub-parts, and are impacted by biologic variability. After attaining the Doctor of Dental Surgery degree, these lessons and standards are well remembered and in most instances implemented. The American College of Dentists, a widely respected honorary organization, has become the standard bearer for these issues. The capacity to accept and meet technical challenges, for example restoring or replacing individual teeth, equilibrating the occlusion, achieving excellent esthetics, and so forth, for a patient who first appears with a complex list of needs provides important satisfaction for the professional. That sense of accomplishment derives from the ability to understand the patients, their needs, their social context, their expectations, and addressing these needs with the skills attained through many hours of education and practice. Providing care to PSHCN, often to a level of excellence far beyond what might initially seem plausible, provides an enormous level of satisfaction. But without preceding experience, especially during one's education in a guided, monitored environment, that sense of satisfaction is rarely attainable. In the ensuing discussion of overcoming barriers, the role of education, its current status, and what needs to be done to enable positive professional experiences with PSHCN will be examined.

ECONOMIC BARRIERS

In analyzing barriers to access to care for PSHCN, chiefly cited among them appears the economic problem. Individuals rarely perform activities that neither promise nor result in any reward, be it psychologic, financial, or otherwise. For health care professionals, this issue is far more complex than simply a Pavlovian stimulus-response paradigm. Financial reimbursements to oral health care providers are typically based not on units of time spent caring for the patient, but rather on the procedures completed with the patient. To spend what could be viewed as "excessive" time completing needed procedures makes these patients less desirable from an economic standpoint. It is clearly recognized that the procedures themselves are typically those provided to the routine patient. A dental restoration for a PSHCN typically is no different from that provided to any other patient, the teeth are not different. For example, in treating a partially destroyed tooth, the usual restoration technique is appropriate. In unusual circumstances, such as after oncology care, there may need to be modifications in procedures, such as preventive protocols. But generally speaking, routine care is simply that: routine care. Educating the practitioner then focuses on two issues: understanding and addressing the patient's specific conditions—physical, psychologic, or medical—and managing the behavior and cooperation of the patient. An individual with cerebral palsy and neuromuscular manifestations, such as spasticity with head and neck involvement or ataxia from central basal ganglion damage, may present uncontrolled motion. Given that the restoration of a carious lesion requires the use of the dental handpiece with a sharp bur at its end typically rotating in excess of 100,000 rpm, and further given that exquisite attention to the margins of the restoration and the shape of the cavity preparation is expected, an inexperienced dentist might easily question his or her ability to perform that service on such a patient. Additionally, the collateral expectation is spending an "excessive" period of time in the provision of that care. But as can be seen in other articles of this issue, with reasonable accommodations these concerns can be significantly ameliorated and a minimum of extra time spent providing the indicated quality care. To the negative side of the equation, fee augmentation for extra preparation time necessary to understand the complexities of the patient is nonexistent. Compensatory, higher than customary private-pay fees, would be interpreted as an added, unfair burden for the patient. Third-party insurers rarely provide additional compensation for extra time to provide services or for similar unusual considerations.

The other financial issue is the source of reimbursement. The issue of fair and reasonable reimbursement for provided services is complex. Usual and customary reimbursement does not seem applicable for PSHCN. Most practitioners establish their own "customary" fees. Third parties do likewise, theoretically relating to practitioner usual and customary reimbursements. Some persons in this patient population have government-sponsored health care benefits, such as Medicaid, MediCal, and others, but Medicaid fees are usually quite modest, both in services covered and in reimbursement rates. Crall[11] recently noted, "Medicaid coverage for adults with special needs, however, is subject to individual financial circumstances and state discretion, and often is less comprehensive in terms of scope and depth of coverage (especially regarding dental benefits)." In many states, it is clearly documented that Medicaid reimbursement, outside of certain carefully specified institutional settings, often provides no better reimbursement than an amount that covers the operational overhead of the practice. Consequently, it is not an uncommon discussion among dentists that they may provide care for Medicaid covered/eligible patients, but do so on a charitable basis, filing no claims for payment. They simply do so pro bono as part of their professional caring for the community and individual patients in need. Clearly, more adequate reimbursement from a variety of possible sources, including the federal and state governments, could change this scenario dramatically. Efforts by all in the profession to secure such change are essential and ongoing, even to patient litigation support against state governments by the profession as amicus curae. Compounding these issues, Medicaid dental support often phases out at age 21, leaving no support alternatives for adult PSHCN.

Funding to support care also must be sought from large foundations, some of which exist expressly to support PSHCN. An excellent example is United Cerebral Palsy (UCP), a national organization that historically sponsored fellowships in medicine and in dentistry for already trained pediatric dentists to further their education in caring for patients with cerebral palsy and related neuromuscular conditions. UCP has a history of comprehensive support, providing counseling and transportation for their clients to sites for care, sponsoring fellowship training and other support services. These coordinated efforts present a strong model or best practice example for the services that a private or public foundation can provide in facilitating access to care for PSHCN.

Edelstein[12] presents a three-point plan for ameliorating the financial access barriers:

- Special needs adult dental coverage in Medicaid: engage state legislatures and Medicaid authorities in electively providing comprehensive adult benefits for PSHCN so they do not age out of coverage at 21, when mandatory dental benefits cease.
- A general anesthesia insurance mandate for PSHCN: use the same approach that has been successful in obtaining anesthesia benefits for young children and extend coverage to older patients who also require anesthesia services.
- Enhanced payment for the care of PSHCN: engage state Medicaid authorities in providing a meaningful add-on payment for the care of PSHCN.

A superb paradigm for a comprehensive approach to addressing any multifactor problem has been presented by Ozar,[13] albeit in another context: that of ethical conduct education. Ozar's problem-solving model can be adapted and applied to the access-to-care problem. The following is such a plan:

Strategic actions to increase PSHCN access

- Increase awareness of dental health importance by the dental profession, medical colleagues, PSHCN's themselves, parents/guardians, legislators, and the public.
- Attain knowledge in each instance of specific individual roles.
- Educate all involved regarding the specific issues.
- Provide mentoring and exemplary best practices:
  - Create/identify an expert corps
  - Create a larger cross-professions cadre of mentors around the expert corps
  - Create a cadre of issue specific leaders and coordinate communication among them

Facilitate practical solutions:
- Address specific barriers

Increase public awareness of issues:
- All stakeholders focus on public relations/education
- Spokesperson training

Identify resources needed and all possible sources.
Examine outcomes, modify approaches and revise actions accordingly.

An important new position is developing that can increase general awareness in a community and communication among all involved, with resultantly better access to care. This superb new concept is being promoted through organized dentistry and by community leaders as well. The focus is a new dental team member, called the Community Dental Health Coordinator (CDHC), a role similar to that of individuals in the Latino community, who are called *promodores de salud* or health promoters. Such trained individuals are increasingly present in very rural settings, as well as in large cities. Depending on the country and the situation, they are often trained by governments to assist individual citizens to access health care. This concept is now being applied to oral health care. In the United States, CDHC may be credentialed and are typically high school graduates who complete approximately 1 year of additional classes in an organized educational setting. These classes include actual clinical experiences and problem-solving approaches. They are sensitized to integrating oral health information with the particular culture or language or value systems of a given community. Community Health Centers and dental colleges would be excellent places to employ such specifically trained individuals. The CDHC would help to organize not only resources for access to care, but also could be a community educator in a wide variety of settings including schools, senior citizen centers, and other community settings.

EDUCATIONAL EFFORTS

As noted previously, educational, psychologic, and emotional barriers exist for less than adequately educated oral health practitioners. It is of note that significant efforts were once in place to increase education to future providers to improve access to care for PSHCN. A specific example is the Robert Wood Johnson Foundation (RWJ) Grant Program in the 1970s. After an extensive request for proposal process, roughly one dozen dental colleges were given large grants to establish programs that would include all graduates in learning to provide care to PSHCN. Different colleges established widely varying styles of programs, but all had a core didactic curriculum followed by a specific guided-care provision for patients. Some of the colleges established special clinical facilities, replete with wheelchair lifts and other ancillary devices, to expedite such care. Other colleges chose to mainstream PSHCN in their general clinics, based on the philosophy that in so doing, a clear message would be sent to students that these patients could be seen in a family practice setting with a minimum of modifications.

Lessons learned from the RWJ programs include challenges in arranging for care reimbursement and the education of families or guardians about the importance of regular oral health care. Grant program start-up problems were found in attempting to identify faculty who were competent in both the didactic and clinical settings to teach students, and secondly in the reluctance of dental students to attempt actual care provision, particularly on patients with neuromuscular or other dyskinetic disorders. Researchers have consistently found that student dentists without such education typically are not prepared to meet the communication and dental care needs of their patients with developmental disabilities.[14] Loan[15] noted in 2005, in a survey of recent graduates about their willingness to care for PHSCN, that the more the respondents agreed that dental education had prepared them well, the more likely they were to treat various types of PSHCN, to set up their practices so they could treat them, and the more they liked treating these patients. Most general dentists did not think their predoctoral dental education had prepared them well to treat special needs patients. The key finding is that the better they reported to have been educated, the more likely they were to treat special needs patients.

In a 2007 survey of special patient care programs in United States and Canadian dental schools, Schwenk and colleagues[16] reported that 40% of the respondent institutions had designated special PSHCN clinics. Those institutions that chose to mainstream patients, instead used existing predoctoral general clinics or, alternatively, referred them to pediatric hospital-based or general practice residencies within the university. Bernick[17] reported that comparing current educational efforts in United States dental schools to the number of hours spent on the same in the 1960s and 70s showed that the numbers had decreased, noting, "surveys suggest only a handful of schools do so and very few provide clinical services for special needs persons."

As a result of such observations, in 2004 the Commission on Dental Accreditation adopted a new standard (Standard 2-26 "Special Needs") that directs dental colleges and dental hygiene programs to prepare dental professionals to care for PSHCN. "Graduates must be competent in assessing the treatment needs of patients with special needs." Implementation was required by January 1, 2006. Compliance with this accreditation guideline during the every 7-year accreditation of each United States dental college is required for full accreditation.[18]

In 2007, McTigue[19] observed, "Clinical education should be incorporated into the dental curriculum in the first year. While Part I of the National Board Dental Examination drives most schools to load didactic courses in the first 2 years, interactions with PSHCN patients where they live or work could do much to educate students about their needs. Exposing students to persons with disabilities early in their training and allowing them to observe those who treat them is as important as their providing the dental treatment themselves. Using community-based clinics remote to the dental school can increase the efficiency of the clinical years (ie, have students go where the patients are, rather than having these patients go to special clinics)." Other educators agree with this approach. Bertolame supported the mentor model as used in medicine for this educational component. A mentor educates a small student group providing care, possibly in a well-run community site. There exists evidence that such settings can increase acceptance of the provider role and the productivity of students.[20]

Certain dental colleges have considerably strengthened their efforts and offer innovative programs. An example is at the University of West Virginia, where a program using a virtual patient model was instituted. "A development team consisting of Pediatric Dentistry faculty members, parents of children with developmental disabilities, an individual with a developmental disability, and educational specialists developed an interactive virtual patient case. The case involved a ten-year-old child with Down Syndrome presenting with a painful tooth. Student dentists were required to make decisions regarding proper interactions with the child, as well as appropriate clinical procedures throughout the treatment protocol. Differences in perceived difficulty level and knowledge change were measured, as well as the student dentists' overall satisfaction with the learning experience. Significantly improved results were obtained in both perceived difficulty level and knowledge-base measures for student dentists. Participants reported overall satisfaction with the modules."[21]

The Columbia University College of Dental Medicine program reflects experiences learned, beginning from the RWJ Foundation grant experience to this date. It was learned that the majority of PSHCN could be treated in the general clinics of the College or in the existing specialty settings, when indicated. But to assure that every student had adequate didactic exposure and subsequent clinical contact with such patients, the College developed a multifaceted program. A critical foundation course in that endeavor, named "Pathophysiology," is a year-long course established to bring information learned in the biomedical core curriculum to bear in patient care. To that end, the medical students of the College of Physicians and Surgeons and the dental students attend core Pathophysiology lectures and then divide into small groups, with faculty from both colleges and, when indicated, biomedical core educators to apply the didactic material directly to the care of patients. Case-based learning is the format. Most patients with complex medical, but nonphysical, manifestations are seen in the general clinics. In addition, new aspects of the curriculum include the creation of video-patient encounters with a core set of individuals with specific conditions. There is a clinical rotation to the United Cerebral Palsy Health care Center on East 23rd Street in Manhattan, where observational and direct patient care experiences are attained. At that site, four part-time dentists discuss treatment needs of individual PSHCN and demonstrate and supervise their care. The numbers of students at the rotation site at one time is limited to two or three to assure appropriate faculty/student/patient interactions. The rotation is for the most clinically advanced students: that is, those in the final, fourth year at the dental college. Contrast the preceding sequenced curriculum with curricula from a study conducted by Wolf and colleagues[22] in 2004. This analysis was based on a survey of recent dental college graduates; it noted that 50% of the students reported no clinical training in the care of PSHCN. Furthermore, 75% reported little-to-no didactic preparation to provide care to this population. When physical plant limitations or a sub-optimal cadre of PSHCNs exist, an innovation is the use of the World Wide Web for the education of current dental students, hygienists, and other office staff. Information technology supports both initial and continuing education. An excellent example is the Birmingham School of Dentistry in the United Kingdom. That faculty has created a large series of computer accessed "E courses" in oral health care. These on-line Web-based courses are quite user-friendly and comprehensive. Many are downloadable free for teaching purposes; others are only accessible for a fee. One of the courses, replete with case-based clinical examples, frequently asked questions, and self-assessment instruments, is for "Dentistry for Patients with Special Healthcare Needs" (http://www.dentistry.bham.ac.uk/ecourse/). Such accessible distance learning via computers is particularly important for sites where the PSHCN population is limited.

The education of other health care professionals, such as physicians, physician assistants, nurses, and so forth is critical to eliminating barriers. The need for collaborative efforts between medicine and dentistry and their supporting professions, such as nursing and dental hygiene, was clearly elaborated by O'Connor and Carr as far back as 1981.[23] The need for the education of those professionals about the implications of poor access to oral health care was clearly delineated by Kane[24] in 2008, who noted, "The relationship between an unmet need for dental care and an unmet need for routine medical care may be of particular relevance to policy and program development. Specifically, this finding underscores the importance of policies and programs that promote inter-disciplinary and inter-professional collaboration and referral mechanisms among medical and dental care providers." Few medical school or resident training curricula include any hours for oral health. As it becomes more clearly documented that oral health relates to systemic disease in a variety of ways, inclusion of accreditation requirements for the same should help to address this current dearth of information presented in medical school.

In educating to increase access to care for PSHCN, it is not only the education of the dentist through improved dental college curricula and access to quality continuing education from national organizations, which is critical. The families and guardians of these patients and their medical caregivers must be educated about the importance of oral health. Through outreach efforts, by improved accreditation and licensure standards, and by legislation, change can occur.

SUMMARY

Access to care for patients with PSHCN clearly can be improved. No one institution or group of individuals alone can address the multiple barriers shown in **Box 1**, nor can they provide the integrated solutions presented in **Box 2**. Through efforts by our federal and state governments, relevant foundations, oral health care organizations, and through the caring and professional dedication of individual leaders among oral health care practitioners, a true difference can occur in access and, further, in the quality of care and therefore of life for these patients.

Cassamassimo noted,[25] "An ideal oral health care system for families of children with SHCN (CSHCN) is one that is accessible, affordable, and staffed by educated and prepared providers and staff. These professionals would safely deliver individualized, compassionate, quality care that includes education, prevention, and treatment. This ideal care system would be well integrated with the overall care system in which children with SHCN participate. In addition to these broad goals, short-term steps can be taken to push oral health into the vision of health for CSHCN and maximize available health services."

Finally, and equally important, the education of those in a position to affect the availability of resources is critical. As noted recently by Edelstein, a major improvement could be garnered through the promotion of best practices. He suggests the need to "identify and replicate examples of integrated care coordination between medical and dental services to local medical and dental provider associations, hospitals, Area Health Education Centers, and/or community health centers in collaboration with local advocacy groups, and additionally, developing social rewards to acknowledge participating dentists."[12] The need for collaborative efforts, and particularly for awareness throughout the community, of these issues is not new. Nowak[26] noted in the early 1980s, "The first problems identified were the appreciation of good dental health and the recognition that good dental health is possible. The solution to these problems is primarily through education." He further noted, "We should use the opportunity in our communities whether in the office, the schools, or the service groups to promote dental health. The doctor and staff of dental assistants and hygienists would be welcomed in community centers, nursing homes, and residential facilities to provide in-service training to the staff and instructional sessions to the clients and residents."

For example, during the 2007 to 2008 fiscal year in New York, over $320,000 in dental services were provided by 286 volunteer dentists. Nationally, the program supported care for 6,578 people at a value of $18.5 million, provided by 12,500 volunteer dentists. Extensive dental laboratory support also exists.[27] Another model best practices program, under the auspices of the National Foundation of Dentistry for the Handicapped is the Donated Dental Services Program began in 1997. Support to the program is from the ADA, state, and local dental societies, and over 30 national dentally related corporations and foundations.

Box 1
Barriers to access to oral health for PSHCN

Psychologic

The dental practitioner

- Lack of experience and resultant anxiety over initiating care for PSHCN

The recipient (patient)

- Underestimating oral health importance
- Underestimating oral health access opportunities

Other health care practitioners

- Underestimating oral health importance
- Inability to coordinate care

Economic

Increased time to provide care

Low reimbursement rate

- Medicaid rates
- Lack of adult Medicaid coverage
- Complexity of required forms

Physical

Office design impediments

Transportation

Education

Minimal dental college curriculum

Accreditation requirements

- Dental colleges—minimal
- Medical colleges—absent
- Dental hygiene, dental assisting, nursing—minimal

Continuing education

Legislators, foundations

Trained faculty

Postdoctoral fellowships

Daily caregivers

The role of dental organizations in the education of the practitioner, fellow health professionals, and the public cannot be overstated. A superb example of such an effort was a symposium held by the American Academy of Pediatric Dentistry (AAPD) on "Lifetime Oral Health Care for Patients with Special Needs." The presentations were published in the March/April 2007 issue of *Pediatric Dentistry*. This volume is a veritable compendium of relevant protocols for addressing access for these patients, and includes suggestions for dental education, for relating to other health professionals, for oral health policies and clinical guidelines, and for financing access

Box 2
Methods to surmount barriers to oral health care for PSHCN

Psychologic

Increased practitioner experience

- Dental curriculum increase
- Postdoctoral clinical fellowships
- Clinical continuing education

Increased patient awareness

- Dental home establishment
- Education by professionals
- Disease prevention education
- Parent/guardian awareness
- Daily caretaker education

Economic

Provide technical education for providers

Increase Medicaid reimbursement and adult coverage

Increase other third-party/foundation involvement

Simplify required filings

Coordinate care among health professionals

Physical

Appropriate office design

Use of information from Americans with Disabilities Act

Coordinate transportation with other service visits

Education

Increased dental college curriculum and experience

- Strengthen accreditation requirements for all related professions

Increase fellowships

Increase continuing education

- Require for licensure
- Expansion of Web-based education

Educate other professionals about the need, access to, and coordination of care

Educate legislators, other resource controllers

Train additional faculty

Educate home or institutional daily caregivers

- Prevention
- Available resources, sites for care

to care. AAPD also is the driving force, now with ADA support, behind the "Dental Home" concept for all children and by extension all PSHCN. The dental home is defined as "the ongoing relationship between the dentist and the patient, inclusive of all aspects of oral health care delivered in a comprehensive, continuously accessible, coordinated, and family centered way."[28] This total approach to oral health is no where more significant than for the PSHCN population.

In summary, the access issue must be viewed in light of the quality of life for individuals with PSHCN and in today's world in light of the relationship between oral health and overall health. Our literature demonstrates evidence that oral health and general health are closely related; this evidence increases daily. Studies of oral health problems and their relationships to cardiovascular health, neonatal outcomes, and other systemic effects are confirming what United States Surgeon General, David Satcher, noted in his report, "Oral Health in America." No individual can truly be healthy without oral health. It is, then, for all the above mentioned parties to work in unison under the leadership of concerned individuals and organizations to increase access to health care for all, especially for those least able in many respects to advocate for themselves and their needs, our patients with special health care needs.

FURTHER READINGS

AAPD Clinical Guideline on Management of Persons with Special Health Care Needs. AAPD Reference Manual 2007–08. Pediatr Dent 2007;29:98–101.

Pediatric Dentistry – The official publication of the American Academy of Pediatric Dentistry, the American Board of Pediatric Dentistry, and the College of Diplomates of the American Board of Pediatric Dentistry. Edited by Steven M Adair. American Academy of pediatric dentistry, 211 E. Chicago Avenue, Suite 1700, Chicago, IL 60611.

Position paper from the Academy of Dentistry for Persons with Disabilities. Preservation of quality health care services for people with developmental disabilities. Spec Care Dentist 1998;18:180–2.

Special Care Dentistry – This journal is published on behalf of the Special Care Dentistry Association, the official journal of the Academy of Dentistry for Persons with Disabilities, the American Association of Hospital Dentists, and the American Society for Geriatric Dentistry. Edited by Ronald L Ettinger. Blackwell Publishing.

REFERENCES

1. Berenson A. Boom time for U.S. dentists, but not for America's teeth. New York Times. October 11, 2007. p. 1.
2. Otto M. For want of a dentist. Washington Post 2007. p. B01.
3. ADA News, Sep 17, 2007, President-Elect Interview.
4. Machen JB. We can be leaders in addressing children's oral healthcare needs. J Am Coll Dent 2004;74(4):7.
5. Waldman HB. Preparing dental graduates to provide care to individuals with special needs. J Dent Educ 2005;69(2):249–54.
6. Lawton L. Providing dental care for special patients: tips for the general dentist. J Am Dent Assoc 2002;133(12):1660–700.
7. Honeycutt A, Dunlap L, al Homsi G, et al. Economic costs associated with mental retardation, cerebral palsy, hearing loss, and vision impairment-United States. MMWR 2004;53(3):57–9.
8. Steinberg BJ. Issues and challenges in special care dentistry. J Dent Educ 2005; 69(3):32–4.

9. Satcher D. Oral Health in America. Rockville (MD): U.S. Department of Health and Human Services, Public Health Service, Office of the Surgeon General. May; 2000.
10. Bonito AJ, Cooper LY. Dental care considerations of disadvantaged and special care populations. Baltimore (MD): U.S. Department of Health and Human Services. Health Resources and Services Administration; April 2001.
11. Crall JJ. Improving oral health care for individuals with special health care needs. Pediatr Dent 2007;29(2):98–104.
12. Edelstein BL. Conceptual frameworks for understanding system capacity in the care of people with health care needs. Pediatr Dent 2007;29(2):108–16.
13. Ozar DT. What to hope for and the challenge of getting there. J Am Coll Dent 2008;75(1):25–9.
14. Fenton SJ, Hood H, Holder M, et al. The American Academy of Developmental Medicine and Dentistry: eliminating health disparities for individuals with mental retardation and other developmental disabilities. J Dent Educ 2003;67: 1337–44.
15. Dao L, Zwetchkenbaum S, Inglehart MR, et al. General dentists and special needs patients: does dental education matter? J Dent Educ 2005;69(10): 1107–15.
16. Schwenk DM, Stoeckel DC, Riemen SE, et al. Survey of special patient care programs at U.S. and Canadian dental schools. J Dent Educ 2007;71(9):1153–9.
17. Bernick SM. Improving dental access (Letters). J Am Dent Assoc 2001;132: 1082–3.
18. Commission on Dental Accreditation. Accreditation standards for dental education programs. Chicago: American Dental Association; July 30, 2004.
19. McTigue D. Dental education and special needs patients: challenges and opportunities. Pediatr Dent 2007;29(2):129–33.
20. Bertolami C. Rationalizing the dental curriculum in light of current disease prevalence and patient demand for treatment: form vs. content. J Dent Educ 2001; 65:725–35.
21. Kleinert HL, Sanders C, Mink J, et al. Improving student dentist competencies and perception of difficulty in delivering care to children with developmental disabilities using a virtual patient module. J Dent Educ 2007;71(2):279–86.
22. Wolff A, Waldman B, Milano M, et al. Dental students' experiences with and attitudes toward people with mental retardation. J Am Dent Assoc 2004;135:353–7.
23. O'Connor CE, Carr S. Interdisciplinary collaboration between nursing and dental hygiene: clinical care for the elderly. J Gerontol Nurs 1981;7(4):233–5.
24. Kane D. Factors associated with access to dental care for children with special health care needs. J Am Dent Assoc 2008;139:326–33.
25. Cassamassimo PS. Children with special healthcare needs: patient, professional, systems issues. Interfaces background paper, Children's Dental Health Project, 2001. Washington, DC.
26. Nowak AJ. The special patient: challenges of the 80's. Special Care Dent 1982;2: 175.
27. New York Donated Dental Services Program Annual Report. 281 Park Ave S. NYC, NY. 10010.
28. Aapd. Dental Home. Available at: http://www.aapd.org/media/policies.asp. Accessed July 2008.

Health Related Issues for Individuals with Special Health Care Needs

H. Barry Waldman, DDS, MPH, PhD[a,*], Rick Rader, MD[b],
Steven P. Perlman, DDS, MScD[c]

KEYWORDS

- Disabilities • Medically underserved • Stigma
- Medical and dental education

More than 50 million individuals in the United States with developmental disabilities, complex medical problems, significant physical limitations, and a vast array of other conditions considered under the rubric of "disabilities" live in our communities, many as a result of deinstitutionalization and mainstreaming. Children and adults with special health care needs have become a much more integral and visible component of everyday life. This process represents an ongoing change in perceptions about individuals with disabilities and subsequent reform of policies concerning the rights and the principles of care for people with special needs. The reform was built upon an increased role for the family and community health practitioners in providing needed care.

THE BEGINNING OF CHANGE: EXPOSING THE "GAP"

In 1999, the President of Special Olympics, Dr. Timothy Shriver, publicized the lack of essential health services for Special Olympics athletes and more generally for people with intellectual disabilities (ID). He recognized that until the public health dimensions of wellbeing for Special Olympics athletes and people with ID were documented and widely communicated to policy makers, there was little chance for improvement. The Special Olympics-sponsored publication, *The Health Status and Needs of Individuals with Mental Retardation*,[1] provided a comprehensive review of the health and social service research literature, which documented the extensive unmet health care needs

[a] Department of General Dentistry, School of Dental Medicine, Stony Brook University, Stony Brook, NY 11794-8706, USA
[b] Morton J. Kent Habilitation Center, Orange Grove Center, Human Development, University of Tennessee, 615 Derby Street, Chattanooga, TN 37404, USA
[c] Department of Pediatric Dentistry, The Boston University School of Dental Medicine, 100 E. Newton Street, Boston, MA 01902, USA
* Corresponding author.
E-mail address: hwaldman@notes.cc.sunysb.edu (H.B. Waldman).

Dent Clin N Am 53 (2009) 183–193
doi:10.1016/j.cden.2008.12.008
dental.theclinics.com
0011-8532/08/$ – see front matter

and extensive risk factors for people with ID. With this study in hand, Shriver convinced Senator Ted Stevens of Alaska to schedule a Special Field Hearing of the United States Senate Committee on Appropriations during the 2001 Special Olympics World Winter Games in Anchorage, Alaska. At this hearing, scores of leaders, scientific and health experts and advocates presented testimony about the health status and needs of people with ID.

During the meeting, Surgeon General David Satcher was informed and made the commitment to focus the attention of his office on the health challenges of people with ID. The Surgeon General Listening Sessions, a national Surgeon General's conference, were followed with the 2002 *Report of the Surgeon General's Conference on Health Disparities and Mental Retardation.* He wrote in the forward of the report that, "It became apparent that, as our system of care for those with mental retardation evolved, our attention to their health needs lessened."[2] The Surgeon General's report directed those who care for persons with developmental disabilities toward six strategic goals that will "close the gap" in the delivery of health care to this population of Americans. Specifically, Goal 4 addressed the lack of professional training in the care of persons with developmental disabilities. Dr. Satcher observed that, "The challenges and rewards of treating individuals with MR are rarely addressed in the training of physicians and other health care professionals. However, anecdotal evidence and limited data indicate that opportunities for clinical experiences with these patients, early in medical and other health professions training, increase the capacity of providers to value and accept these patients into their practices."[2]

For example, specifically, dental education: by the end of the 1990s and into the present century, a series of studies found that during the 4 years of education, more than half of United States dental schools provided fewer than 5 hours of classroom presentation and about 75% of the schools provided from 0% to 5% of patient-care time for the treatment of patients with special needs. In one study, 50% of the students reported no clinical training in the care of patients with special needs. One should not be surprised that only 10% of general dentists in one study said they treated children with cerebral palsy, mental retardation, or medically compromised conditions often or very often. Of those in the study, 75% reported they rarely or never treated children with cerebral palsy in their practice. In addition, a national study of dental hygiene programs reported comparable findings: 48% of 170 programs had 10 hours or less of didactic training (including 14 with 5 hours or less) and 57% of programs reported no clinical experience.[3]

How do you translate the need to both train the next generation of physicians and dentists to care for people with disabilities into innovative curriculums, clinical opportunities, and rewarding careers, and improve the overall heath of individuals with special health care needs? The first step is to "congeal a group of likeminded rogues and someone says, Who wants to be president?."[4] That was the beginning of the American Academy of Developmental Medicine and Dentistry (AADMD). The Academy was established to:

- Assist in reforming the current system of health care so that no person with developmental disabilities is left without access to quality health care.
- Prepare clinicians to face the unique challenges in caring for people with developmental disabilities.
- Provide curriculum to newly established developmental disabilities training programs in medical and dental schools across the nation.
- Increase the body and quality of patient-centered research regarding those with developmental disabilities and to involve parents and caregivers in this process.

Create a forum in which physicians, dentists, families, and caregivers may exchange experiences and ideas with regard to caring for patients with developmental disabilities.
Disseminate specialized developmental medical and dental information to families in language that is easy for the family to understand.
Establish alliances between visionary advocacy and health care organizations for the primary purpose of achieving better health care.

AADMD members present the following series of issues that must be considered if the profession is to improve services for individuals with special health care needs.

Medically Underserved

Satchel Paige, the philosopher and icon ball player, was fond of posing the question, "If no one knows how old you are, how old would you be?" And it's one of the great philosophical questions of the ages. What impact does knowing have on something? In Satchel's lament, perhaps a great deal, but beyond knowing, what you do with that information is what counts. What if no one told you that you were medically underserved? Would that change the way you related to medical care? Would that change your expectations, outcomes, compliance, and sense of personhood? This is not a hypothetical point to ponder.[5]

In the case of citizens with developmental disabilities, this is the point. And it's a point that requires more than pondering—it requires action. In reality, that is the scenario: people with disabilities, despite the evidence, are not considered to be people who are medically underserved.

So what is the evidence? For starters we have the Surgeon General's 2002 report *Closing the Gap, Health Care Disparities for People with Mental Retardation*, exclaiming: "Compared with other populations, individuals of all ages with mental retardation experience poorer health and more difficulty in finding, getting to, and paying for appropriate health care."[6] While this is considered the primary report on health care disparities for people with developmental disabilities, others[7,8] reported that "Children with special health care needs and their families represent an important underserved population. In addition, substantial disparities are present in access, satisfaction, and family impact." More recently, an article[9] opens with the statement, "The literature documents that people with developmental disabilities experience greater difficulty in securing appropriate and affordable health care than do individuals without disabilities." And when all else fails, we also have one of this article's authors (R.R.), as editor of *Exception Parent (EP) Magazine.* R.R. interfaces with thousands of parents each year and although it is totally anecdotal, these interfaces are overwhelmingly revealing. Their kids (across the life span) experience a patchwork quilt form of health care. Certainly, there are many examples of "cultivated care" in which the health care is delivered in a comprehensive, coordinated, caring, culturally competent, and continuous fashion. Great strides have been made through the medical home, case management, physician and dentist training, preventive measures, an expanded knowledge base of secondary conditions, and medical advocacy. But all of this hasn't been enough and one potential (and critical) impediment is the nondeclaration of this population as being medically underserved.

In the 750-page report issued by the Institute of Medicine, *Unequal Treatment - Confronting Racial and Ethnic Disparities in Health Care*, there is not a single mention of "disabilities" in any form or context.[10] Despite the fact that African Americans with Down syndrome have a life expectancy of half that of white individuals (with the same syndrome), this was not cited. Their first finding can serve as both the executive summary of this report as well as the template of this article: "Racial and ethnic disparities in health care exist and, because they are associated with worse outcomes in many cases, are unacceptable."[10]

We simply have to extrapolate the population segments where evidence exists, declaring them to be medically underserved and extend that moniker to individuals with developmental disabilities. But this is not about expanding the subset of citizens who belong to specific racial and ethnic subgroups to another group of those individuals who also have developmental disabilities. This is about recognizing all citizens with developmental disabilities as being both medically disparate and medically underserved, regardless of their racial and ethnic affiliation.

What's All the Fuss About?

There are several reasons for including this marginalized population. For one thing, being declared a medically underserved group immediately calls attention to the group's status. Every study that refers to medically disparate populations always recommends the development of strategies to address this recognized gap. Examples of some of the benefits include the reduction or forgiveness of medical and dental school loans if the graduate gravitates to serving this population. In addition, working with individuals who are medically underserved qualifies international medical graduates (IMGs) to qualify for legal immigration status. An example of the myopia of this scenario is that IMGs, working with specific populations in a given geographic area are granted resident status, while counterparts working with the same population in the adjacent zip code are refused. There are other opportunities that include the expansion of physician and dentist training, benefits for expanded prevention and screening, research agendas and resource allocation, public health initiatives, community health center grants, and the inclusion of people with developmental disabilities in clinical trials. All in all, this is a win-win situation for individuals and families in the special needs arena. In addition the "community" at large can't be far behind in being identified as a collateral winner. And while we can certainly compare the dynamics of citizens with developmental and intellectual disabilities with citizens from distinct racial and ethnic groups, the question of "why" comes to bear. George Santayana[11] offered, "Injustice in this world is not something comparative, the wrong is deep, clear and absolute in each private fate." And that is exactly what the AADMD is trying to achieve with its "Task Force on Health Disparities": that people, individuals, regardless of their zip code, ethnic roots or primary language, should be recognized, where appropriate, as individuals at risk for being medically underserved. The authors feel the evidence is both abundant and compelling that the "where appropriate" translates to individuals with developmental and intellectual disabilities.

Arguments for Inclusion

While the arguments for including citizens with developmental disabilities into the arena of citizens (individually or collectively) that are presently classified as being medically underserved have already been cited, there are additional studies. Two of the most visible and noted "report cards" created to assess disparities are the *Health Accountability 36 Indicators*[12] and the *Integrated Approaches of Laves and Gibbons*.[13] These are offered to defer and defuse anticipated criticisms of arguments generated to question the premise of this presentation. The data (relating to persons with developmental disabilities) can be "inputted" to offset any sociodemographic disparities.

The Data Enter

How would the Health Resources and Services Administration (HRSA) determine and recognize a "medically underserved population of individuals with neurodevelopmental disorders or intellectual disabilities" (ND/ID)? According to HRSA, a population can be considered a medically underserved population if it receives an Index of Medical Underservice (IMU) score of less than 62.0.[14]

The IMU is calculated using the simple addition of four scores. In the case of ND/ID population, it would be calculated by adding scores V1, V2, V3, and V4 as follows:

V1 = The percentage of the ND/ID population living below the poverty line.
V2 = The percentage of the ND/ID population over the age of 65.
V3 = The infant mortality rate among people with ND/ID.
V4 = The ratio of primary care physicians to patients with ND/ID.

Now input:

V1—Roughly 33% of the population of both children and adults with mental retardation live in poverty.[15] Cross referencing this with the HRSA score table give a V1 score of 5.6. The maximum score for this criterion is 25.1.

V2—There are a number of statistics that can be used to calculate the percentage of people with ND/ID that are over the age of 65. Our initial estimates show roughly 10% of the ND/ID population are over the age of 65. This corresponds with a V2 score of 19.8. The maximum score possible for this criterion is 20.2.

V3—The number-one cause of infant mortality in the United States, accounting for 5,623 infant deaths, is classified as congenital malformations, deformations, and chromosomal abnormalities, essentially, the biomedical causes of ND/ID.[16] Because roughly 60,000 to 120,000 people with ND/ID are born every year, the infant mortality for this population is between 47 out of 1,000 and 94 out of 1,000. Both of these scores represent a V3 score of 0.0. The maximum score for this criterion is 26.0.

V4—This is perhaps the most difficult score to calculate, as it is extraordinarily difficult to estimate the number of primary care physicians willing and capable of caring for this population. We know this number to be fairly low. However, we shall use the maximum score, by default, for purposes of completing the IMU calculation. The maximum score for this criterion is 28.7.

To summarize the IMU calculation, we have estimated the following: V1 = 5.6, V2 = 19.8, V3 = 0.0, and V4 = 28.7. The total IMU score for the ND/ID population, then, is 54.1. This falls well below the determination score of 62.0.

Food for Thought

It is obvious that you cannot use formulas to change the face of health care for an individual, a family, a community, or a population. In terms of providing care to citizens with developmental disabilities, there are additional impediments besides the formal declaration of them as being medically underserved. Findings from focus groups conducted by the Institute of Medicine addressing racial disparities in health care have definite transferable applicability to addressing disparities in treating individuals with intellectual disabilities. Attributions included effect of stereotyping, communication barriers, the role of economics, lack of respect, improper diagnosis or treatment, patient's appearance, health care setting, and attitudes of health care providers. Added to that is lack of exposure to this population during training; lack of a shared knowledge base (contributing to questions of motivation, competence, liability and confidence); lackluster reimbursement; questions of informed consent and guardianship; influence of medical model focus on curative mentality; perception of lack of referrals and willing specialists; perception of unrealistic parental expectations; and the ongoing invisibility, marginalization, and devalued personhood of people with developmental disabilities. There are ongoing efforts to address many of these identified obstacles to care. The appropriate recognition of people with developmental and intellectual disabilities as being medically underserved will be a welcome complement to these efforts.

PREPARING MEDICAL AND DENTAL STUDENTS

Writing in the British Medical Journal, Sir Robert Platt[17] commented, "The first staggering fact about medical education is that after two and a half years of being taught on the assumption that everyone is the same, the student has to find out for himself that everyone is different, which is really what his experience has taught him since infancy."

Perhaps Platt's observation that "everyone is different" is no better reflected than in individuals with intellectual and developmental disabilities. Even in the realm of well-documented, researched, and studied specific genetic syndromes, the student has the opportunity to see just how "different" the differences are. One might propose that exposure to patients with developmental disabilities would serve medical and dental students with insights into several clinical fronts. If nothing else, students might see the need to simply appreciate how common conditions and disorders can have puzzling manifestations and presentations and that patients can effectively express their needs, fears and concerns without the use of language. Students can learn valuable lessons about the confluence of multiple-system interface; how one system can alter, impact and disguise the necessary orchestration of other organs. Perhaps the most valuable insight the student can learn from training with patients with intellectual and developmental disabilities, is the opportunity for the student to address his or own levels of subtle stigmatization. So why would medical schools be so reluctant to adopt programs that introduce medical students to the challenges and rewards of treating patients with special health care needs?

The sum total of medical knowledge doubles every 10 years, and thus the body of knowledge with which the student is required to become fluent increases at a formidable rate. The 4-year curriculum is literally bursting at the seams and many educators see the wisdom of expanding the undergraduate medical school curriculum to a fifth year. The adoption of this expansion is doubtful at this time. In addition to the expansion of the body of knowledge, the emergence of new disciplines in medicine and health care has created a competitive field for adding new curriculum modules. Over the last 20 years we have seen the growth of pharmacoeconomics, medical informatics, translational medicine, psychoneuroimmunology, disease management, social medicine, biocultural medicine, and genomic medicine: all making valuable contributions to the health care landscape. How can the medical school curriculum accommodate them all?

Ideally, we should be able to "teach" all of the emerging disciplines as a fluid interplay. W. Russell, Lord Brain[18] wrote in the Canadian Medical Association Journal, "As each new specialty came of age it demanded a front door key to medical education, and a roof of its own in the curriculum and the examinations ... the curriculum should not be that of a honeycomb in which individual bees add cell to cell, but rather that of the cerebral cortex in which all the cells are functionally interrelated." Medical ethics is given a disservice when it is relegated to a Friday afternoon drug-company sponsored "lunch and learn," as if the consideration of ethical thought and protocols are an addendum to mainstream practice. Ethics should be taught at every opportunity, at every bedside, at every case presentation, and at every journal club meeting. Perhaps the same should be said of teaching developmental medicine. As patients are introduced to the students, the patients with intellectual disabilities should be viewed as patients with a presenting complaint or concern against the backdrop of their genetic condition. Two problems counter this ideal teaching scenario. Patients with developmental disabilities are seldom seen in any of the clinics in the clinical years, with the exception of pediatrics. The chances of encountering an adult patient with developmental disabilities in the psychiatry, medicine, ob-gyn, or surgery rotations are remote. In addition to the lack of patient encounters, there are no "faculty champions" to coordinate the background knowledge unique to intellectual and developmental disabilities. But perhaps the ruling reason for the lack of incorporating patients with developmental disabilities into the curriculum of undergraduate medical education lies in Wolf Wolfensberger's thesis of "social role valorization," that marginalized people are devalued by society and thus denied entry into those valued societal portals, specifically health care.[19]

For the time being, the few pockets of medical schools that have faculty champions offering rotations, clerkships, lectures, follow-alongs, and afternoons providing students with the opportunity to encounter patients with developmental and intellectual disabilities will continue to appear to their colleagues as "tilting at windmills."

Why would medical schools be so reluctant to adopt programs that introduce medical students to the challenges and rewards of treating patients with special health care needs, especially when schools of dentistry have adopted curricula change to prepare soon-to-be practitioners to provide care to individuals with special needs?

In 2004, the Commission on Dental Accreditation adopted new standards for dental and dental hygiene education programs to ensure didactic and clinical opportunities to prepare dental professionals for the care of persons with developmental disabilities, complex medical problems, significant physical limitations, and a vast array of other conditions considered under the rubric of "individuals with special needs." The standard states: "Graduates *must* (sic) be competent in assessing the treatment needs of patients with special needs." Implementation of this revised standard was required by January 2006. Specifically, "patients with special needs" has been defined in the standard as "those patients whose medical, physical, psychologic, or social situations make it necessary to modify normal dental routines to provide dental treatment for that individual. These individuals include, but are not limited to, people with developmental disabilities, complex medical problems and significant physical limitations."[20]

Perhaps the major reason for the lack of incorporating patients with developmental disabilities into the curricula of undergraduate medical education lies in the manner in which we tend to consider the individuals with special needs. Many view them in terms of the double pronunciation of the word "invalid," and thus deny them entry into the valued societal portals, specifically health care.

HUMAN RIGHTS

The story of Ashley and her "treatment" recently burst out in the national news.[21] Ashley, who is now 9 years old and has significant and lifelong disabilities, was given "growth attenuation" surgery and medication when she was 6 years old to keep her from growing to a full adult size. Her parents, in a decision that they say on their Web site "was not difficult," found physicians willing to surgically remove Ashley's breast buds, her appendix (even though nothing was wrong with it), and her uterus.

She was then treated with high doses of estrogen to stunt her growth. These procedures were performed without either court or ethics committee approval. Indeed, the institutional ethics committee that the family and physicians consulted before placing Ashley under the knife decided to leave the decision in the parents' hands, rather than engaging in the comprehensive, ethical debate the procedure deserved. As one might expect, the story of the "Ashley Treatment," the name the parents themselves coined for the procedure, generated brief but bitter debate. Things have now quieted down again.

Barely 3 weeks after Ashley's story hit the press, Switzerland's Supreme Court, to virtually no groundswell of public outcry and very little public notice, ruled that it is now permissible in Switzerland to allow assisted suicide for persons with serious mental illness, even if their condition is not otherwise terminal. Switzerland already permitted assisted suicide for people with terminal illnesses at the time this decision was announced.

The "Ashley Treatment" and Swiss assisted suicide stories came along about 15 months after a Netherlands facility announced the creation and implementation of the "Groningen Protocol." The Groningen Protocol, named for the pediatric hospital at which it was devised, described a five-step process physicians are encouraged to follow to sanction the euthanizing of infants who are born with serious, potentially life-threatening disabilities. The end step in the Groningen Protocol is that the physicians inject medication to kill the infants, rather than letting the infants pass away as a result of their disease or defect running its course. The Groningen Protocol physicians, at the time of announcing the Protocol, also announced that they had implemented the Protocol to euthanize four infants even before the Protocol was announced. One of those was a child with Down syndrome. Despite the implications of what the Groningen physicians call "a deliberate, life-ending procedure," the story received no substantive coverage in America outside of the medical community.

History has shown us that children with disabilities have been victims of involuntary sterilization, institutionalization, and widespread abuse, neglect, and death. Historically, society had little or no expectations for children with disabilities, and their families frequently felt shame. In the last 50 years, parents and professionals have united to reject these inhuman practices and to insist that our children have the same opportunity for lives of dignity and achievement that we expect for ourselves.

Over 60 years ago, millions died to rid the world of people who perpetrated these same shameful acts in the name of bogus science. Have we now ignored that sacrifice and the lessons they taught us? It is an outrage that no court or ethics committee engaged in the soul-searching debate a procedure like "Ashley's Treatment" should have generated. It is an outrage that society should countenance extreme surgical procedures and hormone injections as a solution to the challenges of caring for a 6-year-old child with complex disabilities.

Stigma

It is essential to understand the dynamics of stigma as the underlying fabric for disparities.[22] Ideally, physicians and dentists should be the last to be influenced by stigma. Sadly, the reality is that stigma is responsible for women with Down syndrome not being given regular Pap smears, not receiving mammograms, and not being eligible for heart transplants. Stigma is responsible for problems such as:

- Untold numbers of patients not receiving baseline dental radiography;
- Untold numbers of persons receiving inappropriate psychotropic drugs instead of behavioral analysis and behavioral plans;

Dental care being administered without a local anesthetic;
Unnecessary use of sedation or general anesthetics;
The underutilization of hospice and palliative care at the end of life for people with developmental disabilities.

We are also behind in appreciating and treating people with the dual diagnosis of developmental disabilities and psychiatric disorders. We brush off depression, ignore schizophrenia, make cracks at sexual self-abuse, and "ho-hum" suicidal ideation if the patient has a primary diagnosis of mental retardation. Mental retardation is not a diagnosis, it is simply the canvas on which these other footnotes are painted.

Stabilizing Maneuvers

Mothers and fathers have been helping to position, stabilize, and protect their children in medical and dental procedures since William Jenner first vaccinated James Phipps, an 8-year-old boy, for smallpox in 1796. In more recent times, in situations where the parent was unavailable, when the child was brought to the emergency room from a sleep-away camp or from school, the doctor would ask his or her nurse or dental assistant to play that role and compassionately and momentarily restrain the child.[23]

In the twenty-first century, things are pretty much the same, except the child, in addition to having excessive earwax or a broken tooth also has Down syndrome, cerebral palsy, autism, or any number of conditions associated with intellectual and developmental disabilities. Only this time, the dentist and dental assistant performing the same short duration stabilization are charged with physical abuse, improper use of physical restraint, and possibly assault.

This scenario of a dentist or physician facing charges of employing physical restraint on a child or adult with a disability stands as a formidable reason for clinicians to avoid caring for patients with complex disabilities. Sadly, many dentists and physicians who have cared for this population for years have decided that the potential liability is reason enough to exclude them from their practices.

For clarification purposes, the authors are not referring to the use of restraints (of any kind) that are used for the convenience of the staff or because of time-saving or financial considerations. The authors are not speaking of restraints that are used as a first measure before documented trials of desensitization. Specifically, the reference is to the use of short-interval stabilizing maneuvers, including the appropriate use of a papoose board when applicable in critical medical or dental procedures. Of note is that a thorough physical examination (including inspection, palpation, and auscultation) constitutes a "procedure." It often necessitates that a parent or assistant firmly hold a person's arms while they are pushing down on the abdomen to ascertain any abnormality. Without this, the examination becomes ineffectual and invalid.

The use of the word "appropriate" in the appropriate use of restraints and stabilization is key. The astute clinician appreciates that any restraint is part of a multitiered approach to compassionate care. The need for familiarity with desensitizing, distracting, and acclimating techniques must always be the first generation of patient care. For the patient with intuitive or learned fears, sensory issues, low pain thresholds, discomfort in strange environments, apprehension with strangers, or an inability to process the ongoing activity, the need for "steady as we go" needs to be incorporated into all practice cultures and regimens.

This cannot be approached as a "punch list" with half-heartened trials and immediately moving onto the next step. These initial steps are ideally repeated over time in a variety of settings. Even if the medical records demonstrated that previous attempts at desensitization were fruitless and that a restraining maneuver worked well, the dentist or physician has an ethical obligation to begin anew. It is not unusual that contributing factors (pain, time of day, setting, personal approach, uniforms, medications, hydration, bowel or urinary needs, hunger, temperature, music) will result in a different response from the same approach that was unsuccessful weeks before. Again, this requires a unique culture on behalf of the physician, dentists, and staff. Of course, in a life-threatening scenario, the immediate concern is the "fast and furious" life-saving intervention.

The ultimate restraint is of course sending the patient with a developmental disability to the operating room under general anesthesia. While under certain conditions this has its place in the clinical arena, it has its calculus of risk. There is a greater risk in this story: the risk of deferred, deprived, or denied treatment. This is the single biggest consequence of backing clinicians into a threatening corner regarding their ability to employ purposeful, compassionate stabilization.

Parents, caregivers, program administrators, advocacy groups, human rights and ethics committees, direct support professionals, and patients with special needs require education regarding the use of stabilizing and restraining protocols. They must appreciate that these procedures are being used in the continuum of the least restrictive environment, with the end point being the best possible treatment outcome.

As to the future, there is the need for:

- Health Resources and Services Administration to designate people with developmental or intellectual disabilities as a "medically underserved population."
- The Vital and Health Statistics Interview Survey series (for adults and children) to expand the collection of information beyond those individuals with physical disabilities to include individuals with intellectual disabilities.
- Support of demonstration projects designed to provide high quality, community-based dental services for people with developmental or intellectual disabilities.
- Encouragment of continuing education of dental professionals regarding the treatment of people with developmental or intellectual disabilities.
- The creation of a public awareness campaign regarding better oral health for people with developmental or intellectual disabilities.
- The use of Health Resources Administration and National Institute of Health training vehicles to encourage better training of health care professional regarding individuals with developmental or intellectual disabilities.

REFERENCES

1. Horwitz SM, Kerker BD, Owens PL, et al. The health status and needs of individuals with mental retardation. New Haven (CT): Yale University; 2001.
2. Report of the Surgeon General's Conference on Health Disparities and Mental Retardation. A National Action Agenda. Available at: http://www.surgeongeneral.gov/topics/cmh/childreport.html. Accessed September 19, 2008.
3. Waldman HB, Fenton SJ, Perlman SP, et al. Preparing dental graduates to provide care to individuals with special needs. J Dent Educ 2005;69:249–54.
4. Rader R. A legless report gives birth to a new academy. [Editorial]. EP Magazine 2002;32(12):13.
5. Rader R. Satchel Paige on being medically underserved. [Editorial]. EP Magazine 2005;35(1):6–7.
6. Surgeon General's Report. Closing the Gap. A national blueprint to improve the health of persons with mental retardation. Washington, DC: Department of Health and Human Services; 2002.

7. Ziring PR, Kastner T, Friedman DL, et al. Provision of health care for persons with developmental disabilities living in the community. The Morristown model. JAMA 1988;260:1439–44.
8. van Dyck PC, Kogan MD, McPherson MG, et al. Prevalence and characteristics of children with special health care needs. Arch Pediatr Adolesc Med 2004;158(9): 884–90.
9. Reichard A, Sacco TM, Turnbull HR III, et al. Access to health care; developmental disabilities; mental retardation; low income groups; minority groups. Ment Retard 2004;42(6):459–70.
10. Institute of Medicine. Committee on Understanding and Eliminating Racial and Ethnic Disparities in Health Care. Unequal treatment—confronting racial and ethnic disparities in health care. Washington, DC: National Academies Press; 2003.
11. The life of reason: reason in society. In: The letters of George Santayana, Book 4, 1928-1932. Scribner's; 1905.
12. Smith DB. Addressing racial inequities in health care. Civil rights monitoring and report cards. J Health Polit Policy Law 1998;23:75–105.
13. Field MJ, Jette A. The future of disability in America. Washington, DC: Institute of Medicine, Board of Health Sciences policy; 2007.
14. Health Resources and Services Administration. Shortage designation: HPSAs, MUAs & MUPs. Available at: http://bhpr.hrsa.gov/shortage/muaguide.htm. Accessed October 8, 2008.
15. Parish SL. Federal income payments and mental retardation: The political and economic context. Ment Retard 2003;41(6):446–59.
16. Kochanek KD, Murphy SL, Anderson RN, et al. Deaths: final data for 2002. Natl Vital Stat Rep 2004;53(5):1–116.
17. Platt R. Letter. Br Med J 1965;2:551. Available at: http://www.tedi.uq.edu.au/Conferences/teach_conference00/papers/reser.html Accessed October 15, 2008.
18. Brain R. Osler and medicine today. Can Med Assoc J 1960;83(8):349–54.
19. Wolfenberger W. Brief introduction to social role valorisation as a high order concept for addressing the plight of societally devalued people, and for structuring human services. [revised] 3rd edition. Syracuse (NY): Training Institute; 1998.
20. Commission on Dental Accreditation. Accreditation standards for dental education programs. Chicago: American Dental Association; 2004.
21. Valenzano JM Jr, Rader R, Luker T, et al. When the slippery slope becomes a mudslide. EP Magazine 2007;37(5):2–4.
22. Rader R. The emergence of the American Academy of Developmental Medicine and Dentistry: educating clinicians about the challenges and rewards of treating patients with special health care needs. Pediatr Dent 2007;29(2):134–7.
23. Rader R. Before the shot. [Editorial] EP Magazine 2008;38(4):6–7.

Planning Dental Treatment for People with Special Needs

Paul Glassman, DDS, MA, MBA*, Paul Subar, DDS

KEYWORDS

• Treatment planning • Oral health • Disabilities • Special needs
• Complex patients • Management

There are many terms used to describe people who have trouble receiving dental treatment in a routine manner. These include "people with special needs," "children with special health care needs," "people with disabilities," "people with complex needs," and other terms.[1–3] Some of these terms, such as "children with special health care needs" or people with "developmental disabilities" have definitions that are found in federal regulations and used for collection of data and funding purposes.[4,5] Other commonly used terms such as "people with special needs," "people with disabilities," or "people with complex needs" do not have generally agreed upon definitions, but are useful in describing populations who present challenges in providing oral health services. For the purpose of this clinically focused article the terms "people with special needs," "people with disabilities," and "people with complex needs" are used interchangeably and are defined as people who have difficulty accessing dental treatment services because of complicated medical, physical, social, or psychologic conditions.[6] This article discusses considerations in planning dental treatment for people with special needs.

THE POPULATION OF PEOPLE WITH SPECIAL NEEDS IS INCREASING DRAMATICALLY

It has been established that people with chronic medical illnesses, developmental disabilities, and psychosocial issues experience more oral health care problems than others who do not suffer from these conditions.[7–11] Advances in medicine have increased the likelihood that people today live longer with comorbidities that would previously have shortened their lifespan.[12] Patients with special needs have also seen a gain in life expectancy. Thirty years ago, for example, the typical person with Down's syndrome would have a life expectancy of roughly 12 years compared with 60 years today.[13] Because of these advances, the number of people with special

University of the Pacific, Arthur A. Dugoni School of Dentistry, 2155 Webster Street, San Francisco, CA 94115, USA
* Corresponding author.
E-mail address: pglassman@pacific.edu (P. Glassman).

Dent Clin N Am 53 (2009) 195–205
doi:10.1016/j.cden.2008.12.010
dental.theclinics.com
0011-8532/08/$ – see front matter

needs who need oral health services is growing dramatically. According to United States Census 2000, roughly 50 million people, or almost 20% of the population, has a long-standing condition or disability.[14] In addition to those with chronic morbidities or disabilities, the aging population of America also has problems with obtaining basic oral health care services. 3.6% of noninstitutionalized United States citizens over age 65 report needing care but are unable to obtain it.[15] The 2000 Surgeon General's Report on Oral Health indicates that people with developmental disabilities are at a significant disadvantage in obtaining hygiene services, have worse hygiene than their non-disabled counterparts, and have an increased need for periodontal treatment than the general population.[2] Untreated dental disease has been found in at least 25% of people with cerebral palsy, 30% of those with head injuries, and 17% of those with hearing impairment.[7] A study commissioned by the Special Olympics concluded that individuals with intellectual disabilities have poorer oral health, more untreated caries, and a higher prevalence of gingivitis and other periodontal diseases than the general population.[16,17] There is also a relation between disability and income. People from lower socio-economic groups and those covered by Medicaid have more dental disease and receive fewer dental services than the general population and many individuals with disabilities are in these lower socio-economic groups.[2,17,18] The large increase in the number of people with special needs now living in society and seeking dental treatment provides new challenges for dental providers. Among the challenges are those related to developing and implementing appropriate plans of treatment for these individuals (Special Olympics, unpublished data, 1999).

CHALLENGES IN PROVIDING ORAL HEALTH CARE FOR PEOPLE WITH DISABILITIES

There are numerous challenges in providing oral health services for people with special needs that go beyond the normal considerations for other populations. These challenges require oral health professionals to have extraordinary training, empathy, patience, and the desire to be successful. There are a number of areas where providing oral health services for these populations presents unique challenges.

First there is a need to understand and to be prepared to work with people with a wide variety of general health conditions. Although oral health professionals do not need to have complete knowledge of every general health condition that their patients present with, it is essential that they have the knowledge and experience to gather and apply the information they need. This implies the training and ability to function in health care teams and get consultations from physicians, social workers, and other general and social service professionals.

Oral health professionals should be well acquainted with the social service agencies, community living arrangements, and advocacy organizations operating in their community and the social context in which oral health services take place. They also need to understand and use appropriate language when interacting with individuals with special needs and their caregivers. There is a growing movement advocating the use of "People First" language.[19–21] This language emphasizes the fact that disability is a part of the human condition and all people want to be described by their abilities rather than labeled by their disabilities. An oral health professional who does not understand this language and refers to people he treats as "the handicapped patients I see" risks alienating the individual, their caregiver, and those advocating for full inclusion in our society.

Oral health professionals must also realize the extraordinary vulnerability of people with special needs to abuse and neglect in our society.[22,23] They need to understand how to recognize abuse and neglect and their role as mandated reporters. Oral health providers are health professionals and as a part of the health care team they may find that their patients are depressed, suicidal, or unable to cope with various living challenges. They have an obligation to intervene, provide basic diagnosis and counseling and make appropriate referrals for follow-up of these situations.

Oral health professionals need to understand how to prevent oral diseases in people with various disabilities. There are special challenges presented by working with someone where communication and even procedures need to be performed by a third person, the caregiver. Some people have limited physical ability to perform oral hygiene procedures and "partial participation" programs need to be designed and performed. This term refers to having the individual do as much as they are able to, but having a caregiver ensure that needed prevention procedures are completed. There are numerous informational, physical, and behavioral obstacles to be addressed. These are described in detail in "Overcoming Obstacles to Dental Health," a training package for caregivers of people with disabilities.[24] In addition to this package, there is a large body of literature that describes the challenges and techniques for helping people with special needs prevent oral diseases.[25–28]

DEVELOPING A TREATMENT PLAN FOR A PERSON WITH SPECIAL NEEDS

The process of developing a dental treatment plan typically progresses through several phases. The first phase involves gathering data about the individual, which is then used to develop a diagnosis or set of diagnoses. A set of treatment recommendations are then determined, and discussed with the patient and/or their caregiver. After discussion, a plan of treatment is developed to address the various diagnoses. The patient or caregiver must be informed about the benefits, risks, and alternatives to all the treatment options. The process of obtaining informed consent for someone who cannot provide their own consent can be complex, but is beyond the scope of this article.

While the general schema described above for developing dental treatment plans is commonly followed by dentists for all patients, there are important elements within the three phases described above that may receive little attention for healthy patients with uncomplicated histories, yet are critical to consider for people with special needs. This article presents a "Schema for Planning Treatment for Complex Patients" which is diagrammed in **Fig. 1**. The "(4)" after "Treatment Plan" in the diagram indicates that there are four distinct phases of the plan, which are discussed below.

GATHERING DATA

The traditional format for gathering data about an individual's health history follows the schema described in **Box 1**. The process described here follows this format but places much greater emphasis on gathering data about the areas of family history and social history. These areas are often neglected when dentists gather data about patient's health histories. As listed in **Fig. 1**, the emphasis in gathering data for people with complex histories and treatment needs is on medical, physical, and psychologic information; social and personal information; and finally dental information. The order in which these areas are listed is designed to counteract the tendency of dentists to focus on dental history and problems first.

Box 2 presents a series of questions that can guide the oral health provider in gathering data of particular importance for a person with one or more disabilities. The questions are divided into four sections.

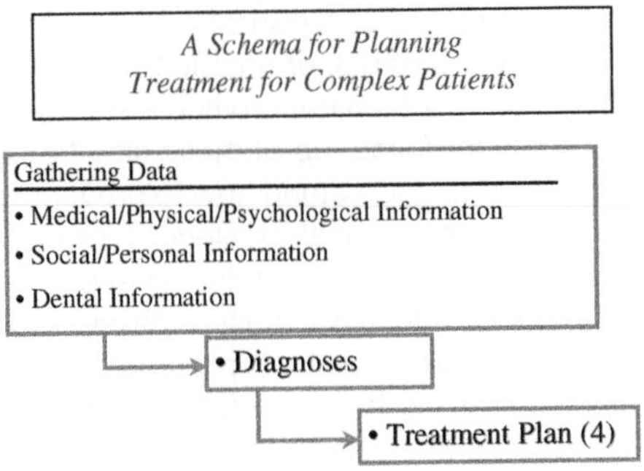

Fig. 1. A schema for planning treatment for complex patients.

Medical Information

The emphasis in gathering medical information, in addition to all the areas listed in **Box 1**, is on understanding the person's disability. It is also important to understand how severe the disability is and its short- and long-term prognosis. A neuromuscular disorder such as cerebral palsy generally does not progress over the individual's lifetime. Other neuromuscular disorders such as Huntington's disease generally result in a rapid functional decline and a fatal outcome. Although at a certain stage of these disorders the clinical manifestations might be similar, long-term prognosis is very different. It's clear that a provider who does not understand this difference in prognosis might make inappropriate treatment recommendations.

In addition to understanding the disability and prognosis, it's essential to understand what treatments are being provided, including medications given, and the short- and long-term effects of those treatments on the provision of dental care and maintenance of oral health.

Social/Personal Information

Once a provider understands the individual's disability and medical treatment, it's important to appreciate how the disability affects their basic areas of functioning, referred to as activities of daily living (ADL) as well as the effect of the disability on the individual's ability to get to dental appointments, sit in the dental chair for treatment, and perform procedures necessary to maintain oral health. An understanding of the effect of the individual's disability on their daily life will allow the provider to

Box 1
Traditional health history format

ID = identifying data (age, ethnicity, source of data)

CC = chief concern

HPI = history of the present illness

MH = medical history

DH = dental history

SH = social history

EX = examination (this includes clinical, radiographic, and laboratory examinations)

DX = diagnosis (or differential diagnosis)

P = plan (including phases, ethical considerations, and further diagnostic steps)

Box 2
Schema for data gathering for developing treatment plans for complex patients

Medical information

a. What is the disability?
b. How severe?
c. What is the long- and short-term prognosis?
d. What treatment is being (or will be) given and what are the side effects?
e. What medications are being taken and what are the side effects?

Social/personal information

a. What is the effect of the disability(-ies) on the patient's life?
b. What are the effects of the dental problems on the patient's life?
c. What would the effect of dental treatment be on the patient's life?
d. What is the person's ability to understand, communicate, and perform procedures?
e. What support persons are available?
f. What are the expectations of the patient and support persons?
g. What financial support is available?

Dental information

a. What dental abnormalities are associated with the disability(-ies)?
   1. Do the abnormalities need treatment?
   2. What considerations are there in treating these abnormalities?
b. What other dental problems exist?
c. How does the person's disability(-ies) affect the delivery of dental services?
   1. What behavioral, psychologic, pharmacologic supports are needed?
   2. What position modifications are needed?
   3. What precautions or special procedures need to be employed?
d. How does the disability and associated problems affect the maintenance of oral health?
   1. What oral hygiene procedures can and will be performed?
   2. How will dental appliances be tolerated and cared for?
   3. Will it be possible to establish a schedule of recall appointments which can be kept?
e. What is the prognosis for the future?
   1. What is the prognosis for dental health and/or dental problems with and without treatment?
   2. What is the risk and benefit of each procedure that might be indicated?

Treatment plan

a. What, when, how, and who for each of the following:
   1. Emergency treatment
   2. Preventive program
   3. Initial treatment
   4. Future maintenance treatment

properly consider the impact of individual's dental problems and dental treatment on their life and achieve a reasonable balance between these considerations. Not all dental problems need treatment. Sometimes the solution is worse than the problem. The provider who has a broad view of the person's life is more likely to recognize these circumstances.

Another social/personal consideration is the individual's ability to understand, communicate, and perform procedures. Some individuals need help from caregivers to perform procedures necessary to maintain oral health. Therefore it is critical to understand what support persons are available for this individual and what can be expected from these support persons. Also, determining the expectations of caregivers, guardians, and family members is key. Some people with disabilities have multiple individuals who are responsible for aspects of their life or care about the outcome of dental treatment. It's much easier for the oral health provider to communicate with all concerned before the dental appointment than to deal with unhappy support persons after treatment has been performed.

Dental Information

While all oral health providers gather detailed information about their patient's dental conditions, there are some particular areas of inquiry that are helpful when gathering data for individual with a complex set of conditions and needs. One area to focus on is whether there are dental conditions that are associated with individual's disabilities and whether these conditions or abnormalities require intervention. An obvious example would be a patient with a seizure disorder who is taking Dilantin. The oral health provider should be aware of the association of this medicine with gingival hyperplasia. If the individual does not yet have this problem, they might be counseled about the increased risk and how to prevent it.

Another important area of inquiry involves the person's ability to participate in dental treatment. It's critical to know whether this individual will require any physical, behavioral, psychologic, or pharmacologic supports to receive dental treatment. The Special Care Dentistry Association (SCDA) has developed guidelines for the indications and use of these treatment adjuncts.[29] It's also important to be aware of any special precautions that need to be taken when providing dental treatment.

When developing a treatment plan, it is critical that the oral health provider take a long-term view. Therefore an essential part of the data gathering process is an understanding about how oral hygiene and oral health prevention procedures will be performed in the future. Consider carefully whether this individual will be able to care for dental prostheses and will be able to establish and keep future continuing care appointments.

Another outcome of taking a long-term view of the individual's oral health is the provider's best guess about which course of treatment is most likely to result in this individual's ability to have a lifetime of oral health. The risks and benefits of each procedure which might be provided should be carefully weighed in light of the individual's disabilities and life circumstances. Sometimes "less is more" in that complex restorations which require maintenance procedures beyond the individual's capability can actually reduce the possibility of an individual maintaining optimal oral health.

THE TREATMENT PLAN

Fig. 2 lists four components of the treatment plan: (1) the plans for immediate or emergency treatment, (2) a plan for a preventive program, (3) a plan for the course of initial

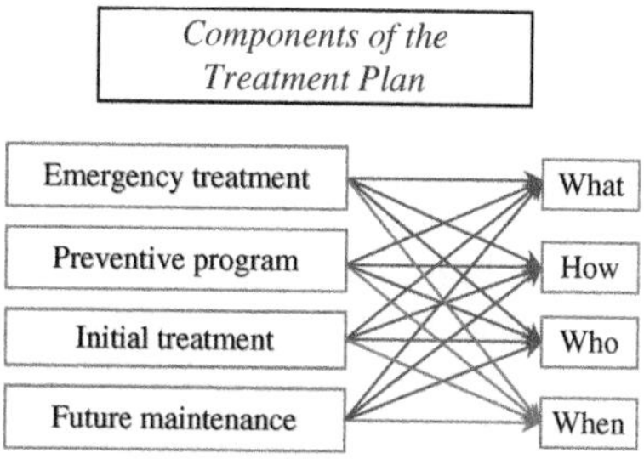

Fig. 2. Components of the treatment plan.

treatment, and (4) a plan for future maintenance. Although these issues are typically included, at least to some degree, in most dental treatment plans, breaking them out into separate components helps to emphasize the unique importance of each area and minimizes the tendency to neglect any of these areas, all of which are critical to a plan to allow people with special needs to have a lifetime of oral health. For each component it is important to decide what services will be provided, how these services will be delivered, who will perform aspects of the treatment, and how the services will be sequenced. The four treatment planning areas are further explored below.

Emergency Treatment

The first phase of any plan is to address areas of pain and acute infection. The goal of these interventions should be to place the individual in a "holding pattern" while the subsequent phases of the treatment plan are developed. In providing emergency treatment the provider should be careful not to carry the treatment to the point where it might differ from the treatment plan that is worked out later. For example, although an initial endodontic access might relieve pain from an infected tooth, it would not be prudent to complete the endodontic treatment and later decide that this tooth should be removed as a part of the overall treatment plan for the patient.

Preventive Program

Activities designed to prevent the occurrence of further dental disease are sometimes considered separate from the dental treatment plan. The preventive program is incorporated here as a second and critical component of the treatment planning process for several reasons. First, when providing oral health services for people with special needs, it is critical to emphasize a preventive approach. For many people with special needs, fixing dental problems once they occur can be much more difficult than with other populations. Second, the preventive program can be thought of as a diagnostic step. It is important that the oral health provider understand the capabilities of the patient and their caregivers to perform preventive procedures. Often this cannot be adequately ascertained without spending some time educating the patient and caregiver, demonstrating plaque removal and other procedures and observing the results of these interventions. Clearly a different treatment plan should be recommended for someone who is able to incorporate preventive recommendations into their daily routine and has stopped the progression of oral disease than the plan that would be recommended for someone who is not able to do so.

It is important to remember that simply having a staff member in a dental office provide "oral hygiene instructions" is not likely to change caregiver or patient behavior if used alone. Interventions designed to improve patient and caregiver knowledge are much more effective when paired with demonstration and mentoring activities.[28]

The Caries Management by Risk Assessment (CAMBRA) evaluation is a system for determining risk for developing dental caries that can apply to people with special needs.[30] The CAMBRA program begins with determining the patient's relative risk for developing caries at present and in the future. To provide additional information about the patient's oral environment, bacterial testing can be done as well. Several testing aids are available that measure relative titers of *Streptococcus mutans* and *Lactobacillus*.[31] A risk score from low to extremely high is then determined based on factors such as food intake and nutrition, home care, professional care, and the existing oral environment. These caries risk indicators are classified as either biologic risk factors or protective factors (both biologic and nonbiologic). Medications can then be prescribed based on the caries score from the indicators and bacterial testing. Medical and other preventive products include antibacterial rinses, fluoride, xylitol mints and gum, sealants, and other adjuncts.

Risk assessment, medical treatments, and health promotion strategies are all necessary parts of the preventive component of the treatment plan. These preventive strategies are described in greater detail elsewhere.[32]

Initial Treatment

The "initial treatment" component of the treatment plan describes the surgical and restorative interventions planned to address individual's identified dental problems. In some cases these interventions are performed in phases, usingthe results of earlier phases to modify the plan for subsequent phases of treatment. This strategy might be particularly important when working with individual where it is not clear to what extent they will be able to tolerate treatment in a dental chair. Initially performing less demanding procedures will give the oral health provider important information about the individual's ability to tolerate more complex treatment.

In addition to determining what procedures will be a part of the initial course of treatment, it's also important to determine how those procedures will be performed. Oral health professionals need to be familiar with a variety of treatment options for providing oral health services for people with special needs. **Fig. 3** describes some of the modalities that are available to help people have dental services. The modalities on the left side of the continuum are those with the least expense and fewest side effects. Oral health professionals who have all these options available personally or by referral are in the best position to provide treatment using the optimal modality for the individual they are seeing. For example, in a given community, if there are no dental offices where behavioral or physical supports are provided, then more people than necessary may end up having dental treatment via sedation or general anesthesia.

The SCDA guidelines referenced earlier describe a range of modalities, similar to those in **Fig. 3**, that can be used to help people with special needs receive dental treatment.[29] These include:

- General anesthesia delivered in hospitals, surgical centers, and dental offices
- Sedation, ranging from minimal sedation to deep sedation
- Behavioral support
- Physical support
- Psychologic support
- Social support
- Prevention strategies

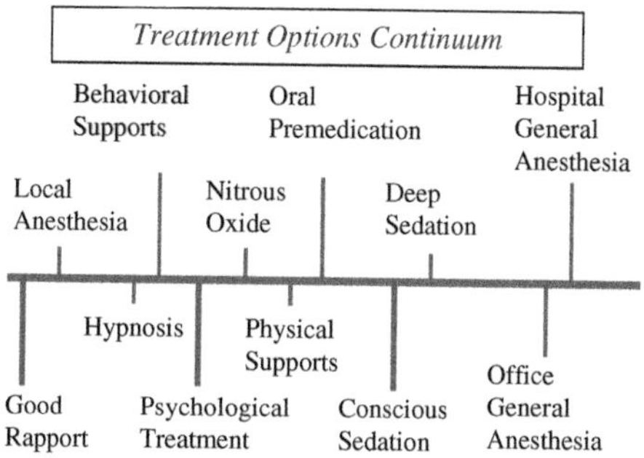

Fig. 3. Treatment options continuum.

The SCDA consensus statement discusses the interplay between these modalities and the possibility that behavioral, physical, psychologic, and social supports and prevention strategies can reduce the need for sedation and general anesthesia.

Future Maintenance

The fourth phase of the recommended treatment plan is the plan for future maintenance of dental health. It is critical to consider a long-term plan before deciding on and performing a course of initial treatment. This involves a careful analysis of the person's medical, physical, social, and psychologic conditions and an analysis of the prognosis of these factors in combination with their oral conditions. For example, it would be inadvisable to construct a complex dental prosthesis that requires meticulous care for an individual who has a neurodegenerative disorder that will predictably result in a significant physical decline and death over the next 3–4 years. The future maintenance plan should be based on recommendations that will have the best chance of allowing the individual to have a lifetime of oral health.

SUMMARY

People with disabilities and other special needs present unique challenges for oral health professionals in planning and carrying out dental treatment. The schema for planning dental treatment presented in this article encourages the oral health provider to fully consider multiple medical, social, psychologic, and dental findings when preparing treatment recommendations for a patient with special needs. If these factors are fully integrated, the resulting treatment recommendations provide the best chance of helping the individual achieve and maintain a lifetime of oral health.

REFERENCES

1. Waldman HB, Perlman SP, Waldman HB, et al. Children with special health care needs: results of a national survey. J Dent Child(Chic) 2006;73(1):57–62.
2. U.S. Department of Health and Human Services. Oral health in America: a report of the surgeon general. U.S. Department of Health and Human Services, National Institute of Dental and Craniofacial Research. Rockville (MD): National Institutes of Health; 2000.
3. Glassman P, Henderson T, Helgeson M, et al. Consensus statement: oral health for people with special needs: consensus statement on implications and recommendations for the dental profession. J Calif Dent Assoc 2005;33(8):619–23.

4. Newacheck PW, Rising JP, Kim SE. Children at risk for special health care needs. Pediatrics 2007;118(1):334–42.
5. Definition of Developmental Disability. 42 US Code, Section 15002(8), 1978.
6. Glassman P, Anderson M, Jacobsen P, et al. Practical protocols for the prevention of dental disease in community settings for people with special needs: the protocols. Spec Care Dentist 2003;23(5):86–90.
7. The disparity cavity: filling America's oral health gap. Oral Health America 2000.
8. Haavio ML. Oral health care of the mentally retarded and other persons with disabilities in the Nordic countries: present situation and plans for the future. Spec Care Dentist 1995;15:65–9.
9. Feldman CA, Giniger M, Sanders M, et al. Special olympics, special smiles: assessing the feasibility of epidemiologic data collection. J Am Dent Assoc. 1997; 128:1687–96.
10. Waldman HB, Perlman SP, Swerdloff M. Use of pediatric dental services in the 1990s: some continuing difficulties. J Dent Child. 2000;67:59–63.
11. Oral health: factors contributing to low use of dental services by low-income populations. United States general accounting office. Report to congressional requesters. September 2000.
12. US Bureau of the Census: Current population reports, series P-25, no 1018, projections of the population of states by age, sex and race: 1988–2010. Washington, US Government Printing Office 1988:29, 94, 95, 97, 99, 100, 01, 03, 05.
13. Bittles AH, Bower C, RH, et al. The four ages of Down syndrome. Eur J Public Health 2006;17(2):221–5.
14. U.S. Department of Commerce, Economics and Statistics Administration, U.S. Census Bureau. Census 2000 Brief. Disability Status 2000. March 2003.
15. Dolan TA, Atchison K, Huynh TN. Access to dental care among older adults in the United States. J Drug Educ 2005;69(9):961–74.
16. Horwitz S, Kerker B, Owens P, et al. The health status and needs of individuals with mental retardation. Special Olympics 2000.
17. U.S. Bureau of the Census: Americans with disabilities: 1994–95. Current Population reports. P70-61. Census Brief, CENBR/97-5 Washington DC: U.S. Department of Commerce, Economics and Statistics Administration, 1997b Dec.
18. Stiefel DJ. Adults with Disabilities. Dental Care Considerations of Disadvantages and Special Care Populations: Proceedings of the Conference held April 18–19, 2001, in Baltimore, Maryland. U.S. Department of Health and Human Services, Health Resources and Services Administration, Bureau of Health Professions, Division of Medicine and Dentistry, Division of Nursing. April 2001.
19. Snow K. People first language. Available at: http://www.disabilityisnatural.com/peoplefirstlanguage.htm. Accessed September 1, 2007.
20. West Virginians with Developmental Disabilities. People first language. Available at: http://www.wvddc.org/people_first.html. Accessed September 1, 2007.
21. The Life Span Institute. Guidelines for reporting and writing about people with disabilities. Available at: http://www.lsi.ku.edu/lsi/internal/guidelines.html. Accessed September 1, 2007.
22. Glassman P, Chavez E, Hawks D. Abuse and neglect of elderly individuals: guidelines for oral health professionals. CDA J 2004;32(4):332–5.
23. Glassman P, Miller C, Ingraham R, et al. The extraordinary vulnerability of people with disabilities: guidelines for oral health professionals. J Calif Dent Assoc 2004; 32(5):379–86.
24. Miller C, Glassman P, Wozniak T, et al. "Overcoming obstacles to dental health—a training program for caregivers of people with disabilities". 4th edition. 1998.

25. Glassman P, Miller C. Dental disease prevention and people with special needs. CDA J 2003;31(2):149–60.
26. Glassman P, et al. Practical protocols for the prevention of dental disease in community settings for people with special needs: the protocols. Spec Care Dentist 2003;23(5):160–4.
27. Glassman P, Miller C. Preventing dental disease for people with special needs: the need for practical preventive protocols for use in community settings. Spec Care Dentist 2003;23(5):165–7.
28. Glassman P, Miller C. Effect of preventive dentistry training program for caregivers in community facilities on caregiver and client behavior and client oral hygiene. NY State Dental J 2006;72(2):38–46.
29. Consensus Statement on Sedation, Anesthesia, and Alternative Techniques for People with Special Needs. J. Spec. Care Dent, in press.
30. Young DA, Featherstone JDB, Roth JR. Curing the silent epidemic: caries management in the 21st century and beyond. J Calif Dent Assoc 2007;35(10): 681–702.
31. Featherstone JDB, Young DA, Jenson L, et al. Caries risk assessment in practice for age 6 through adult. J Calif Dent Assoc 2007;35(10):703–13.
32. Glassman P. Oral health promotion with people with special needs. In: Mostofsky D, Forgione A, Giddon D, editors. Chapter in behavioral dentistry. Ames (IA): Blackwell Munksgaard; 2006. p. 231–42.

Special Needs of Anxious and Phobic Dental Patients

Mark Slovin, DDS[a,b,*], June Falagario-Wasserman, MA, LMHC[c]

KEYWORDS

- Dental anxiety • Dental phobia • Behavioral dentistry
- Dental avoidance • Desensitization • Relaxation therapy
- Sedation • Dental rehabilitation

Modern dentistry has made much progress in providing a patient-friendly environment.[1] Still, despite revolutionary new dental techniques, anxiety toward dentistry has stayed relatively constant over the past 50 years.[2,3] It is said to be ranked fourth among common fears and ninth among intense fears.[4] Severe dental anxiety leading to avoidance is a common occurrence in the United States, where avoidance rates range between 6%–20% of the population. These individuals avoid dental treatment at all costs. Patients who struggle with this debilitating phobia have special needs and, therefore, require special care once they present for dental treatment. Among dental patients who regularly seek care, as many as 50% report some anxiety toward their dental experiences.[5] These individuals can be classified as "casual avoiders" because they frequently postpone necessary dental treatment. In both cases referenced above, the resulting neglect usually leads to dental breakdown. Fearful dental avoiders tend to receive less oral health care, or a lower quality of care, than the general population and may have oral problems that can affect systemic health.[6] Dentists with knowledge and interest in this serious problem can do well to rehabilitate these suffering individuals, whose quality of life is compromised by this troubling phenomenon. For the past 8–10 years, the Commission for Dental Accreditation of the American Dental Association has developed a competency component in the Standard for Dental Education to better address the behavioral aspects of special needs dental care and management issues. The social, psychologic, and physical functional problems of dental phobia have extended this phenomenon to a comprehensive quality of life concern. When oral health is compromised, overall health and

[a] Dental Phobia Program, Stony Brook University School of Dental Medicine, Stony Brook, NY 11794, USA
[b] Department of General Dentistry, Stony Brook University School of Dental Medicine, Stony Brook, NY 11794, USA
[c] Child and Adolescent Services, Advanced Center for Psychotherapy, Jamaica Hospital and Medical Center, 178-10 Wexford Terrace, Jamaica Estates, NY 11432, USA
* Corresponding author.
E-mail address: drslovin@aol.com (M. Slovin).

Dent Clin N Am 53 (2009) 207–219
doi:10.1016/j.cden.2008.12.016

quality of life may be diminished.[7] A study by James[1] found that lack of insurance, finances, or gainful employment had nothing to do with avoidance of dental treatment—it was solely due to fear. A discussion of the subject of dental avoidance due to fear requires a definition of common terms used to describe this issue. Fear is an individual's response to a real threat or danger. The operative word in this definition is "real."[8] Fear is objective, because it is directly linked to something specific, a known danger, and causes a physiologic response.[9] For example, an individual who is going to attempt to ski downhill for the first time following some brief lessons is facing a real threat. One could be seriously injured during this activity. Anxiety is synonymous with fear except that the threat is ill-defined.[8] It is subjective, anticipatory, and often associated with the unknown or ambiguous. Chambers[10] notes that the manifestation of a certain degree of anxiety by the patient toward the dental experience is not only an expected response but also a desirable one. The argument is offered that all situations in life are best approached and executed by the individual when he possesses a measure of anxiety that is optimal for the particular situation. It is important to distinguish between anxiety and phobia. In the example of downhill skiing, an experienced skier who feels uneasy about the activity only on a particular day illustrates anxiety. One often cannot pinpoint the reason for this underlying feeling of uneasiness. A phobia is an overwhelming, irrational feeling of fear which causes one to avoid the threatening stimulus at all costs.[8] Exposure to the feared object provokes an immediate anxiety response that may produce panic-like symptoms. In the case of a skier, an individual cannot even imagine participating in the activity without feeling symptoms of severe anxiety and discomfort. Much of the research in the area of dental phobia shows that "fear" consists of feelings and thoughts that are often expressed through avoidance behavior, and dental fear is learned primarily through aversive experiences.

ETIOLOGY

Fearful dental avoidance stems from either direct or indirect experiences. Direct experiences are those which one experiences personally. A painful dental experience, either past or current,[11] or the belief that painful treatment is inevitable, can initiate the pattern of avoidance.[12] Indirect experiences are those that are vicariously adopted from others (ie, family members, peers, media, etc.). Children are impressionable and often adopt parental fears. Body language and subtle comments can be transferred in such a way that they create a subconscious fear in an "innocent bystander." This phenomenon is not uncommon in adults as well.

Negative interactions with dental staff members can provoke and embarrass a sensitive dental patient into many years of dental treatment avoidance. Many patients who present to the dental office after long periods of avoidance report a feeling of belittlement, which in some way validates their absence. Today's dental staff is cognizant of this serious problem. Staff members are chosen with care and carefully trained to deal with the special needs of the phobic patient. The goal is to ensure that everyone who makes contact with the patient—from the receptionist who takes the initial phone call to the hygienist and dentist, who perform many potentially painful procedures—is adept at welcoming these patients and helping them to relax.[13]

Some dental phobic individuals suffer from a host of psychologic and emotional disorders in addition to their dental phobia. There are many forms of anxiety, and the four major classes of anxiety are: generalized anxiety disorder, obsessive compulsive disorder, phobic anxiety disorder, and panic disorder, which can lead to anxiety crisis or panic syndrome.[14] A panic attack can be a serious and upsetting occurrence during a dental visit, in which one or more of the following physical symptoms may be exhibited: palpitations, sweating, trembling, shortness of breath, feeling like choking, chest pain, nausea, dizziness, derealization, fear of dying, paresthesias, or chills.[15] A comprehensive medical and dental history can elicit the patient's mental health status and possibly prevent this untoward reaction. Consultation with a mental health professional would be in order in these extreme cases.

Most people like to have a sense of control over their circumstances. In the area of dental treatment, phobic individuals report "an intense lack of control,"[16] which exacerbates anxiety and produces a panic-like response. Often patients do not understand the procedure being performed and harbor a general fear of the unknown.[12] Feelings of helplessness may be induced by something as simple as reclining the dental chair. In addition, instrument presentation or manipulation, and the customary hand-piece water spray often cause feelings of choking.

A more comprehensive discussion of the treatment techniques that can be useful in patient management to prevent the previously mentioned etiologic factors are described later in this article.

EVALUATION OF DENTAL FEAR

The evaluation of a dental phobic individual is crucial to the overall management and treatment outcome. Dental phobic adults often manifest their anxiety at its worst in the waiting room, where clinicians are less likely to observe it. Fidgeting, pacing, sitting on the edge of the chair, repetitious limb movement, or startled reactions to noise may be manifested by the anxious patient while waiting for the appointment.[17] A characteristic presentation often includes body language in the form of generalized muscle tension, as noted by clenched hands, causing "white knuckle syndrome." Tension in the facial muscles often causes an eye fixation depicting their fear as a "deer-in-headlights."

Dental phobic individuals tend to cancel or break appointments frequently. In observing this behavior the clinician can ascertain whether these missed appointments are related to the patients' anxiety. One strategy that may be helpful to both patient and practitioner is to work out an agreement with the patient in which the appointment is kept, even if the patient does not want to participate in the planned treatment procedure. In this way, the clinician has the opportunity to further counsel the patient, and the patient has a better sense of control. An added benefit is that the negative reinforcement which would have occurred had the patient not attended the scheduled appointment is thereby averted.

An inquiring dental phobic individual's first contact with the dental office is usually via telephone. It is most important that this patient is greeted by a caring and empathic staff member. This phone call sets the tone for the entire dental experience and should be representative of the office philosophy in regard to the treatment of dental anxiety.

The first face-to-face interview should be an friendly "get-acquainted" meeting with staff members, including dental auxiliaries and clinicians. This may be best accomplished in a location of the office with no dental equipment. In some cases the sights and sounds may trigger memories that increase anxiety. In this interview the patient is encouraged to verbalize in their own words their perception of the origin of their dental fear. This may produce a catharsis, which itself is therapeutic.[13] To enhance the interview process the dentist could ask questions that would elicit more valuable information. Questions such as, "What could a dentist do to make you more comfortable during your procedure?" and "What might a dentist do that would make you more uncomfortable?."[8]

The interview process is often thought to be the foundation of the therapeutic relationship between a health professional and the patient.[18] Whereas communication skills are key to a good relationship, a friendly, smiling face and a reassuring tone are probably more important than getting the dialog correct.[19] Dental phobic individuals are assessing at all times that their dental needs will be met by a sensitive clinician. Effective listening, effective feedback, and clarification also help the professional develop good communication with the patient. Patients who feel that they can communicate with their dentist are more likely to show an improvement in their symptoms, and will return to the same dentist for continued treatment.[20] This rapport establishes a mutual working relationship, whereby the patient builds confidence that their needs are being satisfied, and the clinician enjoys the positive outcomes of the treatment relationship. Non-verbal communication such as touch, proximity, posture and orientation, body movements and gestures, facial expression, gaze and eye contact, and general appearance is an equally essential component to the interview. Dentists are unique practitioners because they have to touch a sensitive part of the body, the oral cavity. The issue of proximity may be threatening to the patient due to the encroachment on their "personal space." It is important for the dentist to face the patient and observe their expressions and reactions during verbal exchange. Rapid movements increase anxiety and should be avoided. The dentist should attempt to offer positive facial expressions which yield optimistic impressions in the patient. Eye contact is essential in conveying respect for the patient. The professional demeanor of the clinician and his or her office staff are substantial elements in establishing overall confidence.[21]

Assessments of dental anxiety have been conducted in various populations around the world. Dental anxiety represents a specific situational and anticipatory state that can be identified and categorized using validated, specially designed questionnaires.[22] The objective assessment of dental anxiety could be made by the Dental Anxiety Scale (**Fig. 1**), developed by Norman Corah, and the Dental Fear Survey (DFS) (**Fig. 2**), developed by Ronald Kleinknecht.[23] Newton and Buck[24] set out to provide an overview of measures of anxiety and pain in dental research over a 10-year period. The authors collected and reviewed the following information: the length of the scale; response format used; data on the reliability of the scale; data on the validity of the scale; and availability of alternate forms of the scale. According to their findings, and consistent with its reputation, the Corah Dental Anxiety Scale is known to maintain high internal consistency and test–retest reliability. Its use as a measurement tool for dental anxiety is well established and evidenced by over 35 articles in which the scale has been used or cited since 1988. The Kleinknecht Dental Fear Survey, measures three dimensions: avoidance of dental treatment, somatic symptoms of anxiety, and anxiety caused by the dental stimuli. They are scored on a 5-point Likert scale ranging from "never" to "nearly every time." Newton & Buck find this scale to be reliable and stable across different groups of respondents. This measurement tool is considered in the field of anxiety research to be the most sensitive and reliable measure for dental anxiety because of the internal consistency of the scale, test–retest reliability and validity of the questionnaire.[25]

In terms of the patients beliefs and perceptions related to dental anxiety, the Dental Beliefs Survey (DBS) (**Fig. 3**) addresses the subjective perceptions of the patient regarding the behavior of the dentist, and the process of how the care is delivered.[26] The purpose of the DBS is to identify to what degree the patient perceives the behavior of dental staff members as contributing to the problem. Therefore, the vital information obtained from this survey can alert the staff to the relative special needs of that patient and enhance the treatment experience.[26]

Corah Dental Anxiety Scale

1. If you had to go to the dentist tomorrow, how would you feel about it?
   a. I would look forward to it as a reasonably enjoyable experience.
   b. I wouldn't care one way or the other.
   c. I would be a little uneasy about it.
   d. I would be afraid that it would be unpleasant and painful.
   e. I would be very frightened of what the dentist might do.
2. When you are waiting in the dentist's office for your turn in the chair, how do you feel?
   a. Relaxed.
   b. A little uneasy.
   c. Tense.
   d. Anxious.
   e. So anxious that I sometimes break out in a sweat or almost feel physically sick.
3. When you are in the dentist's chair waiting while he/she gets the drill ready to begin working on your teeth, how do you feel?
   a. Relaxed.
   b. A little uneasy.
   c. Tense.
   d. Anxious.
   e. So anxious that I sometimes break out in a sweat or almost feel physically sick.
4. You are in the dentist's chair to have your teeth cleaned. While you are waiting and the dentist is getting out the instruments, which he/she will use to scrape your teeth around the gums, how do you feel?
   a. Relaxed.
   b. A little uneasy.
   c. Tense.
   d. Anxious.
   e. So anxious that I sometimes break out in a sweat or almost feel physically sick.

Fig. 1. Corah dental anxiety scale. (*From* Corah NL. Development of a dental anxiety scale. J Dent Res 1969;48:596; with permission.)

Ascertaining the specific foci of threatening dental situations is useful, particularly in developing a hierarchy where the patient can rank on a sliding scale his/her responses toward those experiences. The Mount Sinai Dental Fear Inventory (Mount Sinai Medical Center, 1978) (**Fig. 4**), allows patients to rate themselves on a scale from 0–100, where 0 is so relaxed they might fall asleep, and 100 is the point when fear is at its greatest. The inventory includes many common threatening situations and sensations. It also allows individuals to add their own category if not already included. In reviewing this inventory the dental clinician can develop a treatment plan beginning with the least threatening situation and progressing at a comfortable pace to completion of the treatment.

EXAMINATION AND TREATMENT PLANNING

The governing principles in the psychodynamics of the "dentist–patient relationship" involves the patient's special needs, fears, drives, and defenses that must be considered by the dentist, as well as the dentist's own needs. A set of principles for examining the anxious, fearful, dental patient may be called the "reality approach."[27]

1. The patient is granted the reality of his or her symptoms or complaints. This acknowledgment must be apparent in the attitude and demeanor of the examining doctor. It is not a principle that can be mechanically applied, but must be internally motivated.
2. The patient's anxiety or fear requires a thorough exploration and examination of the symptoms and complaints. Fearful dental patients must be assured

Kleinknecht Dental Fear Survey (DFS)

Name__________________________________

Date_________________________

The items in this questionnaire refer to various situations, feelings, and reactions related to dental work. Please rate your feeling or reaction on these items by *circling the number* (1, 2, 3, 4, or 5) of the category which most closely corresponds to your reaction.

---

1. Has fear of dental work ever caused you to put off making an appointment?

1	2	3	4	5
never	once or twice	a few times	often	nearly every time

2. Has fear of dental work ever caused you to cancel or not appear for an appointment?

1	2	3	4	5
never	once or twice	a few times	often	nearly every time

When having dental work done:

3. My muscles become tense

1	2	3	4	5
never	once or twice	a few times	often	nearly every time

4. My breathing rate increases

1	2	3	4	5
never	once or twice	a few times	often	nearly every time

5. I perspire

1	2	3	4	5
never	once or twice	a few times	often	nearly every time

6. I feel nauseated and sick to my stomach

1	2	3	4	5
never	once or twice	a few times	often	nearly every time

7. My heart beats faster

1	2	3	4	5
never	once or twice	a few times	often	nearly every time

Following, is a list of things and situations that many people mention as being somewhat anxiety or fear producing. Please rate how much fear, anxiety, or unpleasantness each of them causes you. Circle the numbers 1-5, from the following scale, "1" being very relaxed and "5" being so anxious you feel ill. (If it helps, try to imagine yourself in ach of these situations and describe what your common reaction is.)

8. Making an appointment for dentistry	1	2	3	4	5
9. Approaching the dentist's office	1	2	3	4	5
10. Sitting in the waiting room	1	2	3	4	5
11. Being seated in the dental chair	1	2	3	4	5
12. The smell of the dentist's office	1	2	3	4	5
13. Seeing the dentist walk in	1	2	3	4	5
14. Seeing the anesthetic needle	1	2	3	4	5
15. Feeling the needle injected	1	2	3	4	5
16. Seeing the drill	1	2	3	4	5
17. Hearing the drill	1	2	3	4	5
18. Feeling the vibrations of the drill	1	2	3	4	5
19. Having your teeth cleaned	1	2	3	4	5
20. All things considered, how fearful are you of having dental work done?	1	2	3	4	5

Fig. 2. Kleinknecht dental fear survey. (*Courtesy of* P. Milgrom, DDS, Seattle, WA.)

that everything possible is being done to understand the problem and its solution.

3. A positive statement that the problem is understandable helps to overcome the patient's sense of isolation, and fosters a warm human relationship.

Dental Beliefs Survey (DBS)

Developed by Smith, Getz, et. al. 1984

Name__________________________ Sex M / F Date__________

The items in this questionnaire refer to various situations, feelings, and reactions related to dental work. Please rate your feeling or beliefs on these items by *circling the number* (1, 2, 3, 4, or 5) of the category which most closely corresponds to your feelings about dentists in general.

1. I do not think dentists like it when a patient makes a request.

1	2	3	4	5
never	once or twice	a few times	often	nearly every time

2. Dentists are efficient but it often seems they're in a hurry, so I feel rushed.

1	2	3	4	5
never	once or twice	a few times	often	nearly every time

When having dental work done

3. I feel that dentists do not provide clear explanations.

1	2	3	4	5
never	once or twice	a few times	often	nearly every time

4. I feel that the dentists do not really listen to what I say.

1	2	3	4	5
never	once or twice	a few times	often	nearly every time

5. I feel the dentist will do what he/she wants, no matter what I might say I want.

1	2	3	4	5
never	once or twice	a few times	often	nearly every time

6. Dental professionals say things to make me feel guilty about the way I care for my teeth.

1	2	3	4	5
never	once or twice	a few times	often	nearly every time

7. I am not sure I can believe what the dentist says about the work that is needed.

1	2	3	4	5
never	once or twice	a few times	often	nearly every time

Fig. 3. Dental beliefs survey. (*Courtesy of* P. Milgrom, DDS, Seattle, WA.)

4. To remove any aura of omnipotence, the dentist should state that he or she does not know all the answers to the patient's problems. A cooperative approach is necessary between the patient and doctor to achieve optimal results.
5. Finally, a comprehensive treatment plan is developed and presented to the patient.[9]

The importance of these principles is that they acknowledge the patient's fears and allow for a negotiated relationship between the patient and dentist, which will determine desired results with realistic outcomes.

THE SPECIAL NEEDS REQUIREMENTS FOR THE TREATMENT OF DENTAL ANXIETY AND PHOBIA

The many techniques of behavioral modification and pharmacologic intervention can help control fear and anxiety in dental patients.[28] Although a number of behavioral techniques are available for the treatment of dental fear, sedation and general anesthesia are still major modalities of providing dental treatment to phobic patients. The reasons for the slow entry of behavioral methodology are probably very complex and might even reflect sound skepticism as to the true value of behavioral treatment of

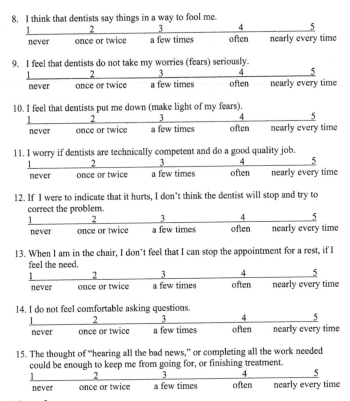

8. I think that dentists say things in a way to fool me.

1	2	3	4	5
never	once or twice	a few times	often	nearly every time

9. I feel that dentists do not take my worries (fears) seriously.

1	2	3	4	5
never	once or twice	a few times	often	nearly every time

10. I feel that dentists put me down (make light of my fears).

1	2	3	4	5
never	once or twice	a few times	often	nearly every time

11. I worry if dentists are technically competent and do a good quality job.

1	2	3	4	5
never	once or twice	a few times	often	nearly every time

12. If I were to indicate that it hurts, I don't think the dentist will stop and try to correct the problem.

1	2	3	4	5
never	once or twice	a few times	often	nearly every time

13. When I am in the chair, I don't feel that I can stop the appointment for a rest, if I feel the need.

1	2	3	4	5
never	once or twice	a few times	often	nearly every time

14. I do not feel comfortable asking questions.

1	2	3	4	5
never	once or twice	a few times	often	nearly every time

15. The thought of "hearing all the bad news," or completing all the work needed could be enough to keep me from going for, or finishing treatment.

1	2	3	4	5
never	once or twice	a few times	often	nearly every time

Fig. 3. (*continued*).

severe dental phobia and avoidance behavior.[29] Dentists, with some additional training in behavioral modification techniques, can successfully meet the special needs of the dental phobic patient.

Relaxation and desensitization techniques as studied by Wolpe[30] concluded that the individual cannot be anxious and relaxed at the same time. Therefore, any technique that relaxes the body and mind will help reduce anxiety. Progressive muscle relaxation as developed by Jacobson in the 1930s involves the instruction of an individual to tense and relax various muscle groups in a progression beginning with lower extremities and continuing through the musculature to the orofacial region. Benson furthered this concept with his contribution of a controlled breathing technique, which he called the "relaxation response." Accordingly, the patient breathes deeply and slowly while reciting a cue word of his own choosing when exhaling. This holistic idea was designed to help the patient focus on slow, deep breathing and to clear the mind of distracting thoughts.[28]

Popular treatment methods for extreme dental fear and avoidance are based on the principals of behavior modification.[31] The use of systematic desensitization has worked well in reducing fear in both child and adult patients, and increasing cooperation during needed treatment.[32] In this technique, there is a progressive exposure of the phobic individual to a hierarchy of threatening dental stimuli. Avoidance increases phobia and anxiety, but exposure reduces them.

Systematic desensitization works to the extent that it increases exposure to the noxious stimulus. The basic notion is that with each successful exposure the

Mount Sinai Dental Fear Inventory

On a scale of 0 to 100, where 0 is so relaxed you could fall asleep and 100 is the point when you are so fearful you might faint, become sick or run out of the treatment room, please rate yourself regarding the following situations:

__________Sitting in the dentist's waiting room

__________Smelling the "smell" of a dentist's office

__________Sitting up in a dental chair

__________Reclining in a dental chair

__________Seeing the needle and syringe for anesthesia

__________Receiving the anesthetic injection

__________Hearing the noise of the dentist's drill

__________Having a tooth drilled

__________Seeing the dental probes or instruments

__________Having the dental instruments manipulated in your mouth

__________The dentist walks into the treatment room

__________Having your teeth cleaned

__________Having dental x-rays taken

__________Other:____________________________________

____

Fig. 4. Mount Sinai dental fear inventory. (*Courtesy of* M. Slovin, MSPharm, DDS, Stony Brook, NY.)

phobic individual develops more confidence and the stimulus becomes less threatening.

Distraction techniques use audio and video formats to remove the focus from the noxious dental stimulus. The use of something as simple as a portable audio device with earbuds can provide a degree of distraction from the dental surroundings, and create an atmosphere of comfort to the patient. This technique can also apply when treating children who may find comfort in a hand-held video game. These devices are particularly effective to fill time and reduce anxiety while the patient is waiting for treatment to continue (ie, anesthesia; radiographs, etc.).

A common fear in all people is loss of control. This is especially true in dentistry. The patient will feel more confident and comfortable if given some control over the dental experience. "Perceived control" addresses this need by allowing the patient to request a "time-out" for any reason. The dentist and patient can develop a signal such as raising the hand and the dentist must comply or the patient's trust will be lost. Because the oral cavity is not visible to the patient, the patient can be given a hand mirror to view the treatment in progress. This decreases the concept of "fear of the unknown," which is so prevalent in anxious dental patients. Chair position is often another threatening factor to dental phobic individuals. Although an ideal chair position for the practitioner may involve a considerable recline, one may realize that this position is anxiety-provoking to the dental phobic individual. A technique which may prove useful is to slowly and incrementally recline the chair while asking for feedback. This is another use of the systematic desensitization technique mentioned earlier. Another form of perceived control involves the dialog itself. Dentists may use phraseology in which the patient responds with approval. For example, the dentist may have plans to perform a particular procedure at the treatment visit. If the dentist were to instruct the patient of the planned treatment, even if done politely, the patient is removed of control. On the other hand, if the dentist asks the patient's permission, then the patient is given control. This fundamental change of dialog style empowers the patient to become part of the treatment team.[13]

Pharmacologic techniques, alone or in combination with behavioral techniques, may be used to help anxious and fearful patients. It is important to note that pharmacologic treatments rely on the use of drugs to depress the central nervous system to various levels to reduce anxiety. Pharmacologic approaches are best used when there is a well-defined need to manage a patient's behavior and the use of behavioral alternatives to accomplish this same goal are not feasible or beneficial.[33] They simultaneously reduce the patient's consciousness and ability to cooperate in the process, which is a prerequisite to long-lasting phobia reduction.[34] Premedication with oral anxiolytic drugs such as Xanax, Valium, and so forth, is often useful to reduce anxiety at dental visits. The patient maintains the ability both to cooperate and concentrate, which is necessary for phobia reduction. Dental phobic individuals often report insomnia before dental visits, which in itself can reduce their level of cooperation. Prescribing this premedication the night before and the day of treatment could be advantageous. Nitrous oxide–oxygen analgesia may be helpful in those patients who comfortably accept the use of a facial mask. However, many dental phobic individuals feel threatened by this confining device.[34] Additional forms of pharmacologic interventions for dental anxiety treatment include oral conscious sedation and the various forms of intravenous sedation. Because the thrust of this article involves the identification of the special behavioral needs for dentally anxious and phobic individuals, the pharmacologic techniques section is brief.

A multidimensional approach which emphasizes the simultaneous consideration of behavioral, pharmacologic, and clinical dental factors appears to be the most rational and effective means for establishing the appropriate therapeutic outcome to meet the personal needs of each individual patient.[35]

Consistent with this notion, the field of dentistry has addressed the special needs of dentally anxious and phobic individuals through the establishment of dental anxiety/phobia programs. In addition, many private dental practices, both general and specialty, have developed programs to accommodate fearful individuals. In this environment, dentists and dental specialists, with additional training in behavioral and pharmacologic techniques, can provide care to this underserved population with consideration to all relative aspects of their treatment needs.

PREVENTION OF DENTAL AVOIDANCE

Dental beliefs may influence the development, manifestation, and treatment of dental fear. There may be a relationship between negative dental beliefs and general psychologic distress.[36] Such a belief system can be established in many ways. Children are impressionable and may vicariously adopt parental fears. Therefore, parents who exhibit dental anxiety need to take precautions not to transfer their dental fear.[37]

There are times when a dental patient may have an untoward treatment experience, which would establish a negative dental belief. Sensitivity of the clinician in this context is crucial. The patient's confidence can often be restored by a quick interaction that should include an apology, an explanation, and a resolution for the discomfort.

Unfortunately, the media often portray dentistry in a way that promotes negative assumptions. Vulnerable individuals may develop anxiety based on misperceptions and misinformation. It is incumbent upon the dental profession to disseminate accurate, positive information to the public to counteract these misleading messages. Outreach related to the latest interventions for patient comfort in dental care will create positive dental beliefs.

SUMMARY

Consideration of the special needs for treatment in dental anxiety is important regarding the patient's ability to receive dental care. Moreover, the patient's sense of accomplishment once treatment is received, especially for those patients who perceived themselves as "lost causes," can translate to a sense of empowerment that often leads to an overall greater level of self-esteem and confidence, which transcends across many life issues.

The treatment of the dentally anxious or phobic individual can turn out to be most gratifying to a dental staff. These patients desperately need comprehensive dental care with an emphasis on their special needs and become most appreciative of the treatment provided by sensitive caregivers. Positive experiences, as those in a successful phobia rehabilitation, produce "good-will ambassadors", referring many prospective patients to the dental practice.[13]

As eloquently stated by Jepsen,[38] "Patient anxiety in the dental office affects both dentists and patients universally. Anxious patients may delay dental treatment or miss appointments without explanation, and treating an anxious patient can add to the everyday stress of dental practice. The dentist is anxious about the patient, the patient is anxious about the dentist, and, in the end, both are exhausted by what might have been, under more relaxed circumstances, a simple procedure."

There has been a considerable amount of research and development in the technologies, which are useful in providing a comfortable experience for dental patients. Examples of these technologies include faster setting impression materials, more comfortable and profound dental injections, and rapid digital x-rays. Research continues in behavioral techniques which would be beneficial in rehabilitating dentally anxious and phobic individuals addressing their special needs.

The 25 million patients who fear the dental experience provide an exciting challenge to the dental staff. With a proper understanding of their special needs and a proper application of the techniques previously discussed, these patients can be successfully and comfortably managed in a modern dental practice.

REFERENCES

1. James A. Fear in the dental chair. About a quarter of adults avoid regular dental examinations as a result of childhood experiences. The dentist who is sensitive to these fears will provide more than just the needed treatment. Oral Health 1997; 87(2):9–14.
2. Hollander J. An assessment of dental fear and anxiety: comparing doctor and patient perceptions. Oral Health 2007;97(12):18–26.
3. Smith T, Heaton L. Fear of dental care: are we making progress? J Am Dent Assoc 2003;134:1101–8.

4. Kvale B, Berg E, Raadal M. The ability of Corah's Dental Anxiety Scale and Spielberger's State Inventory to distinguish between fearful and regular Norwegian dental patients. Acta Odontol Scand 1998;56:105–9.
5. Kleinknecht R, Klepac R, Alexander L. Origins and characteristics of the fear of dentistry. J Am Dent Assoc 1973;86:842–8.
6. University of the Pacific, School of Dentistry 2007. Available at: http://dentalpacific.edu/patientservice. Accessed September 9, 2008.
7. Gift H, Atchison K. Oral health, health, and health related quality of life. Med Care 1995;33(11):557–67.
8. Milgrom P, Weinstein P, Kleinknecht R, et al. Treating fearful dental patients: a patient management handbook. Reston (VA): Reston Publishing Co., Inc., Prentice Hall Co.; 1985. p. 129–30.
9. Rubin J, Slovin M, Krochak M. The psychodynamics of dental anxiety and dental phobia. Dent Clin North Am 1988;32(4):647–56.
10. Chambers D. Managing the anxieties of young dental patients. ASDC J Dent Child 1970;37:364–5.
11. Kulich K, Berggren U, Hallberg L. A qualitative analysis of patient-centered dentistry in consultations with dental phobic patients. J Health Commun 2003;8:171–87.
12. Bare L, Dundes L. Strategies for combating dental anxiety. J Dent Educ 2004;68(11):1172–7.
13. Slovin M. Proven pain and practice management strategies for treating the phobic patient. Dent Econ 1997;2–6.
14. Agras S. Panic: facing fears, phobias, and anxiety. In: Agras S, editor. Palo Alto (CA): The Portable Stanford; 1985.
15. American Psychiatric Association. DSM-IV-TR. Arlington (VA): American Psychiatric Association; 2000. p. 209-27.
16. Willumsen T, Vassend O, Hoffart A. One year follow-up of patients treated for dental fear. Effects of cognitive therapy, applied relaxation, and nitrous oxide sedation. Acta Odontol Scand 2001;59:335–40.
17. Milgrom P, Weinstein P, Rubin J, et al. Assessing patients' fears. Dentistry 1986;86:14–7.
18. Coulehan J, Block M. The medical interview. 4th edition. Philadelphia: Davis; 2001.
19. Chadwick B. Assessing the anxious patient. Dent Update 2002;11:448–54.
20. Gotthelf C. Interviewing – chapter eleven. In: Ayer W, editor. (2000), Psychology and dentistry: mental health aspects of patient care. Binghamton: New York, The Hayworth Press Inc.; 2005. p. 119–31.
21. Ayer W. Psychology and dentistry: mental health aspects of patient care. Binghamton(NY): The Hayworth Press Inc.; 2000.
22. Wolf D, Desjardins P, Black P, et al. Anticipatory anxiety in moderately to highly anxious oral surgery patients as a screening model for anxiolytics: evaluation of alprazolam. J Clin Psychopharmacol 2003;23(1):51–7.
23. Erten H, Akarslan Z, Bodrumlu E. Dental fear and anxiety levels of patients attending a dental clinic. Quintessence Int 2006;4:304–10.
24. Schuurs A, Hoogstraten J. Appraisal of dental anxiety and fear questionnaires: a review. Community Dent Oral Epidemiol 1993;21:329–39.
25. Newton R, Buck D. Anxiety and pain measures in dentistry: a guide to their quality and application. J Am Dent Assoc 2000;131:1449–57.
26. Smith T, Weinstein P, Milgrom P, et al. An evaluation of an institution-based dental fears clinic. J Dent Res 1984;63:271–2.
27. Rubin, Scheman, Protell. Psychodynamics in dentistry. Greater Philadelphia Meeting. Philadelphia, PA, September 1960.

28. Rubin J, Slovin M, Kaplan A. Assessing patients' fears: recognizing and reacting to signs of anxiety. Dent Clin North Am 1986;1:14–8.
29. Berggren U, Linde A. Dental fear and avoidance: a comparison of two models of treatment. J Dent Res 1984;63:123–7.
30. Wolpe J. Psychotherapy by reciprocal inhibition. J Exp Psychol 1947;7:382–90.
31. Berggren U, Linde A. Long-term effects of two different treatments for dental fear and avoidance. J Dent Res 1986;65:874–6.
32. Melamed B, Greenbaum P. Pretreatment modeling: a technique for reducing childrens' fear in the dental operatory. Dent Clin North Am 1988;32(4):693–702.
33. Moore PA, Ramsay DS, Finder RL, et al. Pharmacologic modalities in the management and treatment of dental anxiety. Dent Clin North Am 1988;2:803–16.
34. Slovin M. Managing the anxious and phobic dental patient. N Y State Dent J 1997;36–40.
35. Dorkin S. Intergrating behavioral and pharmacological therapeutic modalities. Paper presentation at American Association of Pediatric Dentistry. Chicago, IL, November 1985.
36. Abrahamsson K, Berggren U, Hallberg L, et al. Dental phobic patients' view of dental anxiety and experiences in dental care: a qualitative study. Scand J Caring Sci 2002;16:188–96.
37. Slovin M, Shakin M. The child dental phobic. N Y State Dent J 1992;39–42.
38. Jepsen C. Controlling anxiety in the dental office. J Am Dent Assoc 1986;113(11):728–35.

Minimal and Moderate Oral Sedation in the Adult Special Needs Patient

John M. Coke, DDS[a,*], Michael D. Edwards, DMD[b,c]

KEYWORDS

• Sedation • Special needs • Management
• Medically complex • Sedation environment

It is well established in the dental and medical literature that fear and anxiety of dental procedures keep a significant portion of the population from receiving timely and effective dental care.[1] It has also has been shown that adult special needs groups are a large portion of this population. As defined, a special needs individual is one who is unable to receive dental care in a traditional dental setting.[2] However, with the cost of hospital-based care increasing yearly, many of these special needs patients are being seen at an increasing rate in the traditional dental outpatient office setting. With the aging of the United States population, it is estimated that special needs patients will increase significantly and further increase the shift toward a traditional office setting.[3,4] Many of these adult special needs patients require sedation, either because of behavioral, communicative, or complex medical problems, for a thorough oral examination and subsequent dental care. An increasing segment of this population needs sedation to lower their stress level in a dental setting because of their reduced physiologic reserve capacity and medical status. Undue stress that can be generated during a dental procedure may in fact precipitate a medical emergency in this population.[5,6]

The use of sedative oral anesthetic agents for dental procedures is well documented, dating back over a century. The use of sedation by appropriately trained dentists continues to enjoy a remarkable record of safety. The use of sedation in dentistry is safe and effective when administered by properly trained individuals.[5]

[a] Department of Diagnostic Sciences, General Dental Residency, University of Alabama-Birmingham School of Dentistry, SDB 39, 1530 3rd Avenue S, Birmingham, AL 35294–0007, USA
[b] Department of Comprehensive Dentistry, University of Alabama-Birmingham School of Dentistry, Birmingham, AL, USA
[c] PO Box 370, Wedowee, AL 36278, USA
* Corresponding author.
E-mail address: jmcoke@uab.edu (J.M. Coke).

Dent Clin N Am 53 (2009) 221–230
doi:10.1016/j.cden.2008.12.005
dental.theclinics.com
0011-8532/08/$ – see front matter

However, because of this continuing shift to a traditional out-patient office setting, the American Dental Association (ADA) convened several workshops between 2003 and 2007 to formalize the guidelines to ensure the delivery of oral conscious sedation safely. In October of 2007, the ADA House of Delegates adopted new guidelines for the use of sedation and general anesthesia by dentists. These guidelines, *ADA Guidelines for the Use of Sedation and General Anesthesia by Dentists*, represent major changes from the 2000 guidelines. Strongly emphasized throughout these new guidelines is the safe delivery of oral conscious sedation through the following:

Defining levels of sedation (regardless of the route of administration)
Educational requirements
Patient evaluation
Preoperative preparation
Personnel and equipment requirements
Monitoring and documentation
Recovery and discharge
Emergency management

It should be noted that separate guidelines exist for the pediatric dental patient (under 12 years of age). In addition, the skill and training requirements have been updated to reflect current practice, as well as the ability of the dentist to "rescue" the patient from a level of sedation beyond the dentist's intent. The goal of the 2007 guidelines, drafted from all communities of interest and regarding sedation and anesthesia, focus now on level of sedation, not route of administration. This will allow guidelines from all communities of medicine and dentistry to translate with common terminology. However, many feel that enteral/oral moderate sedation is the "unique paradigm," especially directed toward modern dental practice because this level of sedation is more commonly used in dentistry for extended procedures. This aspect of enteral/oral sedation is specifically addressed in the 2007 ADA guidelines. Currently, these guidelines have been adopted, in total or modified in part, by the majority of the state dental regulatory agencies in the United States.

This article addresses pertinent changes in the 2007 Guidelines, oral agents to produce minimal and moderate sedation, and modifications recommended for special needs patients. The reader should thoroughly read the 2007 *Guidelines for the Use of Sedation and General Anesthesia by Dentists* and the *ADA Guidelines for the Teaching Pain Control and Sedation to Dentists and Dental Students.* Both can be accessed at www.ADA.org.

LEVEL OF SEDATION

The 2007 ADA Guidelines focus on the level of sedation. The levels are minimal, moderate, and deep sedation general anesthesia. These levels focus on the level of consciousness, status of the airway, and response to stimulation. In addition, cognitive function is addressed, as well as respiratory and cardiovascular function. It must be strongly emphasized that sedation and anesthesia is a continuum, and every level can be reached, regardless of the route of administration. Oral sedation does not assure the patient will remain in a specific level of sedation. The patient may progress into deeper levels of sedation. This is especially true for the special needs patient.

Minimal sedation is a minimally depressed level of consciousness that retains the patient's ability to independently maintain an airway and respond normally to tactile stimulation and verbal command. Although cognitive function and coordination may be modestly impaired, cardiovascular and ventilatory functions are unaffected.

Moderate sedation involves purposefully responding to verbal commands, either alone or accompanied by light tactile stimulation. Respiratory and cardiovascular function remain unaffected without interventions.

The remaining areas of the guidelines address deep sedation and general anesthesia and are beyond the scope of this article. When reviewing the new guidelines, one must remember this is a "living document," subject to change as more research, new drugs, and influences from all communities of interest come into the scope of sedation practice.[7]

PATIENT EVALUATION

A thorough patient evaluation by the dentist before minimal/moderate sedation or general anesthesia is the cornerstone for a safe and effective sedation or general anesthesia experience.[8] The patient evaluation consists of a current medical history, which includes a written review of systems, medication review, and a basic physical inspection. It is emphasized by many authors that the pharmacologic history should include prescription medications, over-the-counter medications, and dietary supplements (herbals, alternative medicines, and so forth). Past experiences with sedation and general anesthesia should also be discussed. The special needs patient often provides a unique challenge in the evaluation process. If this patient is unable to provide his or her own medical history, then a guardian or responsible patient escort is required. Often with the elderly and medically complex, a consult with the physician is needed for more specific information. A basic physical inspection should be completed emphasizing the cardiovascular and respiratory systems. Vital signs should be recorded along with the patient's weight and body structure.

Every patient to undergo minimal or moderate sedation should then be assigned a physical assessment status or risk assessment. The most commonly used classification is the American Society Anesthesiology (ASA) system, first published in 1963.[9] It is recommended those patients with an ASA status of ASA I and ASA II should undergo routine minimal or moderate sedation. Those ASA III and IV patients being considered for minimal or moderate sedation will require consultation from their primary care physician or consulting specialist.[10] Generally speaking, ASA III and IV patients will require a modification in the sedation procedure. Many of the special needs patients fall into ASA III and IV status. It strongly suggested that if the sedating dentist feels uncertain or is uncomfortable with the ASA classification, then appropriate referral to someone with more advance training should occur.[8,10]

PATIENT MONITORING

As required by the 2007 ADA Sedation Guidelines, all minimal and moderate patients must have monitoring of oxygenation, color of mucosa, ventilation, and circulation during the sedative procedure. This to be accomplished by the dentist or an appropriately trained individual.[7] In those special needs patients who are not communicative, it is especially important to maintain a vigilant posture when they are sedated. The standard of care for oxygenation is a by continuous pulse oximetery. It is equally valuable in monitoring the nonsedated special needs patient whose reserve capacity may be compromised. Vital signs are to be taken at specific intervals. All recordings must be documented and become part of the patient's record.

RECOVERY AND DISCHARGE

Special needs patients can often present a challenge in determining when they have sufficiently recovered from the sedation and are ready to be discharged with a responsible adult. Mentally challenged patients may not be aware of the classic questions of name, day of the week, birthday, or other such information. They may also, upon recovering, be uncomfortable with their surroundings and strongly wish to leave. It is imperative that the dentist be satisfied with their level of recovery before discharging them. Elderly patients are often unable to ambulate effectively following a sedation and should be escorted out of the office. It is recommended that a member of the dental staff assure the seat is slightly reclined, seat belt applied, and the importance of airway position reviewed for the trip home and after arrival. For the dentist, this aspect reduces the exposure to liability for the postsedation period.[11] The guardians, escorts, or care givers that often accompany special needs patients should be given specific written instructions regarding postoperative care.

ORAL SEDATIVE AGENTS

Many oral sedative agents have been used in dentistry. The list includes ethyl alcohol, barbiturates, chloral hydrate, ethchlorvynol, opioids, antihistamines, benzodiazepines, and the Z-drugs. These drugs have been used as a single agent or combined with other sedatives or nitrous oxide.[12,13] When choosing a sedative agent, especially for the use in special needs patients, factors that should influence the selection include (1) predictable absorption into systemic circulation, (2) predictable depth of sedation, (3) predictable length of action, (4) low adverse side effects, and (5) reversing of the sedative agent if needed.[14,15] These five factors significantly contribute to the overall safety of the sedative agent. Because of potentially dangerous side effects, unpredictable results, and lack of a reversing agent, the authors do not recommend ethyl alcohol, barbiturates, chloral hydrate, ethchlorvynol, and opioids for the oral sedation of special needs patients. Thus, the discussion will be limited to the benzodiazepines, antihistamines and Z-drugs. It is recommended that all oral sedatives be administered to the patient in the dental office for safer sedations.[12]

Benzodiazepines

The benzodiazepines, first synthesized in 1933 and approved for use in the United States in 1960, have been used extensively as oral sedatives in dentistry.[14] Benzodiazepines act at specific inhibitory receptor sites in the central nervous system and slow down the reuptake of gamma aminobutyric acid (GABA), which in turn reduces anxiety and aggressive behavior, causes muscle relaxation, and exhibits anticonvulsant effects. They have a wide variety of half-lives and some have active metabolites. All benzodiazepines can be reversed by romazicon (Flumazenil). The four benzodiazepine oral agents for minimal and moderate sedation recommended by the authors are alprazolam, lorazepam, triazolam, and midazolam. Each one of these can be used for specific patients depending on the ASA status, depth of sedation desired, and anticipated length of appointment.

Alprazolam (Xanax) is marketed as an antianxiety medication. It has a half-life of 12 to 15 hours and has no active metabolites. It reaches peak plasma levels in 1 to 2 hours. It is used primarily as a minimal sedative agent. The recommended adult dose is 0.25 mg to 1.0 mg.[13,15]

Lorazepam (Ativan) is used a sedative. It has a long half-life of 14 to 19 hours. It has no active metabolites and reaches its peak plasma level in 1 to 2 hours. Lorazepam has been reported to have significant amnesic properties. The recommended adult dose is 1 mg to 2 mg.[13,15]

Triazolam (Halcion) is used extensively as a sedative agent. It has half-life of 2 to 4 hours and has no active metabolites. It reaches peak plasma levels in a relative short time of 1 to 2 hours. Triazolam also provides effective amnesia. The recommended adult dose is 0.125 to 0.5 mg.[13,16]

Midazolam (Versed) is used extensively in intravenous sedation but can also be used as an oral sedative agent. It comes in a liquid form rather than in a tablet. Its half-life is 1 to 2 hours and reaches peak plasma levels in under 1 hour. The recommended dose is 0.5 mg/kg up to a maximum dose of 20 mg.[13]

Antihistamines

Antihistamines (histamine blockers or H1 antagonists) possess sedative properties in addition to their primary purposes of allergies and motion sickness. They are not reversible, unlike the benzodiazepines and Z-drugs, and do not lower seizure threshold but do have a wide margin of safety. The antihistamines are primarily used as combination sedative agents in the pediatric patient but have been reported useful in the adult patient who is a heavy smoker or the asthmatic to cut down on oral secretions.[17]

Hydroxyzine (Atarax, Vistral) has a half-life of 4 to 6 hours and is rapidly absorbed from the gastrointestinal tract and reaches peak plasma level in 30 to 60 minutes. The recommended dose is 50 mg to 100 mg.[12]

Z-Drugs

A new classification of drugs has recently been reported effective in oral minimal and moderate sedation. These are the "Z-drugs" (nonbnenzodiaepine hypnotics or imidazopyridines), so named because of their initial letter. They include zolpidem (Ambien), zaleplon (Sonata), and Eszopiclone (Lunesta). Like the benzodiazepines, they interact with the GABA receptors but appear to selectively affect different subtypes of these receptors. The primary use of the Z-drugs is for the short-term treatment of insomnia. They have a sedative profile similar to the benzodiazepines but have less amnesic, cognitive, or muscle relaxing properties.[18] Both zolpidem and zaleplon have short half-lives, while eszoplicone has a longer half-life. Because of the shorter half-lives, both zolpidem and zaleplon have been used as oral sedative agents in dentistry.

Zolpidem (Ambien) has a half-life of 2.5 hours and reaches peak plasma level in 1.6 hours. It is rapidly absorbed in from the gastrointestinal tract in under 30 minutes and has no active metabolites. The recommended adult dose is 5 mg to 10 mg.[18]

Zaleplon (Sonata) has the shortest half-life of the Z-drugs of 1 hour and reaches peak plasma level in 1 hour. It is rapidly absorbed in under1 hour and has no active metabolites. The recommended adult dose is 5–20 mg.[18]

USE OF NITROUS OXIDE

Keep in mind the most important time in the procedure, the peak effect of the sedation, is usually in the beginning when local anesthesia is to be administered. The concurrent use if nitrous oxide during local anesthesia and other more challenging moments in the procedure allow one to take advantage of some the analgesic properties.[12,19] The dentist can then revert back to 100% oxygen and decrease the risks of nausea that are related to the length of time many patients are carried on nitrous oxide. The authors prefer to use a sedative drug with a half-life that will allow the patient to be recovering from the full effects of the sedation toward the end of the appointment so that the patient may participate more confidently with procedures that require a higher degree of cooperation, such as occlusal records.

SPECIAL NEEDS PATIENT MODIFICATIONS

Mentally Challenged Patients

Perhaps one of the largest adult populations of special needs patients requiring sedation for dental procedure is the mentally challenged. The Association on Intellectual and Developmental Disabilities estimates that 3% of the United States population may be mentally challenged.[20] Because of multiple factors, many of these individuals are seeking or being referred to for dental office-based sedation.[21] The special needs patients can present with challenging dilemmas when contemplating oral minimal and moderate conscious sedation. The initial physical assessment interview is critical. Quite often these patients are not capable of completing a thorough medical history and the dentist must reply on other individuals, sometimes not familiar medically with the patient. It is extremely important to obtain a thorough health history before contemplating any sedation. Mentally challenged patients currently on behavior-modifying medications (benzodiazepines, major tranquilizers, for example) may not be good candidates for oral sedation because of possible drug interactions with the sedative agent. They should be referred for intravenous or general anesthesia.[20]

The adult Down syndrome patient also presents an oral sedation challenge. These patients have a higher incidence of cardiovascular defects and tend to be more obese than the general population.[2] Of particular concern is the large tongue and short neck often associated with Down syndrome. The airway will become more easily obstructed when sedated. These patients should be allowed to recover fully before discharge because of the potential of obstruction.

With mentally challenged patients, it can be quite easy to go from minimal sedation to moderate sedation using oral agents. In the uncooperative patient, often the initial recommended dose seems to have little effect. If subsequent oral doses are then given, the patient may quickly slide into a deeper plane of sedation. The dentist must be aware of the clinical signs of moderate sedation and have training to manage the patient successfully.

Medically Complex Patients

Cardiovascular disease

Fear and anxiety, in addition to painful procedures, increase pulse and blood pressure leading to increased cardiovascular demand for oxygen. Oral minimal and moderate sedation can play a very important role, in addition to excellent local anesthetic technique, in the patient that has a history of cardiovascular (CV) disease. Angina and arrhythmias may occur in the stressed patient with CV disease and are less likely in the relaxed patient. However, one must remember, over-sedation may result in respiratory depression, leading to hypoxia and myocardial ischemia.[5]

Patients with a medical history of CV disease must be thoroughly evaluated in regards to their ASA status. Patients with end-stage CV disease resulting in congestive heart failure should receive a medical consult from their physician or CV specialist concerning sedation.[2] Patients with a history of angina should be questioned concerning the type of angina. A patient with stable angina is an ASA II or III. A patient with unstable angina is an ASA IV and perhaps should be referred for intravenous sedation or general anesthesia. The use of minor sedation with the benzodiazepines is indicated in CV disease patients. Continuous oxygen flow via a nasal canula is also an excellent choice.[20] Excellent pain control during the procedure and postoperative period is very important and should not involve the selection of medications, such as the opioids, that will deepen the level of sedation in an unmonitored environment.[22] Nonsteroidal anti-inflammatory medications are often used.

Respiratory disease

Patients with asthma, chronic obstructive pulmonary disease, and chronic bronchitis are at risk for a medical crisis when exposed to stress in the dental office. Oral sedation using the benzodiazepines, preferably at the minimal level, is safe and effective in this patient group. Consideration of the antihistamines may be very beneficial in these patients because of the anticholinergic effects of these drugs. The benzodiazepines are also very safe choices but do not possess the anticholergenic benefits. Targeted questioning regarding recent episodes of difficulty can greatly assist the dentist in determining the medical eligibility of the patient for the sedation procedure. Close monitoring of the patient's oxygen saturation using a pulse oximetery is essential. Like the CV disease patient, opioid analgesics are cautioned for postoperative pain management.[20]

Hepatic disease

The patient with a history of liver disease should be a concern when considering oral sedation because the sedative agents used are primarily metabolized by the liver. A patient with severe liver disease, cirrhosis, will metabolize the sedative agents at a decreased rate, thus risking a prolonged or exaggerated sedation.[8] The dentist must establish a thorough medical history to gauge the severity of the liver disease. Benzodiazepine and Z-drug oral sedative agents given at minimal doses are recommended for sedation but varying responses should be expected.[20]

The elderly patient

The elderly are an increasing segment of the population in the United States and represent the fastest growing segment of the population age group in the world. It is estimated that there will be over 51 million in the over-65 age group in 2020.[2] Older Americans are at a higher risk for not having a dental contact because of economic barriers. Residents in nursing homes and long-term care facilities generally face additional dental needs because of inadequate nutrition, chronic medical problems, reduced appetite, poor oral health, diminished salivary flow, and inadequate masticatory function.[3] The behavior of elderly patients can also affect the treatment planning and treatment by the dentist. Apart from the physical and psychologic changes often seen in the advanced elderly, physical illness, degenerative brain changes, psychiatric disorders, and psychosocial changes can affect behavior. Physiologically, the elderly undergo changes that can affect the decision on oral sedation. They begin to lose central nervous system receptor cells; they have a decrease in renal clearance; they have decreased plasma protein binding; they experience a decrease in lean body mass; and they have a reduced pulmonary function.[13,23] All of these factors contribute to the philosophy to reduce the dosage of oral sedative agents on patients over 65.[12] The recommended reduction in dose has not been quantified and depends upon the overall medical complexity of the patient.

Because of the increasing incidence of chronic medical conditions encountered while aging, it is assumed that this elder age group will be dependent on increasing numbers of medications, both prescription and over-the-counter. Adverse drug reactions are seen more in the elderly than younger patients.[22] It is, therefore, very important for the dentist to take a very thorough medication history on the elderly and investigate possible drug interactions with the oral sedative drug being considered.

Alzheimer's disease

Alzheimer's disease is a progressive and fatal disorder that results in a degeneration of the central nervous system and is characterized by the loss of intellectual functions, including memory, language, visiospatial skills, problem-solving ability, and abstract reasoning. It is often characterized by behavioral abnormalities.[15] It is estimated that Alzheimer's disease will affect 10% to 15% of the elderly older than 65, and 20% of those above 80 years of age.[24] The disease is staged (1–7) according to the deterioration of cognitive symptoms, and the pharmacologic treatment is dependent upon the stage of the disease. Drugs used in treatment include cholinesterase inhibitors, antipsychotics, antidepressants, and mood stabilizers. The potential adverse drug interaction and oral sedative agents can be very high. Using oral sedative agents on these patients is often a challenge. The decision by the dentist to use minimal or moderate oral sedatives should be based upon the cognitive level of the patient. In the early stages, short-acting benzodiazepines may be used depending on the other medications the patient is taking (antidepressants and antipsychotics).[25] In the late stages of the disease, when there are little or no cognitive skills by the patient, only intravenous sedation may be effective and safely administered.[15,25]

ENVIRONMENTAL FACTORS

It is very important in the office-based dental facility that it appears nonthreatening to the patient. This is especially important for mentally challenged patients. The office should be conducive to efficient flow of the procedure to be done at the sedation appointment. Patients usually desire to maximize the treatment completed at the sedation appointment, so preplanning the sequence and flow of multitask procedures is very important. Transitioning instruments into and out of the operatory must be done so the patient isn't aroused from a comfortable sedation by the sound of banging instrument trays, and other jarring noises. The treatment rooms must have oxygen available, so that nasal oxygen is available for all sedations. The room size must allow adequate use of emergency equipment, if needed, and also for smooth staff transitioning of the operatory for multiple dental procedures. The use of nitrous oxide at strategic times of the sedation appointment, such as during the delivery of local anesthesia or packing retraction cord for impressions for example, should be available for more effective minimal/moderate sedation.[4,13]

SUMMARY

Oral conscious sedation at the minimal or moderate level is an effective adjunct for treatment of the special needs patient. Sedation has proven to reduce anxiety and physiologic stress in patients with a compromised reserve capacity, and to allow dental treatment to be delivered in a safer setting for these patients. Oral sedative agents are available that have minimal adverse effects and can be tailored to the length of the appointment by using their half-lives. Attention to the technique of oral conscious sedation, along with proper determination of the patient's medical status for the procedures must be observed. A keen emphasis on monitoring, airway support, ventilatory, and cardiovascular competence must be observed by the dentist. Proper consenting, documentation, and discharge criteria should be employed in the interest of both patients and dentists. Each dentist should assemble a sedation "tool kit" of sedative drugs that he or she is comfortable with to respond to clinical effects observed and manage the sedated patient safely. Biannual periodic update in training is recommended so the dental team remains aware of improvements and changes occurring in this important aspect of dental practice.

REFERENCES

1. Dionne RA, Yagelia JA, Cote CJ, et al. Balancing efficacy and safety in the use or oral sedation in dental outpatients. J Am Dent Assoc 2006;137(4):502–13.
2. Leyman JW, Mashni M, Trapp LD, et al. Anesthesia for the elderly and special needs patient. Dent Clin North Am 1999;43(2):301–19.
3. Chiappelii F, Bauer J, Spackman S, et al. Dental needs of the elderly in the 21st century. Gen Dent 2002;50:358–63.
4. Yagelia JA. Making patients safe and comfortable for a lifetime of dentistry: frontiers in office-based sedation. J Dent Educ 2001;65(12):1348–56.
5. Donaldson M, Gizzarelli G, Chanpong B. Oral sedation: a primer on anxiolysis for the adult patient. Anesth Prog 2007;54:118–29.
6. Gatchel RJ. The prevalence of dental fear and avoidance: expanded adult and recent adolescent surveys. J Am Dent Assoc 1989;118(5):591–3.
7. American Dental Association: The use of sedation and general anesthesia by dentists. Adopted by House of Delegates, October 2007. Chicago (IL): American Dental Association.
8. Jackson DL, Johnson BS. Conscious sedation for dentistry: risk management and patient selection. Dent Clin North Am 2002;46:767–80.
9. American Society of Anesthesiologists (ASA). New classification of physical status. Anesthesiology 1963;24:111.
10. Malamed SF. Sedation—a guide to patient management. In: Duncan LL, editor. Physical and psychological evaluation. St. Louis: Mosby; 2003. p. 48–51.
11. Seppala K, Korittla K, Hakkinen S, et al. Residual effects and skill related to driving after a single oral administration of diazepam, medazepam, or lorazepam. Br J Clin Pharmacol 1976;3(5):831–41.
12. Haas DA. Oral and inhalation conscious sedation. Dent Clin North Am 1999; 43(2):341–59.
13. Jackson DL, Johnson AS. Inhalation and enteral conscious sedation for the adult dental patient. Dent Clin North Am 2002;46:781–802.
14. Malamed SF. Sedation—a guide to patient management. In: Duncan LL, editor. Oral sedation. St. Louis: Mosby; 2003. p. 89–94, 103–4.
15. Matear DW, Clarke D. Considerations for the use of oral sedation in the institutionalized geriatric patient during dental interventions: a review of the literature. Spec Care Dentist 1999;19(6):275–80.
16. Quarnstrom FW, Donaldson M. Triazolam use in the dental setting: a report of 270 uses over 15 years. Gen Dent 2004;52:496–501.
17. Skidgel RA, Erdos EG. Histamine, bradykinin and their antagonists. In: Brunton Lazo JS, Parker KL, editors. Goodman and Gillman's the pharmacologic basis of therapeutics. 11th edition. New York: McGraw-Hill; 2006. p. 629–51.
18. Wynn RL, Bergman SA. The new Z-drugs as sedatives and hypnotics. Gen Dent 2005;53:174–7.
19. Kaufman E, Hargreaves KM, Dionne RA. Comparison or oral triazolam and nitrous oxide with placebo and intravenous diazepam for outpatient premedication. Oral Surg Oral Med Oral Pathol 1993;75(2):156–64.
20. Malamed SF. Sedation—a guide to patient management. In: Duncan LL, editor. Special considerations. St. Louis: Mosby; 2003. p. 552–89.
21. Yagiela JA. Office-based anesthesia in dentistry. Spec Care Dentist 1999;19(6): 201–15.
22. Shafer SL. The pharmacology of anesthetic drugs in elderly patients. Anesthesiol Clin North America 2000;18(1):1–27.

23. Muravchick S. Preoperative assessment of the elderly patient. Anesthesiol Clin North America 2000;18(1):72–87.
24. Kocaelli H, Yalitrik M, Yargic LI, et al. Alzheimer's disease and dental management. Oral Surg Oral med Oral Pathol Oral Radiol Endod 2002;93(5):521–4.
25. Friedlander AH, Norman DC, Mahler ME, et al. Alzheimer's disease psychopathology, medical management and dental implications. J Am Dent Assoc 2006; 137(9):1240–51.

Treatment of Mentally Disabled Patients with Intravenous Sedation in a Dental Clinic Outpatient Setting

Benjamin H. Solomowitz, DMD[a,b,*]

KEYWORDS

- Intravenous sedation • Mentally disabled • Dentistry
- Preoperative evaluation • Intravenous cannulation
- Intravenous medications • Clinical dentistry techniques

One group of patients is beyond the scope of the general dentist to treat in the office without some form of sedation. Developmental or acquired mental disability is said to affect 3% of our population. Mental disability is a general term, applied when an individual's intellectual development is significantly lower than average and his/her ability to adapt to the environment is consequently limited. The condition varies in cause and severity.[1] Mental retardation is a form of developmental disability that varies in severity and is usually associated with physical problems. It is a disorder of intellectual and adaptive functioning; affected individuals are challenged by the skills they use in everyday life.[2] A method of grouping these patients is by IQ into categories of mild, moderate, severe, and profound mental retardation (**Table 1**). Although patients who fall into the slight category can possibly be treated by a dentist without sedation training, as their mental diagnosis worsens or the complication of their dentistry increases, an option is to treat them with sedation or general anesthesia.

Many handicapped patients, especially higher-functioning patients, live with their families when they are young. As they age, they become more difficult to attend to. Their parents are aging, too, and it is difficult after a period of 10 to 20 years for a parent to manage his/her child, who could still be functioning at a mental age of 5 to 7 years, although the chronologic age could be 20 years. At this point, many are placed into group home facilities where they can be managed by professionals who can address their medical, dental, dietary, and social needs and general welfare and development.

[a] Department of Dentistry, Interfaith Medical Center, 1536 Bedford Avenue, Brooklyn, NY 11216, USA
[b] General Dentistry and Dental Anesthesiology, 407 Ninth Street, Brooklyn, NY 11215, USA
* General Dentistry and Dental Anesthesiology, 407 Ninth Street, Brooklyn, NY 11215, USA.
E-mail address: drsolomowitz@aol.com

Dent Clin N Am 53 (2009) 231–242
doi:10.1016/j.cden.2008.12.017
dental.theclinics.com

Table 1
Classification of mental retardation

Degree of Mental Disability	SB-IV	WISC-III	Communication
Mild	67–52	69–55	Should be able to speak well enough for most communication needs
Moderate	51–36	54–40	Has vocabulary and language skills such that the child can communicate at a basic level with others
Severe or profound	≤35	≤39	Is mute or communicates in grunts; little or no communication skills

Abbreviations: SB-IV, Stanford-Binet Intelligence Scale (IV); WISC-III, Wechsler Intelligence Scale for Children (III).

Data from McDonald RE, Avery DR, Dean JA. Dentistry for the child and adolescent. 8th edition. St. Louis (MO): Mosby; 2004.

These facilities give patients a degree of independence where they can still be supervised.

In group home facilities managed by nonprofit organizations, federal law requires the patients to be seen by a dentist at least once per year. The facility may have more restrictive regulations, requiring more than one visit per year. What the treating dentist recommends regarding recall appointments also needs to be followed by the facility, and this situation could require much more frequent recall appointments for examinations and cleanings.

Once the patient presents to the dental office, the type and quality of the treatment varies, depending on the skills of the dentist and the cooperativeness of the patient.

Patients functioning in the mild-to-moderate categories of mental disability may be cooperative or manageable in the private dental office with minimal treatment modifications. A full range of dental treatment can be offered.

As the degree of disability worsens, a private dental office might not be the optimal setting for the delivery of care. Uncooperative or violent patients may require more staff, with additional training, to control their behavior. Other equipment, such as a papoose board (Olympic Medical Corp., Seattle, Washington) to restrain the patient from hurting him/herself or the dental staff, might be necessary. The severe-to-profound developmentally disabled patient can yell or scream, run through the office, physically hurt others or him/herself, or damage equipment. Other patients in the office, or neighbors, might not understand what the commotion in the office is all about.

A partial solution is to treat the developmentally disabled patients at a specific time of the day when only they will be treated, which is not always possible.

If patients are unamenable to treatment in the conventional manner and need referral, many dentists are unaware of to whom or where to refer this set of patients for further care.

Referral to an office or to a hospital dental clinic outpatient setting geared for treating the developmentally disabled might be the solution. In a hospital setting, especially one with a general practice residency program, dental specialists are available to treat the needs of these individuals. Dentist anesthesiologists can help with behavior management by administering sedation in the clinic. An option of general anesthesia in the operating room is always available for patients unmanageable with sedation or for those needing extensive dental treatment.

Many group residencies are interested in providing the maximum treatment in the fewest possible visits. Although the patient will need to be physically evaluated as if undergoing general anesthesia, treatment with intravenous (IV) sedation will need less laboratory work, requiring fewer visits. The day of treatment will require less treatment time than general anesthesia in the operating room, making IV sedation an attractive option for the group residency staff.

PREOPERATIVE EVALUATION

On the day the patient presents for preoperative evaluation, the evaluation starts before the patient sits in the chair. The cooperativeness of the patient on entering the dental operatory (if he/she comes at all) is assessed.

The medical history must be reviewed, including medications, allergies, reason for wanting/needing sedation, dental history, physical examination, American Society of Anesthesiology (ASA) classification (**Table 2**),[3] surgical history, and any general anesthetics or sedations for past treatments. Referrals for laboratory work and for physician evaluation should be given as needed.

The dental history is elicited from the aide or parents who brought the patient. This history may be known (parents) or not known. What was done in the past and how it was done (with or without sedation/general anesthesia) will help give the practitioner a better understanding of how to manage the patient.

The aide/parent will know how cooperative and thorough the patient is in brushing his/her teeth or if he/she lets another caretaker brush for him/her.

An oral evaluation at this point can be attempted. If the patient will sit in the dental chair and allow an examination, a more accurate treatment plan can be formulated. If the patient will not sit in the dental chair, he/she might sit in a regular chair and open his/her mouth. At times, the patient will not be cooperative at all. At this point, two options are available. The patient can be placed in a papoose board, the head stabilized, and an examination done using manual manipulation and mouth props. Alternatively, the patient might allow just the lower lip to be pulled down. Even if the patient refuses to open fully, much can be learned from observing the lower anterior dentition. The practitioner will determine if the patient has teeth and will evaluate his/her oral hygiene and periodontal condition.

Mental disability can be associated with other forms of physical disabilities, illnesses, and genetic disorders. Examples of these are Down syndrome, pervasive developmental disorder under which autism falls, cerebral palsy, fragile X syndrome, and other genetic disorders. The specific dental component of these entities, and the medical conditions that might affect dental treatment and IV sedation, need to be evaluated before treatment commences.

Table 2
American Society of Anesthesiology physical status classification system

ASA I	A patient without systemic disease; a normal healthy patient
ASA II	A patient with mild systemic disease
ASA III	A patient with severe systemic disease that limits activity but is not incapacitating
ASA IV	A patient with incapacitating systemic disease that is a constant threat to life
ASA V	A moribund patient not expected to survive 24 hours with or without operation

Data from Malamed SF. Sedation: a guide to patient management. St. Louis (MO): Mosby; 2003.

In evaluating proposed dental treatment, consideration should be made to try to save teeth wherever possible. Periodontally involved teeth that are mobile but not infected, should not be extracted. Many times, the mentally handicapped will have an uncorrected malocclusion or severely decimated dentition caused by extractions, which places an increased occlusal force on the remaining teeth and actually increases the mobility of the teeth in occlusion.

Another situation to consider is the parent who wants his/her child's dentition restored after an extraction. This situation frequently occurs when dealing with the upper anterior teeth. Before an extraction in this area, inquiries to the parent or aide should be made to determine if the patient would be a candidate for a removable partial denture. A patient might not tolerate a removable appliance in his/her mouth. He/she may also be unable to remove it to clean it or to allow an aide to do it. Some might take it out and throw it away. An implant might not be the solution either because the surgical site might be mutilated by the patient, not allowing proper healing or the maintenance of oral hygiene. A fixed partial denture might be a better option if enough teeth remain to support a bridge, and oral hygiene and occlusion are favorable. This option will also necessitate multiple sedations for treatment. Because many mentally disabled patients are covered under state-sponsored insurance programs, costs for fixed bridgework and implants are usually not covered. If this treatment is desired, the costs would have to be financed privately.

The practitioner will have to take all of these considerations into account in formulating a dental treatment plan customized to each individual patient's situation.

Medical consultation or laboratory work, if needed, can be ordered at this time. Based on the collected information, a sedation and dental treatment plan can be formulated.

Consent forms for sedation can be given to the aide accompanying the patient or mailed directly to the legal guardian/parent if the legal guardian/parent will not be present on the day of sedation. Group homes can forward the consent to the legal guardian/parent for signature too. In the treatment section of the consent, the area can be written as "oral rehabilitation under IV sedation, which may include examination, radiographs, cleaning, fillings, extractions, root canals as needed," which will cover most treatment when a presedation treatment plan cannot be fully assessed. The original consent form is returned on or before the day of treatment.

Points to be noted include the following: How extensive is the dentistry that needs to be done? Can the patient's treatment plan be completed in one to three 2-hour sedation visits or will the treatment take a longer amount of time? How manageable is the patient? Is the patient cooperative enough to get into the dental chair with a papoose board on his/her own or with gentle urging by the residency staff, or is the patient combative and does he/she pose a physical danger to you, your staff, or him/herself? What is the medical and physical condition of the patient? Is the patient obese and unable to fit into a papoose board? Is the patient considered an ASA III patient and not a candidate for outpatient IV sedation?

If the dentistry is extensive or delicate, the patient might better be served if treated under general anesthesia in the operating room. Also, patients who are combative can be premedicated with intramuscular ketamine to make them more manageable for starting an IV. This treatment will depend on the training of the dentist and the recovery facilities available because the recovery time could be much longer than with IV sedation alone. In the author's clinic setting, they like to have the patients move in and out quickly, so having the longer recovery period usually seen with ketamine is not appealing. If medical or physical issues are a problem or if the patient has an ASA III classification or higher, he/she will be disqualified for IV sedation as an outpatient in the author's dental clinic and will be worked up for the operating room.

Written preoperative instructions are given, which include nothing by mouth status for 8 hours preoperatively for adult patients (except for their usual medications with a small sip of water), comfortable loose clothing, and no jewelry.

DAY OF TREATMENT

The day of treatment begins with a telephone call to the patient's legal guardian. Although a written signed consent form is brought to the clinic by the person accompanying the patient, the legal guardian of adult patients in group homes usually does not accompany them. The legal guardians are informed of the date of the sedation in advance and are asked to be available for a phone call on that morning. Informed consent is discussed, including proposed procedures and other options. An opportunity to ask questions is given. The conversation is witnessed by a second person and a note to this effect is placed in the dental chart and signed before treatment.

The aide accompanying the patient is then asked, "What did the patient eat or drink today?" as opposed to "Did the patient eat?" It requires more than a yes/no response. Patients are allowed to take their usual medications with a small sip of water.

The patient is placed on a papoose board over the dental chair. The chair is in a flat position and the patient is told to "lie down on the bed." If the patient is cooperative, blood pressure and EKG leads are placed at this time. An oxygen saturation reading can be taken. Lungs are auscultated for bilaterally clear breath sounds. If the patient is noncooperative, he/she is placed on the papoose board without the monitors. The patient is wrapped in the papoose with one arm left out. A tourniquet is placed medial to the antecubital fossa. When the patient lies down on the chair, the chair should be at its lowest point to make it more appealing for the patient to lie down and minimize any injury should the patient fall or jump off the chair before being secured by the papoose board. After the patient is secured, the head is tilted up from the flat position.

With one arm out of the papoose, two people can then start the IV. The second person stabilizes the arm by leaning it on the arm of the chair or on his/her leg as a fulcrum. One of the stabilizer's hands is placed under the patient's arm, with the second hand above the forearm (**Fig. 1**). With the tourniquet medial to the antecubital fossa, the whole length of the arm can be examined at one time for an appropriate vein. To aid in IV cannulation, the following steps are taken. First, the vein needs to be below the level of the heart for it to fill up, which is accomplished by tipping the head of the chair up and then raising the chair so the patient's arm hangs down.

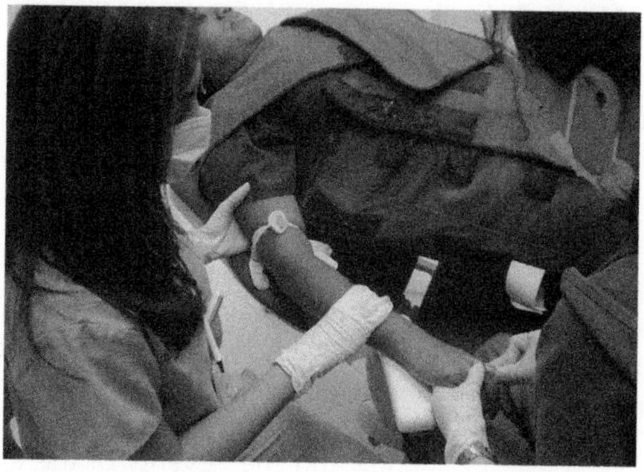

Fig. 1. Demonstration of a patient in a papoose board with one arm being stabilized for IV cannulation.

Second, adequate light at a 45° angle is needed to help visualize the vein. The back of the practitioner's finger is used to tap the vein to irritate it and have it engorge with blood. Slapping the hand or arm with a full open hand, as some practitioners do, can appear aggressive to the patient (especially a child). The vein is cannulated by first injecting a small amount of lidocaine (for infiltration and nerve-block; not with epinephrine) subcutaneously with a small 25-gauge needle.[4] This procedure is accomplished by placing the needle on the skin with the bevel pointing downwards, maintaining a "seal" of the needle flush with the skin (**Fig. 2**). The syringe is then forced in a downward and backward direction while pressing on the plunger, forcing anesthetic solution through the skin without needle penetration. The solution is pushed subcutaneously through the skin's semipermeable membrane to develop a skin wheal. With practice, it can be done painlessly. The needle from the lidocaine syringe is removed and is replaced by the IV catheter. This whole unit is easier to manipulate than holding the catheter by itself. The catheter is slightly bent at 45°, allowing a different approach to the vein (**Fig. 3**). The catheter tip penetrates the skin through the skin wheal of local anesthesia, with no sensation felt by the patient. After venous cannulation, the plunger is aspirated to check for a blood backflow confirming successful venous access. If a vein is small or has collapsed and no backflow is noted, 0.5 mL of lidocaine can be injected to see that no extravasation of the solution occurs, which serves as confirmation of a successful cannulation. The lidocaine is a vasodilator that enlarges the vein and also decreases the sensation of the venous injection of certain drugs, which can irritate the vein. It is important to never remove one's hand from the IV catheter after it is successfully inserted until after it is secured with tape, to prevent loss of the IV catheter by movement of the patient's hand or by the patient managing to pull it out. A microdrip IV tubing of 60 drops/mL is attached to the catheter. A microdrip, as opposed to an adult IV line of 15 drops/min, will assure that the patient is not overloaded with fluid quickly, and the microdrip will allow a slower, more even drug release.

After securing the IV line, the pulse oximeter is placed on the same hand and the arm is secured with Velcro straps to the outside of the papoose board.

INTRAVENOUS MEDICATIONS

Appropriate drugs are given through IV at this time. The drugs should be appropriate to the practitioner's comfort level and match what is being done from a dental

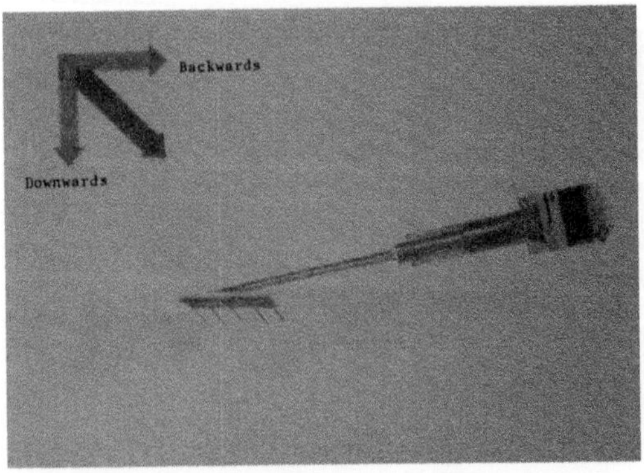

Fig. 2. The 25-gauge needle, with its bevel facing the skin, is pulled in a downward and backward direction to inject local anesthesia without perforating the skin.

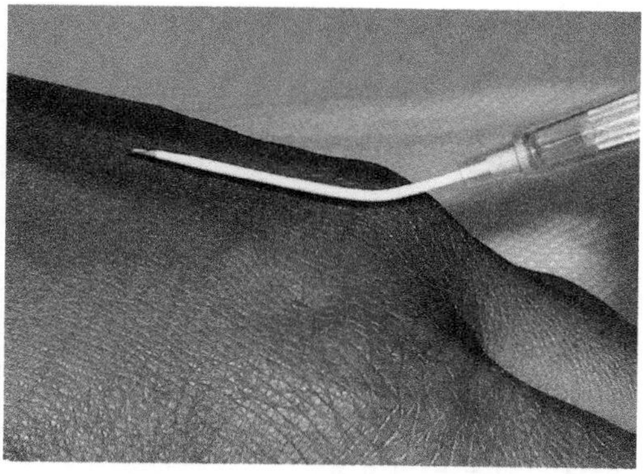

Fig. 3. The IV catheter is slightly bent at a 45° angle, allowing an easier approach to IV cannulation.

treatment and time perspective. The drug combinations mentioned here are considered moderate-to-deep sedation[5] and should be used with the proper anesthetic training (**Table 3**). A minimum of three people should be at chair side treating the patient under this level of sedation. Common categories of drugs used for sedation are benzodiazepines, narcotics, propofol, and adjunct drugs such as an antisialagogue. In addition, many practitioners have their own cocktails of drugs they are comfortable administering.

Benzodiazepines, such as midazolam (Versed) and diazepam (Valium), have many properties that are appropriate for IV sedation, such as anxiolysis, sedation, muscle relaxation, and amnesia. Benzodiazepines are also anticonvulsant medications, which is good for the mentally disabled who might have seizure activity.

Although all the drugs in this category have all of the properties of the benzodiazepines, some are better at certain properties than others. For instance, midazolam causes a more profound amnesia, whereas diazepam causes an appearance of deeper sedation and anxiolysis. Diazepam gives a longer clinical effect than midazolam and therefore, in longer cases, diazepam might be a more beneficial drug choice. Diazepam's clinical duration of action is approximately 45 minutes, whereas midazolam's clinical duration of action is approximately half that time.

Diazepam, a lipid-soluble medication, is formulated with propylene glycol. It stings on injection and is responsible for one of the side effects of diazepam use, thrombophlebitis. To minimize this complication, diazepam should be injected slowly into a fast-running IV fluid drip. Midazolam is water soluble and does not burn on administration. It should be administered in a slow-moving IV drip. Both drugs, though, should be titrated to effect.

Fentanyl is a short-acting narcotic with a clinical duration of action of approximately 0.5 to 1 hour. Narcotics are used in sedation to raise the pain threshold level so the procedure is more tolerable for the patient. Although local anesthetics are one of the best forms of pain control in dentistry, giving local anesthesia is not practical at times. Narcotics, therefore, would be helpful in these instances: taking radiographs during which the patient might feel the edge of the film on his/her mucosa and either be unable or not capable of expressing him/herself except by movement, and in scaling and root planning.

An inferior alveolar block injection is not always a good choice for the mentally disabled patient. The feeling of numbness that persist after the sedation is completed

Table 3
Methods of anxiety and pain control

Level of Sedation	Level of Consciousness	Airway	Response to Tactile Stimulation and Verbal Command	Cardiovascular Function
Minimal sedation	Minimally depressed	Is able to maintain independently and continuously	Normal	Unaffected
Moderate sedation	Depressed	Maintains a patent airway; ventilations adequate	Responds purposefully to verbal commands, either alone or with light tactile stimulation	Usually maintained
Deep sedation	Depressed	Ability to independently maintain ventilatory function, may be impaired; may require assistance in maintaining a patent airway and spontaneous ventilation may be inadequate	Cannot be aroused easily but responds purposefully after repeated or painful stimulation	Usually maintained
General anesthesia	Loss of	Ability to independently maintain function, often impaired; often require assistance in maintaining a patent airway and positive pressure ventilation may be required	Not arousable	May be impaired

Data from the American Dental Association. Guidelines for the use of sedation and general anesthesia by dentists. Available at: http://www.ada.org/prof/resources/positions/statements/anesthesia_guidelines.pdf. Accessed September 26, 2008.

can sometimes baffle the patient, thereby increasing the likelihood of the patient biting his/her lip, tongue, or cheek, necessitating resedation to suture the wound. An intraosseous injection, which can numb one tooth and wears off quickly and might not affect the lip or tongue, is a better choice when anesthesia is needed but is not always practical when large sections of the mandible need to be anesthetized. Using the IV drugs appropriately can help with this problem. If a nerve block injection is needed, a short-acting local anesthetic, such as Carbocaine 3%, without a vasoconstrictor might be a good choice.

Propofol is a short-acting versatile drug. Clinically, its duration of action is approximately 5 minutes. It can be used for short-term IV sedations or to induce and maintain general anesthesia. The response from the patient, whether in sedation or general anesthesia, depends on the dosage and how quickly the drug is administered. The drug is formulated in an emulsion of soy bean oil and egg whites. The medical history needs to be reviewed for allergies to these foods. On administration, it is painful and can cause the patient to react to the sensation, usually by moving his/her arm. Injecting lidocaine beforehand can reduce this sensation. In addition, administering a benzodiazepine, such as midazolam, will prevent the patient from remembering the burning sensation.

Propofol can be given by a continuous infusion pump or by bolus injections, usually at 10 mg increments. By using the microdrip infusion line, the drug can be placed in the line and will slowly be infused, simulating a continuous infusion pump. An easy way to keep track of the time for the administration of additional drugs is to listen for the automated blood pressure machine to start its inflation cycle, which is set to 5-minute intervals. When it goes off, an additional bolus increment is given.

The aforementioned drugs have additive central nervous system depressive effects. As such, their dosage in combination with each other should be reduced occasionally up to 30% from the dose of the individual drug alone. Titration is the key to safe administration of all IV sedative medications.

An adjunct drug is glycopyrrolate (Robinul), which can be used as an antisialagogue. When patients are placed in the supine position for treatment, saliva can run down the back of their pharynx, and the patients will start coughing, which can be manifest as an actual cough or rock of the patient's head and chest ("bucking"). In either case, the practitioner will be unable to work until the coughing stops. Using an antisialagogue alleviates this problem and gives a dry field for restorative treatment.

Nitrous oxide and oxygen through a nasal mask are other medications that help in sedating the patient. Many in the severe and profound levels of mental disability will not tolerate the mask on their faces first without IV medications. On many occasions, those who have the mild-to-moderate range of disability will let a nasal mask be placed first if it is shown to them and its function explained.

If the nasal mask is tolerated first, nitrous oxide and oxygen can be used to allay any fear and anxiety involved with the insertion of the IV catheter. In either situation, nitrous oxide and oxygen are excellent adjuncts to IV medications. Breathing gases through the nasal hood will decrease the amount of IV medications that need to be administered because of the additive effect of all the sedative drugs. Oxygen will raise the oxygen saturation of the blood, one of the vital signs monitored through pulse oximetry, decreasing the likelihood of hypoxia.

Nitrous oxide and oxygen are beneficial to patients who have specific medical conditions such as bronchial asthma, because they are nonirritating to the bronchial mucosa and can help decrease the stress that may exacerbate an acute asthmatic episode. Other conditions that may benefit from the increased oxygen concentration are seizure disorders and sickle cell disease, in which acute episodes can be brought on by hypoxia and stress.

An emergency drug kit with medications to handle the most common emergencies needs to be available. The practitioner should have training in dealing with emergencies and should feel comfortable administering the drugs in his/her kit. A customized emergency drug kit put together by the practitioner is preferable over a generic kit. Emergency reversal drugs for the sedatives used should be part of the kit. Flumazenil (Romazicon) is a benzodiazepine antagonist. Naloxone (Narcan) reverses the effects of fentanyl (opioids).[6]

CLINICAL DENTISTRY TECHNIQUES

If radiographs need to be taken, an easy way to accomplish this is with the Rinn x-ray system (Dentsply Rinn, Elgin, Illinois). The radiograph is placed in the patient's mouth in the usual fashion. Tape used for securing the IV is placed in the midline of the patient's neck, going vertically over the patients chin and to the side of the patient's nose. The tape is crimped so it does not stick to the patient's hair going over his/her head and is secured behind the headrest (**Fig. 4**). This technique allows the patient to bite on the Rinn x-ray holder, and supports the head in a position that opens the airway. Because the x-radiograph tube is aligned with the Rinn ring outside the mouth, no matter where the head lays after the taping, a clinically excellent radiograph can be taken.

A Molt bite block (Hufriedy, Chicago, Illinois) (**Fig. 5**), as opposed to a rubber bite block, is a preferable choice to open the patient's mouth. It uses a reverse scissor ratchet mechanism. If the patient is resistive and only opens partway, as long as the arms of the bite block can be slipped into the patient's mouth, the mouth will be able to be opened to an appropriate degree for treatment (**Fig. 6**). The Molt can be held in place by the person responsible for stabilizing the head, with the same hand with which he/she lifts the chin. To change the position of the Molt, it is closed and turned while its arms remain in the patient's mouth, and is then reopened, which prevents the patient from clamping closed, and then having to fight with him/her to get his/her mouth reopened. In the event this should occur, the mouth can be opened by taking the operator's thumb and pressing down on the lower labial anterior frenum.

For several reasons, it is important during sedation to protect the patient's airway. The patient being sedated is supine in the dental chair and is at risk for aspiration of dental filling materials, debris from preparation of the tooth, an extracted tooth, or calculus being scaled. Saliva can be produced in copious amounts and can flow backward, too, causing coughing. A third consideration is the use of water for cooling instruments. Hand scaling over the cavitron (Dentsply International, York, Pennsylvania) is

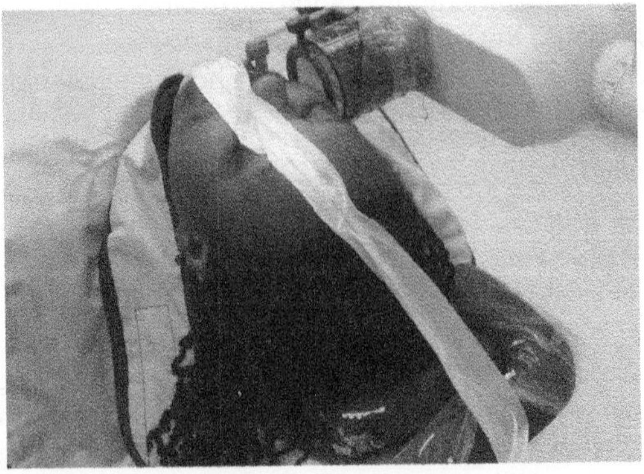

Fig. 4. Demonstration of radiographs being taken with the Rinn system and IV tape stabilizing the head and airway.

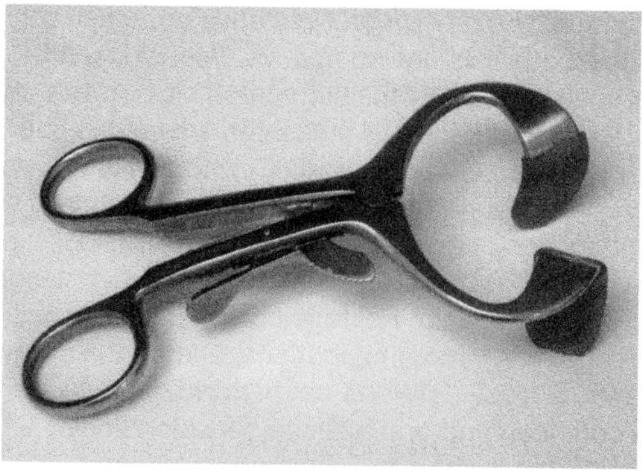

Fig. 5. Molt bite bock with reverse scissor ratchet action.

preferred. No matter how well suctioned, water and blood will still manage to flow backward and result in coughing. Minimal to no water in tooth preparation should be considered. If water is needed for lavage, minimal amounts in short duration with as much suction as available should be considered.

A throat shield should always be used to protect the airway when a rubber dam is not in use. The throat shield can be a piece of 4 × 4 gauze opened and strategically located behind the area being worked on to catch debris, excess amalgam, blood, water, and so forth. It should be changed frequently as it gets wet or full of debris. A rubber dam is an excellent way of confining debris to the area being worked on, protecting the airway and maintaining a dry field.

POSTOPERATIVE EVALUATION

Ideally, the sedation should be timed to end with the conclusion of treatment. With the sedative medications used today, the patient will usually recover within a short time. When treating special care patients who might not be able to obey or respond to verbal commands, it is better to keep the patient in the chair wrapped in the papoose board until consciousness is fully restored and the patient can ambulate. Many patients are intolerant of having an IV or monitors attached once alert. Therefore, they should be removed beforehand.

The patient's aide should be called to stay with the patient in the recovery area because he/she is best able to control the patient's behavior. The patient should

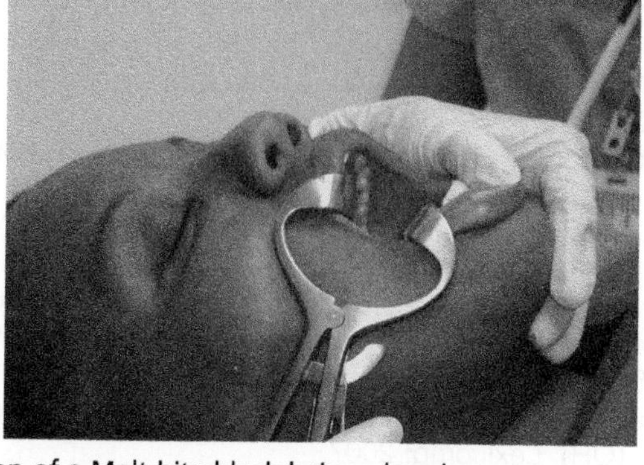

Fig. 6. Demonstration of a Molt bite block being placed.

remain until he/she is back to the preoperative condition, which can be a period of less than a half hour. If the patient is not combative, vital signs should be taken before discharge. If the patient will not allow the automated blood pressure cuff to be placed, or will not sit still for the reading, manual measurements of the pulse, and perhaps the blood pressure, may be taken. A fighting patient who can ambulate usually has good vital signs and is probably returned to preoperative condition. The chart should be noted as such. Written postoperative instructions are given, along with a written note of what treatment was accomplished, the dental recommendations for the next IV sedation appointment to continue treatment or for recall appointment, any medications prescribed, oral hygiene recommendations, and dental diagnosis.

Recall appointments, after all needed treatment is completed, should be based on medical and dental condition and oral hygiene considerations.

SUMMARY

Following the protocols and clinical tips presented will allow a dental clinic facility to treat special care patients in a safe and efficient manner. These suggestions will benefit a dental clinic that may not currently be treating special care patients but desires to increase provided services. It also will be beneficial for facilities already treating special needs patients that may want to compare their treatment regimens to those presented here. The special needs patients will benefit the most by having a greater choice of access to care for their dental needs.

Treating the special care patient is challenging for the treating dentist and for the dentist anesthesiologist. The goal is to have a patient free of disease and pain restored with esthetic and functional use of his/her oral cavity. The challenge is to incorporate the patient's medical, physical, behavioral, financial, and oral hygiene considerations into this goal. It can sometimes be a frustrating process for the dentist, caregiver, and patient. The health benefits of successful treatment of the patient are tremendous. The satisfaction for the dentist is seeing a healthy smile.

ACKNOWLEDGMENTS

Special thanks to Drs. Edward Lustbader and Lynn Gargano, who proofread this article.

REFERENCES

1. Weddell JA, Sanders BJ, Jones JE. Dental problems of children with disabilities. In: McDonald RE, Avery DR, Dean JA, editors. Dentistry for the child and adolescent. 8th edition. St. Louis (MO): Mosby; 2004. p. 540–1.
2. NIH Publication No. 07–5194. Practical oral care for people with mental retardation. National Institute of Dental and Craniofacial Research. Bethesda (MD). Reprinted July 2007.
3. Malamed SF. Sedation: a guide to patient management. St. Louis (MO): Mosby; 2003.
4. Solomowitz BH. Intravenous cannulation: a different approach. Anesth Prog 1993; 40:20–2.
5. ADA guidelines for the use of sedation and general anesthesia by dentists. Available at: http://www.ada.org/prof/resources/positions/statements/anesthesia_guidelines.pdf. Accessed September 26, 2008.
6. Wynn RL, Meiller TF, Crossley HL. Drug information handbook for dentistry. 13th edition. Hudson (OH): Lexicomp; 2007.

Evaluation, Scheduling, and Management of Dental Care Under General Anesthesia for Special Needs Patients

Mary L. Voytus, DDS

KEYWORDS

- Criteria for dental operating room for special needs patients
- Residents and operating room
- Preoperative dental screening for general anesthesia

Provision of dental care under general anesthesia for special needs patients requires evaluation of the patient both from a dental and a medical perspective. The dental patient must be screened for the necessity of dental care since there are inherent risks associated with the administration of general anesthesia. The goals of the medical assessment include comprehensive review of the past medical history, previous surgical history, and review of current and past medications. The dental assessment requires obtaining enough information concerning dental pathology to justify the provision of dental care under general anesthesia if the patient is not cooperative for care under local anesthesia in the outpatient setting.

The registration process can be time-consuming and disruptive for an uncooperative patient. In an established practice that facilitates the provision of care for the special needs patient it is more efficient to obtain copies of the demographic and insurance information, medical history, and necessary general consents before the initial dental screening visit. Information about the guardianship status is also needed. Forms may be mailed to the families/caregivers following the initial contact. Once the registration paperwork is completed and returned, the appointment can be scheduled. Of course, when there is an emergent situation every attempt must be made to expedite this process.

MEDICAL HISTORY

It is essential to obtain an accurate medical history. An evaluation for pre-existing medical conditions must be performed before any therapeutic measures.[1] Because patients may

Dental Residency Program, Division of Dentistry, Department of Medical Education, Mountainside Hospital, 1 Bay Avenue, Montclair, NJ 07042, USA
E-mail address: mary.voytus@mountainsidehosp.com

Dent Clin N Am 53 (2009) 243–254
doi:10.1016/j.cden.2008.12.018

be living apart from family, obtaining the history may require collating information from multiple sources. Patients who live at home with parents/family often have had ongoing medical care from physicians with whom the family has developed a close relationship. In that case, obtaining accurate information is easier because there is continuity. When patients are living in group homes or with a sponsor, the individual who is transporting the patient to the dental office often has little or no information concerning the patient. Acquiring information from primary sources is critical to ensure accuracy. Patients residing in group home settings often have a large medical journal that is brought to each dental visit. Copies of the annual physical, current medications, and recent consultations provided in this journal are an excellent resource for the dentist to obtain an accurate medical history, medication reconciliation, and list of current medical providers.

CRITERIA FOR DENTAL CARE UNDER GENERAL ANESTHESIA

Patients with special needs require the same level of assessment as regular patients. The assessment includes a comprehensive dental examination of hard and soft tissues, complete radiographs, periodontal charting, and assessment of function and occlusion. If there is limited cooperation from the patient while reviewing the medical history and initiating the assessment, it is important to obtain as much information as possible even if treatment cannot be completed under local anesthesia in the outpatient setting. Sometimes a panoramic film can be taken that provides some insight into treatment requirements. In addition, especially for patients who are in their 20s and 30s, the presence of impacted teeth may necessitate the presence of an oral surgeon for the completion of care under anesthesia.

If patients have not received treatment for a considerable period of time there may be an overwhelming amount of dental care that needs to be provided while the patient is under general anesthesia. Often the oral hygiene is limited or non-existent and the periodontal treatment needs are extensive. Specific documentation about presence of caries, nonrestorable teeth, impactions, significant calculus assists in planning the time for the scheduled care under general anesthesia.

PREOPERATIVE FLOW SHEET

Once it is determined that care under anesthesia is required, an organized approach to scheduling reduces the time required for the support staff, and is essential for procedures taking place in the operating room (OR).

The flow sheet should include

1. Patient name, date of birth, and medical record number
2. Current address and phone number of home or facility where patient resides
3. Contact person and phone/cell phone number
4. Guardian name, address, and phone number
5. Insurance company, address, phone number, plus copy of insurance card
6. Date and time scheduled for the OR
7. Confirmation number from the OR
8. Name of dentist
9. Name, address, and phone number of primary care physician
10. Place for additional notes concerning the case

Providing all of the above information on one form assists every individual who is involved in the case. If the person who does the scheduling is not available, having this information accessible for another staff person to review is invaluable.

Since the advent of precertification by insurance companies, preformatted forms for additional information can reduce the need to write individual letters and descriptions. The second part of the preoperative evaluation includes a checklist of medical diagnoses/conditions, dental diagnoses, behaviors in the dental setting, and a tentative treatment plan. When signed by the providing dentist. this document can be used for precertification for facility charges as well as the dental charges. **Figs. 1** and **2** provide examples of a preoperative flow sheet and a preoperative medical/dental checklist.

☐ Dentistry for the Disabled
☐ Pediatric
☐ Adult
☐ OS

PLEASE COMPLETE AT TIME OF CLINIC VISTIT

Date: ____________

Patient Name ____________ **DOB** ____________

Address ____________ **City** ____________ **State** ____________ **Zip** ____________

Telephone ____________ **Alternate Phone** ____________ **Contact** ____________

Physician Name ____________ **Office Phone** ____________

____ **Preoperative Guidelines Given to Caretaker**

Legal Guardian Name ____________ **Relationship** ____________

Address ____________ **City** ____________ **State** ____________ **Zip** ____________

Phone ____________

Consent: _____ Sent to Guardian (Date: ___________)
_____ Signed

Scheduled in Operating Room: Date: ______________
Time: ______________

Notification of Scheduled Date: ____ Patient (Spoke with: ______________)
--Discussed arrival time; NPO status; reporting to SDS
____ DR. ______________ (Dentist Caring for patient)
____ Medical Clinic ____ Private Physician (if applicable)

Request for Medical Clearance Sent: ______________________
Insurance Verification:
Medicaid #: ____________________ Verified: __________________
Private Insurance Co & #________________________ Verified: __________________
Pre-Certification (Private or HMO): ______________ Verified: __________________
Payment: __________
Notes: ____

Fig. 1. Preoperative flow sheet. (*Courtesy of* Mountainside Hospital, Montclair, NJ; with permission.)

Patient Name: ____________

DOB: ____________

Medical Diagnoses	Check	Dental Diagnoses	Check	Behaviors	Check
Acute Situational Anxiety		Abscessed teeth		Bites on Dental Instruments	
Age 5 or below		Bone Loss		Refuses Dental Treatment	
ALS		Caries		Refuses Panorex	
Anticoagulation Therapy		Dental Pain		Refuses intra-oral radiographs	
Anxiety		Fistula		Refuses family/staff to brush teeth	
Arthritis		Fractured Teeth		Refuses to come to dental operatory	
Asthma		Gingivitis		Refuses to open mouth	
ADD/ADHD		Impacted teeth		Refuses to sit in Chair	
Autism		Malposed teeth		Several Dental Phobia	
Bipolar Disorder		Nursing Bottle Caries		Severe gag reflex	
Brain injury		Periodontal Disease		Spastic Behavior	
Cerebral Palsy		Poor oral hygiene		Unable to brush teeth	
Dementia		Retained Roots		Unable to fully examine	
Depression		Severe calculus			
Diabetes					
Down Syndrome					
Enlarged prostate		**Tentative Treatment**	**Check**		
Explosive personality disorder		Exam			
Fragile X Syndrome		X-rays			
GERD		Prophylaxis			
Hearing impaired		SC/RP			
HIV/AIDS		Gingivectomy			
Mental Retardation				**Tooth #**	
Minimally Verbal		Extractions			
Mitral valve prolapse		Pulpotomy/RCT			
Multiple Sclerosis		Stainless Steel Crown			
Non-verbal				**Tooth and Surface**	
Obsessive-compulsive disorder		Amalgam			
Pervasive developmental disorder		Composite			
Psychosis					
Seizure Disorder		Other pertinent information:			
Self-injurious behavior					
Spina Bifida					
Thrombocytopenia					
Visually impaired					

Bisphosphonate Therapy ☐ Yes ☐ No Medication name: ____________ How taken: ☐ Oral ☐ IV

Dates taken: From ___/___/___ To:___/___/___

Resident Signature: ____________ Attending Signature: ____________

Date: ________

Fig. 2. Department of dentistry preoperative checklist. (*Courtesy of* Mountainside Hospital, Montclair, NJ; with permission.)

PATIENT SCHEDULING

Each institution that provides dental care under general anesthesia has rules and regulations concerning appropriate timing of hospital, surgical, and anesthesia consent, medical clearance, and laboratory testing.

Consent

The risks, benefits and alternatives to treatment—including no treatment—must be included as part of the discussion for the consent.

It is imperative to determine who gives consent for the procedures. If guardianship has been established, a copy of the guardianship papers should be obtained. Higher functioning patients may be able to sign their own consents. Because many patients are accompanied by staff if they are residing in a group home setting, it is appropriate to ask if the patient has any relatives whom they want to inform about the scheduled procedures. With HIPAA regulations it is mandatory to get the patient/guardian's consent before discussing the details of care with other individuals. In addition, the consent is only valid for a finite period of time, which is stipulated by the rules and regulations of the hospital/surgical center where the procedure is taking place.

Among older patients and their elderly parents it is sometimes difficult to obtain consent. The discussion about who gives consent and how readily it can be obtained needs to occur during the presurgical screening. If a face-to-face discussion and signing of the consent is not possible, attempts should be made to call the guardian to discuss the proposed procedure. If that fails, then a cover letter describing the procedure in detail with information on how to contact the treating dentist for questions should be sent to the guardian along with the consent forms. The group home staff often has detailed information on the availability of the guardians and whether the consent should be mailed directly to the guardian or given to the group home staff for signature when the guardian visits the patient. Again, a written description of proposed procedures is required.

Medical Clearance

A preoperative history and physical must be obtained within a defined period of time before the surgical procedure. Again, the hospital/surgical center will stipulate that time frame in their rules and regulations. If the hospital has guidelines for presurgical testing, this should be included in the packet of materials that are given to the patient and any guardians/staff who accompany the patient to the medical visit.

Anesthesia Consent

Depending on the facility there may be a separate anesthesia consent that must be signed before the initiation of the dental case.

Facility Scheduling

Arrangements must be made with the facility where the dental case is to be completed.

Information for elective dental cases require

1. The requested date and time of the operation
2. Condition of patient
3. Type of operative procedure
4. Length of operation
5. Type of anesthesia
6. Type of admission (eg, inpatient, outpatient, day surgery)
7. Special equipment

Once this information is obtained a specific time/date is scheduled.[2]

SAME DAY SURGICAL MANAGEMENT

Preoperative Management

Consideration must be given to the availability of the dentist to perform the procedure and the availability of OR time. Patients with low cognitive function may not understand the directive to have nothing to eat or drink after midnight before the procedure. Therefore it is important to schedule this patient as the first case of the day so they are not with others who are eating and drinking. If a patient eats during the same day as the procedure, the case must be cancelled and rescheduled. This results in a tremendous loss of time for the dentist, the anesthesiologist, the OR scheduling and OR staff, as well as the individuals who are transporting the patient to the hospital. When calling the scheduling office to book the case, demographic information from the preoperative flow sheet listed above is needed. In addition, precertification from the medical insurance company that is covering the facility charges and the dental insurance company that is covering the dental charges must be obtained. It is important to leave enough time between scheduling the case and obtaining the precertification required unless it is an emergency situation.

Any special equipment needed during the procedure should be noted when booking the case. This may include surgical or endodontic equipment. Any special medical concerns (eg, latex allergy) should also be conveyed to the staff who is booking the case.

In addition, if there are special circumstances for a particular patient, the manager and the nursing staff who will be caring for the patient should be notified. This may include not mentioning "needles" in front of the patient, allowing the patient to bring a favorite toy into the OR, or other tips that the family/caregivers may have that will assist with general management of the patient.

Once the case is booked a written confirmation is sent to the patient/family/group home indicating:

1. Date and time of the procedure
2. Time the patient needs to arrive at the facility
3. Exact location where the patient needs to report (this may be different from the dental facility where the patient was initially seen)
4. Instructions concerning food and liquid intake before the procedure
5. Instructions concerning medications that may be taken the day of the procedure

Intraoperative Management

Preparation for the dental case assists in the timely and efficient management of the patient. Equipment and supplies that may be required should be set out before anesthetic induction so that time is not wasted looking for required dental supplies. If radiographs will be taken with holders, these should be prepared for use before the beginning of the case. Two posterior holders can be set up so that time is not wasted switching the holders for correct positioning during the case. If digital radiographs and a dental software program are used, connections should be made through the hospital/surgical center's information systems department to allow the radiographs to be viewed in the OR setting.

All other dental materials, cassettes, and handpieces should be prepared and ready. Materials such as amalgam, composite, bands, wedges, bonding agents, fluoride varnish, and sealants should be easily accessible for all cases. Because the OR staff may not be trained dental assistants, inservice education for the OR staff on a periodic basis provides an opportunity for development of a close working relationship and increased efficiency. Opportunities for inservice education can be arranged through the managers of the OR.

It is important for the dentist to be available to communicate with the anesthesia and nursing staff. Because the dentist is probably the only person whom the patient and their family/caregivers have seen preoperatively, and with whom they are comfortable, the dentist may be able to provide a calming environment for the anxious patient, and can provide assurance to the family/caregivers about the status of the patient undergoing general anesthesia. Again, because the relationship has been established preoperatively the dentist can ease any anxiety that is present.

OPERATIVE TECHNIQUES

Intraoperative Dental Care

Because the data required for completion of the treatment plan often cannot be obtained until the patient is under anesthesia, it is essential that data collection and an appropriate treatment plan be established once the radiographs and dental charting are completed. Site marking is required by National Patient Safety Goal 1B and is one requirement of the Universal Protocol. "The ADA acknowledges that there does not appear to be a practical or reliable method to actually mark the teeth that are intended for extraction. Therefore, dental procedures are considered exempt from the site marking requirement. In lieu of directly marking the teeth, the ADA recommends—and The Joint Commission concurs with—the following:

- Review the dental record including the medical history, laboratory findings, appropriate charts and dental radiographs. Indicate the tooth number(s) or mark the tooth site or surgical site on the diagram or radiograph to be included as part of the patient record.
- Ensure that radiographs are properly oriented and visually confirm that the correct teeth or tissues have been charted.
- Conduct a "time out" to verify patient, tooth, and procedure with assistant present at the time of the extraction (two-person rule)." [Reviewed 1/09][3]

Forms can be developed to provide data collection and development of a treatment plan. These forms should include existing restorations, required restorations, and other procedures including tooth and surface, and a place to indicate the date completed.

Examples of other procedures that should be included on the form include examination, periodontal charting, number and type of radiographs, prophylaxis and fluoride, scaling and root planing and gingivectomy by quadrant, and biopsies, amalgam or composite restorations, and extractions. Samples of dental forms are shown in **Figs. 3–5**. The forms must be included as part of the medical record.

Many patients have extensive dental needs and it is not uncommon for a treatment plan to include comprehensive examination, full mouth series of radiographs, dental prophylaxis, four quadrants of scaling and root planning, and multiple restorations and extractions. The list developed and written in the OR ensures accurate progress and completion of the dental treatment plan.

ROLE OF RESIDENTS IN PATIENT CARE

Whether they are general practice, pediatric dentistry, or oral surgery, residents must develop the skills to evaluate, schedule, and manage special needs patients under anesthesia. By involving the residents at the patient's initial screening visit, such as having them complete the preoperative flow sheet and the medical/dental screening form, they can discuss the options for care with their supervising attending physicians and assist in outlining the specific dental care plan. It must be understood by the residents that the attending makes the final decision for care and the attending must always sign the forms for the initiation of the procedure for scheduling in the OR. Residents must learn the documentation requirements for care under anesthesia. The required documentation listed below can be completed by the resident as per hospital protocol with appropriate countersignature.

Patient Sticker

Procedure	Check if Required	Date Completed	Additional Description
Exam			
FMS			
4 BW			
2 BW			
Periapical X-ray #			
Prophylaxis			
Fluoride			
SCRP UR			
SCRP UL			
SCRP LR			
SCRP LL			
Gingivectomy UR			
Gingivectomy UL			
Gingivectomy LR			
Gingivectomy LL			
Biopsy			

Fig. 3. OR dental procedure charting. (*Courtesy of* Mountainside Hospital, Montclair, NJ; with permission.)

Patient Sticker

			NEEDS						NEEDS		
Tooth #		Existing	Procedure	Surface/Q	Date Completed	Tooth #		Existing	Procedure	Surface/Q	Date Completed
	1						17				
	2						18				
	3						19				
A	4					K	20				
B	5					L	21				
C	6					M	22				
D	7					N	23				
E	8					O	24				
F	9					P	25				
G	10					Q	26				
H	11					R	27				
I	12					S	28				
J	13					T	29				
	14						30				
	15						31				
	16						32				

Legend: X= Missing
U= Unerupted

Signature: ______________________ Date: ______________

Fig. 4. OR dental tooth charting. (*Courtesy of* Mountainside Hospital, Montclair, NJ; with permission.)

Patient Sticker

	Date:			
	Buccal	Lingual	Recession	Mobility
Tooth #	distal mid mesial	distal mid mesial		
1				
2				
3				
4				
5				
6				
7				
8				
	mesial mid distal	mesial mid distal		
9				
10				
11				
12				
13				
14				
15				
16				
	distal mid mesial	distal mid mesial		
17				
18				
19				
20				
21				
22				
23				
24				
	mesial mid distal	mesial mid distal		
25				
26				
27				
28				
29				
30				
31				
32				

OH ☐ Excellent ☐ Good ☐ Fair ☐ Poor
Calculus ☐ Severe ☐ Moderate ☐ Mild ☐ None
Gingival Inflammation ☐ Severe bleeds easily ☐ moderate red ☐ mild redness ☐ none

Signature: __________ Date: __________

Fig. 5. OR periodontal charting. (*Courtesy of* Mountainside Hospital, Montclair, NJ; with permission.)

Chart Completion

These include

1. Preoperative Note
2. Postoperative orders
3. Postoperative note
4. Dictated operative report
5. Discharge instructions
6. Discharge order
7. Medication reconciliation
8. A preoperative note written by both the resident and the attending physician that contains
    a. Brief summary of the patient including:
    b. Age
    c. Past medical history
    d. Current medications
9. Justification for treatment in the OR, including preoperative clinical dental findings and radiographic findings (if able to take radiographs in the outpatient setting)

Following the procedure, postoperative orders must be written describing any specific requirements for the patient such as observation for postoperative bleeding following extractions, whether the head of the bed should be elevated. and so forth.

A postoperative note should include the name of the surgeon and OR assistants, anesthesiologist, specimens taken, drains in place, procedures completed and a note describing the current condition of the patient in the postanesthesia care unit, including vital signs, presence of bleeding, whether gauze is in place, and so forth.

An operative report must be dictated the day of the procedure by either the resident or the supervising dentist, and must include:

1. Patient's name
2. Medical record number
3. Preoperative diagnosis
4. Postoperative diagnosis
5. Procedure
6. Surgeon
7. Assistant surgeons

Patient Name ______________________

Date of birth __________ MR # ____________

Information Source: ☐ Patient / family ☐ Rx bottles ☐ List of meds ☐ MD ☐ Pharmacy

AT HOME Medications Includes OTC / vitamins / herbal supplements	**Dose**	**Route**	**How Often**	The reconciliation and decision to change or discontinue the use of these medications has been made by the Licensed Independent Practitioner and communicated to the patient. **DIRECTIONS**
☐ Patient takes no meds				
Listed by:	Verified by:			

☐ The medication list has been reviewed and no changes were made. Signature ______________ Date ________

STOP **STOP**	Date	Time	**RE - START**

ADD	Dose	Route	How Often	**DIRECTIONS**

☐ The medication list has been reviewed and the above changes were made. MD Signature ______________ Date ________

Fig. 6. Postprocedure medication instructions. (*Courtesy of* Mountainside Hospital, Montclair, NJ; with permission.)

8. Type of anesthesia
9. Anesthesiologist
10. Operative technique, which is a detailed description of the procedures that were performed
11. Estimated blood loss
12. Specimens taken and sent for pathologic review
13. Presence of drains

Once the report is transcribed, it must be signed by the supervising dentist.

PATIENT NAME ____________ DOB______
Dentist Name ________________

DEPARTMENT OF DENTISTRY
SAME DAY SURGERY GENERAL / PEDIATRIC DENTISTRY POST-OPERATIVE INSTRUCTIONS

PLEASE REVIEW ITEMS THAT ARE CHECKED

- ❑ Dental treatment has been performed under general anesthesia. You may experience a mild sore throat and general drowsiness for the next few days.
- ❑ A comprehensive dental examination, x-rays and general cleaning have been completed.
- ❑ Fillings were placed
- ❑ A deep cleaning and gum treatment was completed.
  Some oozing or mild bleeding from gums may occur over the next few days. This is to be expected. Begin brushing gently the day following surgery.
- ❑ Extractions have been completed in the following location: circle where required
  Lower right Lower left Upper right Upper left Upper front Lower front
  All sites should be treated with care for the 3 days. No hot liquids, no spitting, no smoking and no drinking with a straw for the next 3 days.
  - ➢ No rinsing the day of surgery. Begin rinsing the day after surgery with warm salt water (1/2 teaspoon salt in a large glass of warm water) four times a day for 4 days.
  - ➢ Place ice packs on the cheeks next to the extraction sites (Right / Left / Front) if the patient will tolerate. Place on and off every 20 minutes for the next 6 hours.
  - ➢ Some bleeding or mild oozing is to be expected. If sutures were placed they will dissolve within a few weeks
  - ➢ Resume toothbrushing the day following surgery

- ❑ <u>**Diet**</u>
  - o Liquid diet for ____days
  - o Chopped / Soft (e.g. cereal, eggs, yogurt) for _____ days
  - o Regular
  - o Avoid spicy food for 3 days (e.g. orange juice, tomato sauce)

☐ If there is heavy bleeding bite on gauze for 20 minutes with continuous pressure. If the bleeding does not stop call your dentist.

- ❑ Call for a follow-up appointment in _____ weeks
- ❑ Take prescriptions as prescribed, call if any concerns regarding this.
- ❑ Call your doctor for any unusual symptoms or fever greater than 100 degrees.

Dentist name__________________**Phone #**________________

Fig. 7. General/pediatric dentistry postoperative instructions. (*Courtesy of* Mountainside Hospital, Montclair, NJ; with permission.)

Residents are advised to keep copies of the operative reports for the patients with whom they were involved so that they will have a record of cases completed if in the future they apply for privileges at a hospital or surgical center.

In addition to the information noted previously, patients must complete a medication reconciliation form. The form lists all of the medications that the patient was taking before the surgical procedure, what should be stopped after the procedure, and what should be added after the procedure (**Fig. 6**).

A sample of dental postoperative instructions is shown in **Fig. 7**. By using a check-off sheet, the information required for the patient can be customized.

Assessment of Intervals for Care Under General Anesthesia

Following the completion of dental care under general anesthesia, a postoperative visit is scheduled. This visit provides the dentist the ability to inspect the oral cavity for evaluation of healing, function of restorations, and adequacy of oral hygiene practices; to answer patient and/or guardian questions; and to review oral hygiene and dietary guidelines for prevention of future dental problems.[4]

In addition, aids to dental care such as rotary toothbrushes, prescription fluoride, or mouthwashes may be prescribed.

At this time it is important to review in detail all the information about the patient, particularly the number of required operative procedures, and the periodontal charting that was completed under anesthesia. The oral hygiene pre- and postanesthesia should also be assessed. All of these factors need to be considered when suggesting an interval for any further treatment requiring general anesthesia. Although the patient may be evaluated in the outpatient setting in 6–12 months, deciding to have the patient undergo general anesthesia again must be made with a review of the previous dental examination and the degree of care that was provided. If the patient's caries is minimal and the periodontal status is healthy, the patient may not require care under anesthesia for several years. On the other hand, a patient who had multiple extractions and restorations due to severely carious lesions, scaling, and root planning due to severe periodontal pocketing and poor oral hygiene may require dental care under anesthesia within 1 year. In addition, some patients may exhibit limited cooperation for dental care in the outpatient setting. If these patients can be scheduled with a hygienist at regular 3-4 month intervals, the timing for care under anesthesia may be extended. Also, the amount of intraoperative time may be diminished.

Dental care for the special needs patient under general anesthesia requires a competent, well-trained dentist who can facilitate the care in order to maximize the essential treatment and minimize the fear, anxiety, and complications for the patient and their family and caregivers. In addition, the dentist can assist the surgical staff in providing the highest level of care for these special patients.

REFERENCES

1. Sonis S, Fazio R, Fang L. Principles and practice of oral medicine. Philadelphia: W.B. Saunders; 1995. p. 3.
2. Kwon P, Laskin D. Clinician's manual of oral and maxillofacial surgery. IL: Quintessence Publishing Co., Inc.; 1997. p. 208.
3. The Joint Commission. Available at: http://www.jointcommission.org/AccreditationPrograms/Hospital/Standards/Faqs/DentalProcedures. Accessed January 2009.
4. Sani RJ, Spence RO. Integrating hospital dentistry into general dental practice. J Calif Dent Assoc 2001;29(6):433–44.

Treatment Planning Considerations for Adult Oral Rehabilitation Cases in the Operating Room

Allen Wong, DDS, FACD

KEYWORDS

- Intellectual disability • Developmental disability
- Caries management by risk assessment • Dental varnish
- Glass ionomer • Desensitize • Triage
- Monitored anesthesia care • General anesthesia

Patients referred for general anesthesia dentistry usually need oral rehabilitation. This article addresses care of adult patients who have exhausted options for treatment in a routine setting, assuming that all means to achieve dental care have been tried and that oral pathology requiring attention exists in the mouth. This article discusses adult patients who are cooperative but cannot tolerate the dentistry because of medical compromise, psychologic reasons, or developmental or intellectual disabilities (DD/ID).

Treatment planning for dental general anesthesia cases has many considerations for patients, dentists, and facilities. Hippocrates stated, "[you] cannot treat what you cannot diagnose." A dental diagnosis is dependent on medical and psychologic diagnoses. There are many approaches and philosophies to planning treatment for a case. A surgeon's responsibility is to be accountable and responsible in delivering care. Knowing the endpoint of the dental care requires attention and observation of patients. Patients, caregivers, and legal guardians who are well informed of the whole hospital process and expectations are key to a pleasant and memorable experience. This article does not suggest that any described process is the standard of care, but allows practitioners to make their own best-suited plans for their patients.

OPERATING ROOM PREPARATION

The art of treatment planning for operating rooms requires quick, decisive thinking and awareness of limitations. Suggested treatment planning considerations and some

Department of Dental Practice, University of the Pacific Arthur A. Dugoni School of Dentistry, 2155 Webster Street, San Francisco, CA 94115, USA
E-mail address: awong@pacific.edu

Dent Clin N Am 53 (2009) 255–267
doi:10.1016/j.cden.2008.12.007

current techniques that have been beneficial are discussed. Treatment planning has benefited from recent advances in technology and science in terms of equipment and materials. The limiting factors of operating room consideration are time and finances. Considerations of postoperative care immediately after efficient and predictable operating room dentistry are provided.

Patient Considerations

There is a wide range of adult patients who present for oral rehabilitation using general anesthesia or monitored anesthesia care. Some are medically compromised, some are developmentally delayed, and some exhibit extreme dental fear. Patients who have current radiographs and can tolerate preoperative examinations provide practitioners a distinct advantage in preparing for oral rehabilitation cases and coordination of other disciplines. When patients are noncooperative and require sedation, however, dentists must be able adapt to those situations. Every attempt should be made to evaluate a patient's oral condition in order to proceed to scheduling the hospital visit. Practitioners must be able to create a treatment plan, deliver services, and have assurance that what is done will achieve a positive outcome.

In the past, oral rehabilitation under general anesthesia meant extracting everything that had pathology or may have had pathology. Now, many patients and their care providers desire restorative options or even conventionally restoring their mouth to preserve dignity. Increasing numbers of persons who have DD/ID and are integrated in the community are part of the work force. Teeth are important not only for eating but also for employment and self-esteem.

The age of adult patients, from adolescent to geriatric, can be a major determinant of final treatment. As the population ages, there are more complicated health concerns, including dementia and polypharmacy. Patil and Patil outline some of those concerns: "The dentist is concerned with the emotional and psychological state of the patient, for it is an essential component of treatment and the success of the treatment often depends on the emotional state of the patient. It is thus important for the dentist to be aware of practical- problem-oriented approach that helps in patient management and in maintaining and improving dental health as part of total healthcare services available to the elderly."[1]

Practitioner Concerns

Oral health is essential for total health of the body, according to the Surgeon General's report of 2000. Practitioners deciding whether or not general anesthesia or monitored anesthesia care is the suitable method to safely treat a patient cannot focus solely on the oral cavity. If a patient is noncompliant in a routine setting for dentistry, the same noncooperation may exist for the patient's other medical disciplines. Annual examinations often are abbreviated for patients who have special needs because of a physician's inability to attain full cooperation from those patients. Consultation with a patient's primary care provider may generate a collaboration of additional services while the patient is under anesthesia. Additional services may be as simple as blood tests or more complex, including otolaryngologic, optical, gynecologic, podiatric, or cardiac examinations or procedures, such as transesophageal echocardiograms, cardioversions, and EKGs. Treatment planning for multidisciplinary cases requires coordination of medical and dental specialists for dates and times.

The dental case is the primary admission, with the various subspecialties interposed accordingly. Practitioners may decide to bring to the operating room dental specialists, such as a periodontist, endodontist, orthodontist, and oral surgeon, for procedures beyond their comfort level. Each specialist needs to be on medical staff or obtain temporary privileges, secure informed consents, and make financial arrangements in advance. Cases need to reflect any additional time required and the modification of table set-up.

Hospital Limitations

For hospitals that have oral maxillofacial and dental services, there may be a portable dental cart, X-ray head, and developer. In some cases, hospitals may have digital radiography software and hardware connected to a computer. If a hospital does not have an X-ray head, practitioners must supply their own. Most hospitals have a radiology department that can provide head films, such as lateral cephalometric, Waters view, or submental vertex. Equipment availability at hospitals can vary for dental procedures. Some hospitals store and share their instrument set-ups and have all the instruments necessary for procedures from oral surgery to restorative dentistry, whereas others have only a few instruments for emergency oral surgery. Dental cart, dental hand pieces, ultrasonic scaler, and dental instruments and supplies may be items that a practitioner needs to supply.

Hospital staffing for an operating room requires that a scrub nurse and circulating nurse be present in addition to an anesthesiologist and surgeon. In some hospitals, the scrub nurse is well versed in dental procedures but not in others. A trained dental assistant who meets the criteria for assisting in an operating room usually can be brought in to work as a scrub nurse if permission and paperwork are completed in advance. A trained dental assistant is advantageous in dealing with dental materials and assisting.

Time

Hospital dentists of today must carefully weigh the time it takes for dental procedures and the prognosis of the teeth that are treated. Providing hospital dentistry services requires a substantial amount of time, especially if there is coordination with financial concerns, medical subspecialties, and care providers. The paperwork and financial arrangements for the hospital, preoperative work-up, additional physicians' appointments, and laboratory work are significant. For practitioners who bring in their own staff and equipment to the operating room, there is additional paperwork, setting up the operating room, breaking down the room, and maintaining the supplies and equipment. Practitioners also are responsible for preoperative and postoperative evaluation of patients, dictation, and making sure proper consent and medical clearance are available. Preoperative work-up and waiting for an operating room can add additional hours to a case.

In order to see patients at set times and minimize the possibility of being bumped from time slots, clinicians who have a substantial number of hospital cases desire block time. Block time is reserved time allocated in the schedule for surgeons to fill with their patients, providing they use the time in a regular manner. A utilization review committee reviews these requests and assigns the block times. Time utilization in an operating room is important in order to be considered for future block time. If a surgeon fails to keep the schedule full or uses the block time inadequately, that surgeon loses the privilege. Therefore, a reasonable estimation of time is approximated from patient evaluation information.

Patients and caregivers must prepare in advance for the time required for preoperative appointments and day of surgery and postoperative visits. Transportation of patients and coordination of withholding oral food and fluids status must be assured. There should be no misunderstanding that operating room times require a serious commitment. On rare instances, patients may stay overnight for observation after a procedure.

Consent

Before scheduling a case, a dentist must have a good working relationship with patient, caregiver, and legal guardian. Not only is it a legal requirement of hospitals to secure informed consent, it is essential for patients or legal guardians to understand the importance of surgical consent and the need to follow-up with instructions, such as medical clearance and presurgical instructions. Each hospital has specific guidelines on dealing with patients who are not able to sign for themselves and are not conserved. Patients or legal guardians should be well informed of the philosophy and potential treatment options prior to scheduling an operating room. For patients who are having radiographs taken while under general anesthesia, some practitioners are requested to leave the operating room once radiographs are taken to discuss a case with a caregiver or guardian. Leaving an operating room to discuss a case can take time from an operator and extend the time a patient is under general anesthesia. If the philosophy is explained in advance, such as fixing teeth that can be fixed and extracting teeth that no longer are restorable, there should not be a need to come out to discuss the case.

Preparing for the Assessment Appointment

Make sure patients or caregivers are aware of the need for an assessment appointment. The goal is to explain the actual hospital dentistry process, evaluate dental and medical needs, and review postoperative care instructions. If possible, dental radiographs should be attempted and a thorough examination performed. If a patient is fearful or has DD/ID, it may be helpful to have a caregiver or parent familiarize the patient by introducing the concepts of counting teeth and having the patient practice opening the mouth and brushing. Having patients practice these at home helps desensitize them for similar activities in a dental office hospital. They should bring their current medications, medical records, dental X-rays, and notes and information on previous surgeries. In addition, they can bring something that comforts them or allows them to be distracted, such as a familiar toy or music.

Assessing Patients

Treatment planning for the operating room does not start at the hospital—it starts at the initial assessment. Patients are assessed beginning with external characteristics and continuing with internal characteristics. Patients' physical coordination and dexterity may provide insight to their physical agility for postoperative preventive dental care. Much of the dentistry to be accomplished requires practitioners to have a good estimation of how the dental work will survive in successive years. Some major considerations are a patient's tolerance to following-up dental care in a routine setting; the patient's ability to have preventive care; and physiologic changes in the oral cavity with respect to habit, medications, and stability of the medical condition.

There are several ways of determining compliance, using direct observation and asking probing questions of caregivers of patients who are unable to cognitively understand. Generally, the more compliant a patient, the more elaborate a treatment plan can be, such as a fixed crown and bridge or implants. For patients who are less compliant or more medically complex, less sophisticated dental care is considered. Quality dental care is provided for all patients in a customized approach.

A careful dental, medical, and cooperation risk assessment helps minimize multiple hospital visits for the same procedures. The goal of the oral rehabilitation visit should be to bring patients to optimal dental health and a strategy to maintain their oral health.

Working with Patients Who Have Special Needs

When working with patients who have specials needs, dentists must take adequate time to review medical health history, dental history, and current medications. Patients who have special needs may include those in the geriatric population and those who have Alzheimer's disease. Smith and colleagues[2] summarize, "The assessment of dental treatment needs must take account of the clinical dental status of the subjects, their demands for treatment and their oral handicaps." Whenever possible, patients are the most direct and reliable source in obtaining detailed information; the next best source is caregivers or guardians. Find out what makes patients feel nervous or uncomfortable; sharing a patient's dental experience is a good way to get to know the patient.

Whether or not patients are cooperative and cognitive or uncooperative and combative, approach patients carefully and do not make sudden movements. Do not do anything to patients without getting their permission. The adage, "inform before you perform," is a good rule of thumb. Safety to patients and dental teams should dictate how care is delivered. In situations where patients are combative, a team should not be put in a position in which they feel endangered. There are no absolute protocols in dental assessment except to try to make a good assessment. When in doubt, ask, "What is in the best interest of the patient?" It may be that a caregiver or parent is present to calm a patient or can assist in having a patient cooperate until the patient is more familiar with the surroundings. The clinical examination may take place in a private area of the waiting room while the patient is watching television. There is an emphasis on the importance of obtaining a thorough examination in order to properly plan a case from the time estimate to deciding which other subspecialties need to be involved. A patient's cooperation level determines the level of treatment options.

Preparing the Dentist

Dentistry in an operating room is not much different from dentistry in an office, other than limitations of operating room bed position. Dentists should be familiar with the equipment available if they are new to a hospital. Any electrical items brought to an operating room area may require a hospital engineering department for clearance (sometimes a week in advance), and any medications, such as local anesthetic, brought into an operating room also must be cleared with an operating room supervisor. If there are essential instruments required, it is best to take them for sterilization and disinfection in advance. Disposable items, such as gauze, sutures, local anesthetics, dressing, and sutures, and equipment, such as surgical hand pieces and electrosurgery units, may be available but the sizes or delivery system may not be a dentist's preference. A preference card usually is established for surgeons so that nurses can supply the room and set it up according to preferences.

As professionals, dentists should practice only within their comfort level and training. Hospital dentists who offer an array of services must be proficient and kept abreast of the various techniques, including endodontic, periodontic, restorative, and oral surgical, or refer to specialists. As Carrotte[3,4] notes, for instance, pertaining to root canal treatment: "[its] techniques probably develop and change more frequently than any other area of dental practice and it can be hard for the busy general dental practitioner to keep up to date." Being a safe practitioner means knowing limits and having contingency plans. It is prudent to classify treatments as those most necessary having first priority and those least necessary having last priority. Do not overcommit or promise what may not be able to be delivered.

Preparations for unexpected situations may be (1) restorative: unsupported tooth structure leading to extraction, inability to isolate for composite restorations, or unexpected odontogenic fractures; (2) endodontic: perforation, missed canal, separated instrument, or poor obturation; or (3) surgical: inability to remove entire portion of root, dislodging fragment into the sinus cavity, or iatrogenic outcomes of hard or soft tissue.

Recovery Room

Postoperative considerations should include minimizing pain, swelling, nausea, postextraction alveolitis (dry socket), and fractured restorations. In the recovery room (postanesthesia care unit), pain and nausea are managed by anesthesiologists through a systemic approach, usually using narcotic and antiemetics, respectively. Numazaki and colleagues[5] provide a recommendation: "Prophylactic dexamethasone 8 mg is effective for the prevention of nausea and vomiting after dental surgery and in the management of postoperative pain. Increasing the dose to 16 mg provides no further benefit." Pain can be from a nasal tube, laryngeal discomfort, or the procedures. Nausea may be from medications, swallowed blood, or low blood sugar. Most noncooperative patients who require oral surgery for dental care are more likely to need sutures that dissolve. Ice packs to the side of the face help with facial swelling, depending on a patient's tolerance of cold packs.

Financial Considerations

For most procedures, consideration of finances is a concern. Insurance limitations can affect ideal treatment and should be addressed prior to surgery. The business of doing dentistry cannot be ignored; otherwise, a practice is stressful and unsatisfactory. Planning time in an operating room includes determining where financial arrangements and insurance paperwork are cleared. Failure to have the necessary paperwork completed in advance may result in large bills to patients or practitioners.

Costs for patients

In order for patients to have restorative treatment, there are fixed costs of the dental procedures. Those procedures must be maintained through frequent visits to a dentist; patients need to tolerate prevention procedures. If insurance or patients do not support the prevention model, such as paying for additional cleanings or chemotherapeutic supplies, restorations are at risk for premature failure. Premature failure in a restoration can result in another hospital dentistry encounter and possibly an extraction. Therefore, it is imperative that patients or caregivers be fully aware that prevention requires care that is not always a covered benefit. The more elaborate the dental procedure, the more investment in time and preventive visits is required. In order for patients to have a fixed bridge, for example, patients must be able to tolerate prophylaxis and flossing under the fixed prosthesis. In the case of implants, patients must be able to tolerate periodic radiographs and possible adjustments in a clinic. Patients who wear removable prostheses must be able to communicate fit and function and have the ability to remove their appliance and clean their mouth.

Most outpatient "come and go" surgeries proceed as planned. On occasion, patients may be admitted overnight for observation, with corresponding increased overnight costs for patients and additional costs for caregivers.

Costs for dentists

Dentists who are at a hospital without an established dental or oral surgery department may need to equip their own practice at the hospital. Dental supplies and equipment are obvious cost items for dentists to consider. The return on investment on dental supplies and equipment must have criteria that give the best final long-term results. Quality equipment may last longer than economical equipment, especially if the items are mobile. When possible, time-saving measures are a cost-containing ingredient; for example, a digital X-ray system may be a large initial investment but when it saves operators waiting times of 30 to 40 minutes per case and reduces frustrations of waiting while having the benefit of enhanced radiography, the cost is justified. Parks agrees: "The expenses associated with converting to digital radiographic imaging are considerable."[6] Saving time equates to efficiency in patient care, with less time under anesthesia and, for cases that are paid with Medicaid, it means greater chance of breaking even.

The choice of dental materials for restorative dentistry should match the needs of patients as it relates to their risk assessment.

Costs to the hospital

In order for dentists to maintain hospital privileges, cases should flow in an expedient manner. Each hospital case incurs an hourly cost for the hospital; if reimbursement for that care is dramatically less than the cost of the care, there results a challenge in seeing more patients. Therefore, a clinician's responsibility is to aide in the process of a smooth and efficient course of hospital admission. A smooth case is one in which a patient has all paperwork completed and shows up to the hospital early, not late. In addition, a procedure should finish at the time anticipated at scheduling, patients should have a "painless" recovery period, and discharge should be within a reasonable time without too much excitement. Working closely with an anesthesiologist to assure adequate pain and nausea control in the recovery room is important for expedient discharge.

IMPLEMENTING A TREATMENT PLAN FOR THE OPERATING ROOM

Having reviewed considerations of competency, time, and finances, a treatment plan for the hospital operating room can be made. As discussed previously, dental radiographs in advance provide a good starting point. If possible, a panoramic X-ray is encouraged to rule out dental pathology and visualize important landmarks, such as sinus floors, inferior alveolar nerves, mental nerve, temporal mandibular joint, and ridge thickness.

If preoperative radiographs are not possible, a full set of radiographs should be taken after patients are under general anesthesia. In situations where dental radiographic equipment is not available, the radiology department of a hospital can be notified to take various head films. Hard tissue and soft tissue charting then is recorded and diagnosis is made. A caries risk assessment that identifies factors that influence recurrent periodontal disease and caries is done. Young and colleagues emphasize, "A risk-based approach to managing caries targets those in greatest jeopardy for contracting the disease, as well as provides evidence-based decisions to treat current disease and control it in the future."[7] The assessment includes a salivary evaluation of acidity and flow. The more xerostomic a patient, the more likely dental restorations are needed. In patients who have medical compromise and DD/ID, they are common secondary to the medications prescribed and, in some, a mouth-breathing habit.

With knowledge of risk factors, a dentist can go through a systematic approach of six stages.

Stage One: Periodontal Stability

Teeth that exhibit a poor periodontal prognosis may be removed except in conditions when bisphosphonates are used. Teeth with mobility grade 3 should be removed as a source of infection and potential swallowing or aspiration hazard. If there are enough teeth that occlude, function, and can be maintained, then restorative dentistry can be considered; if not, removing the teeth is a viable option. If there are periodontal pockets that exceed 4 mm and have significant inflammation, hyperplasia, or redundancy, gingival surgery may be necessary in addition to the initial nonsurgical periodontal therapy.

Stage Two: Restorative Stability

Patients whose teeth have small to large carious lesions and normal saliva may have a choice of restorative material. Any teeth with compromise in hygiene or saliva may be limited to a glass ionomer restoration. The teeth to be restored should have adequate healthy tooth structure and be able to resist the occlusal forces. Posterior teeth that do not have anterior guidance are in jeopardy of excessive occlusal function and should be restored appropriately and, if tolerated, perhaps a night guard appliance should be used.

For teeth that have deep grooves and have a risk factor for caries, sealants and varnishes should be considered. Glass ionomer sealants are easy to use, economical, and efficacious. A study in 2006 demonstrated that glass ionomer sealant maintained its integrity better than a resin sealant.[8]

Stainless steel crowns that are well adapted to the tooth are a good option for significantly broken down teeth, with large restorations that need coronal protection in teeth for which cast crowns are not suitable.

Restorations should use materials that can withstand the environment in which they reside. Composite restorations are best for restoring teeth with healthy enamel margins and moisture control. Less enamel in a preparation requires a restoration with physical retention, such as amalgam, or chemical retention, such as glass ionomer. Dentin-bonding agents are not as predictable in large areas of dentin exposure or root surfaces.

Fixed restorative options should be considered only when patients can maintain the hygiene and standard concepts of occlusion and when crown-to-root ratio is maintained. Keep margins of restorations supragingival and check occlusion. Fixed prosthodontic preparations under general anesthesia must be done with nasotracheal intubation or monitored anesthesia care in order to manage occlusion and take impressions. Depending on location and cooperation of patients, the delivery of an appliance may be done with general anesthesia again, monitored anesthesia, or possible oral sedation in a routine dental setting.

Stage Three: Endodontics

Occasionally, a deep carious lesion may reach the pulp or a presence of a necrotic tooth may require endodontic therapy. Carotte notes, "Some information may be gleaned from the pre-operative radiograph, but much will be part of the practitioner's own knowledge. An understanding of the root canal morphology is also essential when cutting efficient and effective access cavities, remembering the endodontic cliché that 'access is success.'"[9] As with all endodontic procedures, diagnostic radiographs that depict the canal morphology must be visible in order to proceed. Patency of the canal must be visualized so that a favorable outcome is attained. The electronic apex locator is a helpful tool in establishing canal working length. Traditionally, the options for irreversible pulpitis and necrotic pulps usually were extraction or, in unique situations, treatment with endodontic therapy. Prior to rotary endodontics, time was a major factor in deciding if a tooth would be treated endodontically along with a multiple-appointment philosophy. With the advent of rotary endodontics and the acceptable practice of single-visit endodontics, practitioners may be able to safely and efficiently prepare and obturate teeth in order to restore teeth, function, and dignity.

A growing population of patients on bisphosphonates is emerging. Bisphosphonates are used to treat osteoporosis and cancer. The incidence of bisphosphonate-related osteonecrosis of the jaw (BONJ) can be a serious situation wherein a person can have a nonhealed extraction site for years as a result of necrosis, with the result of resection of the jaw bone. To avoid possible osteonecrosis, the recommendation is an endodontic procedure to avoid potential bone exposure. Most reported BONJs are from an intravenous route but the oral route is still suspect.

Patients who present for oral rehabilitation requiring extractions should consult with their physician to have a blood test—morning fasting serum C-terminal telopeptides—as baseline to evaluate their tissue turnover rate. If the level is above 150 pg/mL, preliminary studies suggest minimal risk for BONJ; if less, a consideration of a 3-month drug holiday from bisphosphonate use can be tried. After the 3 months, another blood test is done to evaluate the new levels of C-terminal telopeptides.[10]

Stage Four: Oral Surgery

The last stages are surgical consideration. As discussed previously, the presurgical consideration for bleeding concerns and prior bisphosphonate use should be cleared by a patient's specialist before a case is scheduled. McLeod and colleagues note, "The risk associated with oral therapy is in the order of 0.01% although with parenteral therapy it may be as high as 10%."[11] Less cooperative or more mentally or physically impaired patients require a surgeon to practice an atraumatic surgical technique and use good hemostatic strategies. Good hemostatic strategies may include resorbable sutures, such as gut or chromic gut; surgical dressings, such as Gel foam (Absorbable Gelatin), Surgicel (NU-KNIT Hemostat), or Avitene (Microfibrillar collagen hemostat); and achieving a primary closure. Oral pathology that is questionable should be documented properly and biopsied.

In the DD/ID population, patients tend to explore with their fingers and tongue. It is prudent to secure and stabilize the extraction sites with primary closure and sutures in order to minimize the possibility of postextraction alveolitis. Ucontrolled bleeding in postoperative patients may result in another admission to resolve the situation.

Postradiation therapy

A good preoperative work-up from an oncologist is necessary before treating a patient after radiation who may require extractions. Radiation oncologists can let surgeons know the ports of radiation and the amount of exposure and make necessary recommendations. Kanatas and colleagues[12] note specific concerns: "When contemplating exodontias or minor oral surgery in the irradiated patient, special consideration should be given to issues such as radiotherapy history, surgical assessment, surgical procedure and the role of antibiotics and hyperbaric oxygen."

HIV and bleeding disorders

Patients who have potential risks for healing problems and bleeding problems should have their condition evaluated with current tests along with atraumatic dental procedures. Scully and colleagues, in a study of complications in HIV patients, reported increased incidence of oral surgical complications: "Dental extractions and other oral surgical procedures, including local analgesic injections, potentially can cause problems in haemophiliac and HIV infected persons. There are few data on treatment results in HIV-infected haemophiliacs compared with non-HIV-infected haemophiliacs. The oral surgery treatment results in 48 patients with special needs, including HIV-infected haemophiliacs, non-HIV-infected haemophiliacs, HIV-infected non-haemophiliacs, and a group with other medical problems were therefore studied. Around 20% of the haemophiliacs developed post-oral surgical complications, which was not significantly different whether or not they were HIV-infected. However, complications were less frequent (8%) in HIV-infected non-haemophiliacs or other patients with special needs. Although the patient groups are not large, it would appear that haemophiliacs had more postoperative complications but that the presence of HIV infection had no notable influence on treatment outcome."[13] In a population that is not able to tolerate routine settings, strong consideration for minimizing all postextraction alveolitis sequelae should ensue. The most predictable methods of minimizing postextraction alveolitis are to make sure caregivers understand and are cognizant of the postoperative instructions and to use a good surgical approach. Deep local anesthetic injections, such as the inferior alveolar injection, should be avoided as a traumatized vessel may cause a major hematoma or be a significant bleeder. The approach is to minimize trauma to the hard and soft tissues, irrigate the sockets well, place hemostatic agents while giving a secure primary closure, and provide postoperative care instructions.

Impactions and difficult extractions

Never attempt any surgical procedure that can put patients in jeopardy of jaw fracture. Clinicians should never practice beyond their educational training. If a patient presents with pericoronitis on a partially impacted tooth at the angle of the ramus with inferior alveolar canal proximity and thin bone, a referral to an oral surgeon for possible bone plates should be considered. Proper postoperative instruction is essential to avoid further damage to patients.

As more adult oral rehabilitation cases are scheduled, it will be necessary to start a triaging system to help prioritize dental care. Cases and colleagues[14] describe the benefits of triage: "Use of the prioritization system demonstrated improved timeliness of treatment for urgent cases and the effects of additional measures taken to reduce the waiting list."

Transplant patients

Transplant patients should be cleared properly with their physicians prior to surgery.

Liver and kidney Bleeding concerns are managed best in advance with planned contingencies. Infusion of platelets or factors may be required preoperatively. Unless all teeth have poor prognosis, studies suggest that a full-mouth edentulation (sanitation) can present problems. A study in Germany by Niederhagen and colleagues reported 15.4% secondary bleeding (severe in some cases) after edentulation in pretransplant liver patients and advised, "given the high rate of complications found in this study after sanitation prior to transplantation, the demand for radical prophylactic dental sanitation should be reconsidered."[15] An atraumatic surgical technique and hemostatic control are essential (described previously).

Patients who are on renal dialysis should be scheduled on off days and their physician consulted regarding antibiotic coverage.

Heart Stress tests, echocardiogram, EKG, and blood work are important tests for evaluating the cardiac condition. In rare instances where the heart condition is dubious, an overnight stay may be necessary. Many patients who have heart conditions are on blood thinners, such as clopidrigol and aspirin, or other cardiac medications. It is prudent to discuss the anticoagulation therapy with a physician to work out a safe strategy prior to dental treatment.

Nasogastric tube/stoma

Patients who are fed through a tube or breathe through a port in the neck rather than the mouth may have extreme xerostomia. When the salivary glands are not stimulated with food or swallowing, the buffering capabilities may lessen. Prevention strategies in these patients are important to lessen a potential acidic environment, dental caries, and periodontal disease. Oral hygiene is important whether or not food enters the mouth, as bacteria continue to develop in the oral cavity.

Stage Five: Removable Appliances

Removable appliances are considered only if they do not endanger patient health by accidental choking or aspiration and if patients can remove the appliance themselves without complication. If patients are able to understand the proper care and use of an appliance, an attempt to make an appliance is made.

Fit and function need to be evaluated carefully and regularly and any sharp clasps minimized, if applicable. Yeast can grow easily on removable appliances if they are not cleaned and soaked properly.

In cases where there is a strong tongue thrust or impression taking is futile, there is no way to take an impression in a chair. For those patients or caregivers insistent on making a set of dentures for a noncooperative patient, a plastic disposable impression tray can be given to a caregiver to use as a desensitizer. An impression can be taken after the caregiver can assure that a patient is able to tolerate an impression tray in the patient's mouth for 10 minutes.

The myth about edentulous patients not being able to eat compels caregivers and loved ones to demand replacement teeth. The fact is that many times edentulous patients gain weight and have fewer gastrointestinal problems once diet is modified.

Stage Six: Postoperative Instruction and Recare

On completion of oral rehabilitation, it is important to document and inform patients and caregivers as to the proper care and maintenance of restorations and healing sites. Frequent postoperative visits and prevention protocol for caries and periodontal risk assessment should be started immediately to maintain good oral health. The higher the risk, the more frequent the recare visits. Nonalcoholic mouth rinses, pH control rinses, fluoride (gel or high-concentration toothpaste), amorphous calcium phosphate, xylitol therapy, chlorhexidine, and doxycycline are various agents that can be prescribed to treat teeth. Varnishes, sealants, preventive resin restorations, salivary tests, and bleaching trays are procedures practitioners may perform.

TREATMENT PLANNING FOR DISCHARGE

The last part of the treatment planning process is predicting the level of discomfort expected for patients. Because patients are asleep and under systemic pain control, they are not able to communicate discomfort well and, in the case of patients who have DD/ID, they may not be able to communicate afterwards. Postoperative pain often is treated in a recovery room (postanesthesia care units) with a narcotic, such as morphine or fentanyl, which can affect the length of recovery time in sensitive patients. If the length of recovery is longer than 3 hours, there is a good chance that the local anesthesia, if used, has worn off. Therefore, the anticipated area of pain could be addressed with long-acting local anesthesia to supplement the systemic pain control that is wearing off. Restorations in general are not considered to result in much postoperative pain, but oral and periodontal surgery and, in some cases, endodontic therapy may generate moderate to severe pain. If patients are not allergic to aspirin products, a strong nonsteroidal anti-inflammatory drug may be given intravenously or intramuscularly to reduce pain. Pain should be controlled so that patients can sense their lips, tongue, and cheek in order to avoid cheek- or lip-biting trauma. By managing pain in advance locally, patients are able to reach the discharge criteria quickly and be discharged from the hospital.

Nausea, as discussed previously, may result from sensitivity to medications, swallowed blood, or low blood sugar. Bland foods, such as saltine crackers and yogurt, and liquids, such as apple juice or orange juice, may help patients feel better. Patients should avoid spicy and hot foods, especially if there is suspected local anesthesia on board. Also avoid mechanical disruption of healing sites in the mouth with aggressive suctioning or use of straws.

SUMMARY

Treatment planning for adult dental cases of oral rehabilitation is a challenge. Treatment planning is not the same as providing actual care. When in doubt, it always is best to consider a more conservative approach and recruit help. Once patients are involved in their dental care, short maintenance appointments that are painless help them break the cycle of dental neglect and protect the investments of time and dental procedures through prevention.

REFERENCES

1. Patil MS, Patil SB. Geriatric patient—psychological and emotional considerations during dental treatment. Gerodontology 2008; epub ahead of print.
2. Smith JM, Steele LP, Sheiham A. Delivery programmes for elderly and isolated populations. Int Dent J 1983;33(3):301–7.
3. Page RC, Martin JA, Loeb CF. Use of risk assessment in attaining and maintaining oral health. Compend Contin Educ Dent 2004;25(9):657–60, 663–656, 669; quiz 670.
4. Carrotte P. 21st century endodontics. Part 1. Int Dent J 2005;55(2):105–9.
5. Numazaki M, Fujii Y. Reduction of postoperative emetic episodes and analgesic requirements with dexamethasone in patients scheduled for dental surgery. J Clin Anesth 2005;17(3):182–6.
6. Parks ET. Digital radiographic imaging: is the dental practice ready? J Am Dent Assoc 2008;139(4):477–81.
7. Young DA, Featherstone JD, Roth JR. Curing the silent epidemic: caries management in the 21st century and beyond. J Calif Dent Assoc 2007;35(10):681–5.
8. Antonson SA, Wanuck J, Antonson DE. Surface protection for newly erupting first molars. Compend Contin Educ Dent 2006;27(1):46–52.
9. Carrotte P. 21st century endodontics. Part 2. Int Dent J 2005;55(3):162–7.
10. Marx RE, Cillo JE Jr, Ulloa JJ. Oral bisphosphonate-induced osteonecrosis: risk factors, prediction of risk using serum CTX testing, prevention, and treatment. J Oral Maxillofac Surg 2007;65(12):2397–410.
11. McLeod NM, Davies BJ, Brennan PA. Bisphosphonate osteonecrosis of the jaws; an increasing problem for the dental practitioner. Braz Dent J 2007;203(11): 641–4.

12. Kanatas AN, Rogers SN, Martin MV. A practical guide for patients undergoing exodontia following radiotherapy to the oral cavity. Dent Update 2002;29(10): 498–503.
13. Scully C, Watt-Smith P, Dios RD, et al. Complications in HIV-infected and non-HIV-infected haemophiliacs and other patients after oral surgery. Int J Oral Maxillofac Surg 2002;31(6):634–40.
14. Casas MJ, Kenny DJ, Barett EJ, et al. Prioritization for elective dental treatment under general anesthesia. J Can Dent Assoc 2007;73(4):321.
15. Niederhagen B, Wolff M, Appel T, et al. Location and sanitation of dental foci in liver transplantation. Transpl Int 2003;16(3):173–8.

Managing Older Patients Who Have Neurologic Disease: Alzheimer Disease and Cerebrovascular Accident

Robert G. Henry, DMD, MPH[a,b,c,*], Barbara J. Smith, PhD, RDH, MPH[d]

KEYWORDS

- Alzheimer disease • Cerebrovascular accidents • Stroke
- Neurologic disease • Neurologic conditions • Geriatric
- Elderly • Management

Neurologic diseases/conditions in older age can be classified into three primary categories.[1] The first, degenerative disorders, implies some type of degeneration in the central nervous system or an accelerated aging process. Alzheimer disease (AD) is the most prevalent example of this type of disorder. The second category encompasses structural abnormalities in the brain or central nervous system, such as brain tumors, which may lead to seizures and may occur at any age. However, tumors that occur in the elderly have different implications, manifestations, treatment, and prognosis. The third category is cerebrovascular disorders. These disorders occur with greater frequency in older age and are associated with risk factors such as hypertension and atherosclerosis. Cerebrovascular accidents (CVA), or strokes, would represent this type of neurologic condition.[1]

In contrast to these three categories, several neurologic conditions are not characteristic in the elderly. Conditions including epilepsy, the muscular dystrophies, demyelinating conditions such as multiple sclerosis, and migraine generally occur at young or middle ages. These patients live into older age with "acquired" disabilities. More

[a] Department of Dental Services, Veterans Affairs Medical Center, Lexington, KY 40502, USA
[b] University of Kentucky College of Dentistry, Lexington, KY 40506, USA
[c] Sanders-Brown Center on Aging, Lexington, KY 40506, USA
[d] Geriatric and Special Needs Populations, Council on Access, Prevention, & Interprofessional Relations, American Dental Association, 211 E. Chicago Avenue, Chicago, IL 60611, USA
* Corresponding author. Department of Dental Services (160), Veterans Affairs Medical Center, Cooper Dr. Division, 1001 Veterans Drive, Lexington, KY 40502, USA.
E-mail address: robert.henry@va.gov (R.G. Henry).

Dent Clin N Am 53 (2009) 269–294
doi:10.1016/j.cden.2008.12.011
0011-8532/08/$ – see front matter. Published by Elsevier Inc.

and more elderly patients who have primary or acquired neurologic conditions are being seen today in dental offices because effective interventions and therapies for treating these diseases/conditions are adding years to life. This article reviews the two most common neurologic diseases affecting the elderly, AD and stroke, focusing on oral and dental concerns and providing suggestions for dental personnel to manage patients who have these conditions.

ALZHEIMER DISEASE

Definition and Cause of Alzheimer Disease

AD is the most common form of dementia, which is the loss of intellectual and social abilities severe enough to interfere with daily functioning. AD is a progressive, degenerative disease that attacks the brain and results in impaired memory, thinking, and behavior[2] It typically occurs after age 65 with prevalence increasing with advanced age. From age 70, prevalence doubles every 5 years. By age 85, more than 40% of individuals will have developed AD. Although an estimated 5.2 million people in the United States have AD, the prevalence is predicted to triple by the year 2050.[3] An average dental practice of 2000 adult patients is predicted to include about 46 patients who have AD.[4]

The cause of AD is unknown, although the following have been shown to be associated risk factors: advanced age (85+),[5] having trisomy 21 (Down's syndrome),[6] a history of severe head trauma,[7] or having a first-degree relative who has the disorder.[8,9] Recent findings suggest that unidentified factors trigger the deposition of beta-amyloid plaques, initiating an inflammatory response that results in neurofibrillary tangles and the loss of cortical neurons. This process begins in the hippocampus and entorhinal cortex and spreads to the areas in the brain responsible for memory and learning (the temporal, parietal, and frontal lobes). Eventually, continued destruction of neurons leads to atrophy of the cerebral cortex and enlargement of the ventricles. However, motor, visual, and somatosensory portions of the cerebral cortex generally remain intact.[4]

Genetic predisposition, known as familial Alzheimer disease, contributes less than 20% of all cases. Numerous environmental factors, such as aluminum, mercury, and viruses have been proposed as causes of AD but none have been proved as causative factors.[8,9] Risk factors for AD are seen in **Box 1**.

Mild cognitive impairment is the decline in memory function that may occur in normal aging, or be a precursor to AD.[10] The focus of studies on mild cognitive impairment is to discover factors that may decrease the risk for AD.[11] Current findings are listed in **Box 2**. Further research is needed to determine the importance of each in controlling/preventing AD.

Dementia and Alzheimer Disease

Dementia is the loss of intellectual functions (such as thinking, remembering, and reasoning) to such an extent that it interferes with a person's daily life and activities.[12] Dementia is not a disease in itself, but a group of symptoms that often accompanies a disease or condition. More than 70 different diseases or conditions can cause dementia, some of which are treatable, whereas others are less responsive or not possible to treat. **Table 1** lists causes of dementias, including those that are less responsive to treatment or are incurable.[13]

AD is the most prevalent form of dementia and is considered progressive and incurable. The cost of caring for a person who has AD either at home or in a skilled nursing facility was estimated to be $47,000 per year in 1996 and is estimated to have risen to

Box 1
Risk factors for Alzheimer disease

Advanced age (the older the person, the greater the risk)

Genes: families with history of AD

- Distributed according to autosomal-dominant gene
- Early-onset familial AD involves mutation in at least three genes on chromosomes 14, 1, 21 (20%)
- Strong relationship between gene for apolipoprotein E (APOE) on chromosome 19 and sporadic and familial late-onset Alzheimer disease
- Persons homozygous for APOE 4 allele have 10 times the risk for AD
- Persons heterozygous for APOE 4 allele have 4 times the risk for AD

Trisomy 21 (Down syndrome) family history (increases risk for AD 2–3 times)

- Down syndrome gene and AD gene are associated with chromosome 21

Head injury or trauma

Limited education or limited linguistic ability early in life

Gender predilection (controversial): greater prevalence of AD in women may be attributed to increase in survivorship of women into older age

Data from Refs.[6–10]

$75,000 per year in 2002. The total cost to society at present is estimated at $100 billion, ranking behind heart disease ($183 billion) and cancer ($109) as the third costliest disease in the United States.[14]

The human costs of caring for patients who have AD (and dementias) are incalculable and include the burdens born by family members who act as the primary

Box 2
Factors that decrease the risk for Alzheimer disease

Genes: presence of ApoE2/ApoE2 genotype

Attainment of higher educational levels

Moderate (no more than two glasses/day) red wine consumption

Regular exercise

Good control of high blood pressure

Medications (under investigation):

- Use of statins (for cholesterol)
- Use of anti-inflammatory medications (nonsteroidal anti-inflammatory agents)
- Use of histamine (H2) blockers
- Use of antioxidants (vitamin E and selegiline) (may actually decrease the progression of AD if given in high doses)
- Ginkgo (extract believed to have antioxidant properties): remains unclear
- Estrogen

Data from Refs.[11–16]

Table 1 Meta-analysis of dementia causes: 1987–2002	
Alzheimer disease	56.3%
Vascular dementias (multi-infarct dementia/strokes)	20.3%
Mixed	6.2%
Infectious	0.3%
Metabolic	1.1%
Tumor	0.9%
Normal pressure hydrocephaly	1.0%
Subdural hematoma	0.3%
Depression	0.9%
Medications	0.1%
Trauma	0.2%
Anoxic	0.2%
Huntington's	0.1%
Parkinson's	1.6%
Alcohol	0.6%
Miscellaneous	7.6%

Data from Clarfied A. The degreasing prevalence of reversible dementia: an updated meta-analysis. Arch Intern Med 2003;163:2219.

caregivers and health care personnel (nurses and nursing assistants/licensed practical nurses) who provide daily care such as cleaning the oral cavity and teeth. Emotional burdens are often overwhelming for family members who struggle with symptoms of a loved one (patient) for a disease that has no cure and becomes progressively worse.[15] The Alzheimer Association (www.alz.org) estimates that for every person who has AD, at least two to three family members see their lives significantly affected by caring for that individual.[3]

Clinical Signs and Symptoms

The clinical course of AD can be divided into three stages.[1] The early stage usually begins subtly, with the first sign generally being recent memory loss. To many older adults, this occurrence is frightening, because they may feel they are experiencing symptoms of AD. However, normal aging changes can also lead to recent memory loss (benign senescence) and may not be a sign of AD. In AD, however, memory problems increase, ultimately interfering with a person's ability to keep up with daily activities such as balancing a checkbook or finances, finding his/her way around, or remembering where he/she put things. Other signs of AD in the early stage include a gradual and steady deterioration in the ability to remember names, recent events, and conversations; misplacing items; missing appointments; and repeating questions or answers during conversations. In this stage, the person prefers familiarity and can be easily upset when confronted with new situations. Family members, relatives, or coworkers may report strange behaviors (eg, getting lost on the way home or to work), which may be accompanied by the onset of emotional outbursts when confronted. Some patients remain unaware of these problems, and others are aware of them and become frustrated and anxious.

The middle, or moderate, stage may occur within a few months or years. In this stage, the person is unable to work, becomes easily lost and confused, and has lost the ability to care for him/herself. Patients become agitated easily and have disturbances in language use, learning skills, judgment, and decision making. Although they remain ambulatory, they are at significant risk for falls or accidents secondary to confusion. Behavioral problems include agitation, hostility, uncooperativeness, or physical aggressiveness. During this stage, the patient has lost all sense of time and place and begins to have perceptual problems (may not recognize his/her own face in a mirror).[1]

The late, or severe, stage finds the patient profoundly apathetic, disoriented, incontinent, and totally dependent. Recent and remote memory are completely lost. Aggressiveness and anxious behavior are common, and a typical behavioral complication is for patients to reach and grasp objects that are close by. Patients in this stage are at risk for pneumonia, malnutrition, aspiration, and pressure necrosis of the skin. The progression of the disease is gradual, with some patient's symptoms seeming to plateau for a time. The end stage is coma and death.[1]

DIAGNOSING ALZHEIMER DISEASE

Definitive diagnosis of AD is determined by autopsy confirmation of changes in the brain. Microscopic features include cerebral cortical atrophy and ventricular enlargement, and microscopic features include cerebral cortical atrophy and ventricular enlargement of the microscopic features, inluding neurofibrillary tangles and neuritic plaques containing beta-amyloid in abnormally high proportions for a normal aging brain.[12] However, clinical diagnosis of AD can be made with more than 90% accuracy based on patient history and clinical findings alone.[16] The patient and family must be questioned, with a thorough history to establish if the patient demonstrates any sign or symptom of dementia. A thorough history can identify other causes of dementia that are not AD and may be treatable, including infections, injuries, anoxia, cardiovascular problems, alcohol abuse, illegal drugs, or prescription medications. Diagnosis of probable AD is given based on meeting six criteria:

- Dementia established by clinical examination and documented with testing
- Deficits in two or more areas of cognition
- Progressive worsening of memory and other cognitive functions
- No disturbance of consciousness
- Onset between ages 40 and 90
- Absence of systemic disorders or other brain diseases that could account for the progressive memory and cognitive changes[17]

Essentially, the clinical diagnosis of AD is one by exclusion following a complete assessment, including a health history and physical examination, neurologic and mental status assessments (such as the Mini-Mental State Examination), and other diagnostic tests including blood studies, urinalysis, ECG, chest radiographs, CT scan, electroencephalograms, medication removal, and sometimes spinal tap. If all tests are considered normal, and the six criteria for probable AD are met, then the clinical diagnosis of AD is given.

MEDICAL MANAGEMENT OF PATIENTS WHO HAVE ALZHEIMER DISEASE

No definitive treatment of AD exists, although drugs have been developed recently that can reduce or delay certain symptoms of AD.[18–22] Cholinesterase inhibitors (donepezil/Aricept, tacrine/Cognex, rivastigmine/Exelon, galantamine/Reminyl) are drugs that inhibit the enzyme acetyl cholinesterase from degrading acetylcholine (a key neurotransmitter between neurons). Using these agents has resulted in short-term (1–5 years) cognitive improvement (especially in memory and attention) and improvement in daily function and behavior in some patients who have mild-to-moderate AD. Unfortunately, fewer than 50% of patients who have AD who are prescribed these drugs appear to benefit from their use.[4] Side effects are dose related and may include nausea, vomiting, diarrhea, anorexia, weight loss, muscle cramps, bradycardia, heart block, syncope, and fatigue. The first drug developed in this class (Tacrine/Cognex) is infrequently prescribed today because it requires frequent dosing and can be hepatoxic.[20]

Only one medication, memantine (Axura) has been approved by the Food and Drug Administration to manage symptoms of people who have moderate-to-severe AD.[23,24] Memantine (an N-Methyl-D-Aspartate receptor antagonist) prevents elevated concentrations of glutamate, the principal excitatory neurotransmitter in the central nervous system, from destroying cholinergic neurons. Studies[23–25] suggest that memantine may preserve or improve memory and learning. When given with cholinesterase inhibitors, memantine appears not only to improve cognitive function but also to reduce the person's decline in activities of daily living (dressing, bathing, and so forth) and reduce the frequency of new behavioral symptoms.[25] Adverse effects of memantine include dizziness, headaches, hypertension, and confusion.[26] No information suggests that any special precautions are required when using local anesthetics with a vasoconstrictor for any of the cholinesterase inhibitors or memantine.[4,26]

Vitamin E is often added as another AD-specific treatment for its antioxidant effect and role in neuroprotection. One study suggested that vitamin E delayed the development of severe dementia, placement in a nursing home, and death.[27]

Symptom-specific medications are used when behavioral approaches such as providing a predictable routine, modifying the environment, and simplifying tasks, fail. For anxiety, depression, irritability, and sleep disturbances, medications such as short-acting benzodiazepines (eg, lorazepam/Ativan), antidepressants (eg, tricyclics/Elavil), and antipsychotics (eg, haloperidol/Haldol) are prescribed with unpredictable degrees of success.[4,26] AD is the number one cause of nursing home placement in the United States, because of caregiver's inability to manage a loved one at home in the severe stage of the disease.[28]

DENTAL MANAGEMENT OF PATIENTS WHO HAVE ALZHEIMER DISEASE

Patients who have AD in the moderate-to-severe stages will generally require assistance in daily oral hygiene from a caregiver (spouse, child, nursing assistant, nurse) because of a progressive neglect and lack of interest in caring for themselves.[29] Assistance may range from gently reminding the person to brush, to stand-by assistance, to ultimately providing hands-on daily care. Beginning in the moderate stage, the unique combination of impaired cognition, apathy, and apraxia (difficulty in ordered movement) results in not only a disinterest in oral care but also an inability to perform oral hygiene techniques.[26] Compromised daily oral hygiene leads to destruction of the dentition by coronal and root caries and periodontal disease.[30,31] For patients who wear dentures or partials, AD changes may result in patients forgetting to remove the appliances for days at a time. Dentures are often not removed from the mouth unless directed by others. Dentures are frequently broken or lost.[32] Medications that are commonly used to control symptoms often cause hyposalivation, resulting in dry mouth, furthering oral deterioration.[33–35] Caregivers report that oral hygiene becomes too difficult when the patient becomes resistant or combative.[36,37] Finally, caregivers stop taking patients who have AD to the dental office because of the overwhelming and increasing problems required from them to manage day-to-day living.[38]

As a result, when the patient who has AD is seen by a dentist, extensive oral disease is present.[37–40]

General Suggestions for Patients who have Alzheimer Disease

Most patients who have AD will have been clinically diagnosed before their dental visit. If not, dentists should be able to recognize the signs and symptoms of dementia, such as a decline in recent memory, inability to follow directions, or obvious personality changes, and refer them for medical evaluation and treatment.[41]

The patient who has AD should always be treated with respect and approached in an empathetic way. A humane way to view the patient who has AD is as someone who has a progressive terminal disease, not as a child who has no autonomy or abilities.

Regardless of the stage of dementia, the dentist should begin with a careful medical and dental history, including a review of medications. Communication should always take place in the presence of a family caregiver (spouse, child, or responsible adult). If the patient is able to understand and respond to questions, the dentist should address the patient directly. Verbal directions should be presented in short, simple phrases, giving only one direction at a time. It may be appropriate to address the patient by his/her first name or nickname, because they may forget their own last name at times. One should be prepared to repeat comments or questions frequently, and to repeat the words exactly in a calm, slow, and clear voice, at a low pitch. Rephrasing questions leads to confusion. One should only ask/respond to one question/comment at a time and wait for a response. Nonverbal communication is even more important in these patients and includes a relaxed, calm, and confident manner, using direct eye contact. Firm but gentle touching on the patient's hand, arm, or shoulder can be used as a sign of encouragement. Demonstrating procedures before performing them is a good management strategy.[42–45]

The presence of a caregiver (likely a family member) will often alleviate a dementia patient's anxiety. Because dementia interferes with the patient's ability to communicate, it is important to have the caregiver's input to verify reported symptoms such as dental pain.[32,45] Often, caregivers will be able to interpret the meaning behind a sudden worsening of behavior, moaning, or increased restlessness as an indicator of dental pain.[45] Facial expressions appear to be helpful in assessing dental pain in dementia patients.[46]

Informed Consent

The dentist and staff should always determine whether the patient is legally able to make informed decisions. The elements of informed consent include the capability of the patient to make decisions by the demonstration of (1) understanding relevant information, (2) understanding the situation and consequences, (3) manipulating the information rationally, and (4) communicating a choice.[47] If the patient who has AD is verbally aggressive (cursing), resistant (moving away, refusing to open), or combative (striking out), the important questions to ask are, "Does the patient really not want dental care?" and if so, "Is the informed consent process in place?" If the patient is legally competent and capable of making decisions, he/she should sign his/her own consent. If unable to sign his/her own consent, the legal guardian or health care proxy has the authority to give permission. If no proxy is identified, state law takes precedence and usually the person in the closest, loving relationship can give consent.[45,47]

If patients wander or curse, or are restless, resistant, or combative, nonpharmacologic and pharmacologic approaches of management should be considered. Nonpharmacologic approaches include having the caregiver hold the patients hand or hands, keeping the caregiver in the operatory for familiarity and helping with management, reducing background noise, reducing excess activity, using an extraoral mouth prop (eg, Molt prop), cradling the head to reduce movements, having the patient hold onto a soft textured object (stuffed animal), and moving with the patient.[32,41,43] If a soft (cloth) restraint is used to hold a patient in the chair to keep him/her from wandering/getting up during treatment, it is important to follow the guidelines for restraint use.[48,49] It is important to document clearly why the restraint was used, where it was placed and for how long a period of time, and whether a separate consent was given for its use.

Dental Treatment by Stage

Table 2 provides some suggestions for dental management of the patient who has AD at different stages.[41,43] In a patient who has mild dementia, good oral health should be attained aggressively, with restorative work completed and early lesions restored (no "watches"). Restorations should be long lasting and easily maintained. Crowns would be preferable to large restorative buildups, in most cases. Materials selected should be based on the ability to manage the patient and to maintain a dry operating field (eg, can you use a rubber dam?). Glass ionomers are good materials for root surfaces because of their ability to release fluoride and prevent recurrent decay.

For moderately demented patients, subsequent care should concentrate on preventing dental disease through aggressive home care and frequent recalls (every 3 months).[30,41,43] Complex dental procedures should rarely be performed (if at all) before the disease has reached the advanced stage.[32] If a patient loses a partial or denture, it is hard to predict whether or not new removable prostheses should be made. General guidelines include discussing this with the caregiver and making the decision based on the perceived risk/benefit. An understanding should be reached with the caregivers that the patient will not likely be able to wear prostheses in the future. If the caregiver is willing to assume the risk and cost, a new partial/denture can be fabricated, but the long-term prognosis is questionable at best.

Patients in the advanced stage often display behavior problems such as anxiety, hostility, wandering, and inability to sit still and open their mouths, and are generally

Table 2
Managing Alzheimer disease in the dental office

Early	Moderate	Severe
Aggressive prevention including caregiver involvement: daily oral hygiene, topical fluorides, caregiver education are all critical beginning in the early stage and continuing through severe		
Minimal changes needed	Shorter visits More frequent recalls Possible oral or intravenous sedation	
Treatment plan anticipating decline	Treatment plan with minimal changes in mind	Treatment plan to maintain dentition if possible
Restore ASAP!	Simpler interventions: Extract versus complex restore Reline/repair versus new denture Partials versus fixed crown and bridge	Palliative care: Maintain comfort, dignity Treat infection Treat symptomatic problems

Data from Refs.[41,43,48]; and Shuman S, personal communication; and continuous education lecture October 2007.

uncooperative. These patients are difficult to treat but likely will require short appointments for simple procedures (like fluoride treatments or treatment planning) and sedation (oral or intravenous) for everything else. Nitrous oxide is not indicated because of the inability of the patient to understand and cooperate, but short-acting oral benzodiazepines (lorazepam/Ativan or triazolam/Halcion) work well for some procedures. Intravenous sedation works well for longer or complex procedures such as oral surgery and restorative care.[4,30,45] However, Midazolam/Versed should be used with extreme caution in older patients who have AD because it has a profound effect at low doses. Rarely should more than 1 mg be given as an incremental dose, with a maximum total dose for a 1 hour procedure totaling to no more than 5 mg in most cases.

Several specially adapted preventive products are helpful for caregivers to use with patients who have AD. A foam mouth prop called the Open-Wide Plus (Specialized Care Com., Edison, New Jersey) is designed for caregivers to use to keep the mouth open during oral hygiene. A specialized toothbrush, the Collis Curve (Collis Curve, Inc., Brownsville, Texas) has three rows of bristles that, when placed correctly, can clean the lingual, facial, and occlusal surfaces of teeth at the same time. Approved by the American Dental Association for assisted brushing, the Collis Curve uses a simplified scrubbing motion, making it easier for caregivers to use than conventional or electric brushes.[30,50]

Other conventional preventive products may be helpful for caregivers to maintain oral hygiene in patients who have AD. For cleaning between teeth, proxabrushes work well. Caregivers need to be reminded to keep their fingers from between the teeth of their patients because of the danger of biting. Finally, fluoride use is an essential preventive tool. Toothpaste, mouth rinses (if the patient is not late stage and at risk for aspiration), the use of gels at home or varnish in the office should all be considered as part of a daily plan to prevent new caries.[4,30,32]

DEFINITION AND CAUSE OF STROKE

The term "stroke" is used to refer to a CVA, which is defined as a serious and often fatal neurologic event occurring when a part of the brain is suddenly deprived of oxygenated blood.[4,51] This event results in tissue necrosis in the part of the brain affected and can range from mild to severe disabilities, and even death. In recent years, the term "acute stroke" is rapidly being replaced by the term "brain attack," to indicate that a stroke is similar to a heart attack: It is a medical emergency in which immediate intervention can prevent and even reverse the effects of early brain damage.[52]

The two main causes of stroke are a blockage of an artery that supplies blood to a part of the brain (ischemic), or bleeding (hemorrhagic) into the brain because an artery has burst. If the blockage of the artery is temporary and blood flow is quickly restored, the brain may recover quickly. A transient ischemic attack (TIA) is defined as a stroke that lasts less than 24 hours and has no residual effect.[53] Some people think of a TIA as a ministroke. Although most TIAs last less than 10 minutes, up to one third of patients will have noticeable changes on brain imaging studies that indicate injury to the brain.[54] If the blockage of the artery is long lasting, the part of the brain supplied by that artery is permanently damaged and dies. The damaged area is said to be infarcted, so ischemic strokes are also called brain infarctions, or cerebral infarctions (similar to myocardial infarctions in the heart).[55]

Ischemic strokes result from occlusion of a cerebral artery by a blood clot formed on the arterial wall obstructing blood flow (thrombus) or by having the clot break off (embolus) from the arterial wall and travel through the bloodstream until it becomes lodged. Obstruction of the blood flow distal to the embolus results in infarction. The primary factors associated with thromboembolic strokes are atherosclerosis and cardiac pathology, such as a previous myocardial infarction and atrial fibrillation. Approximately 10% of persons who have had a myocardial infarction will have a stroke within 6 years.[56]

In hemorrhagic stroke, bleeding occurs into the brain (intracerebral) or into the space between the brain and the inner lining of the skull (subarachnoid). Hypertension is the most important risk factor for intracerebral hemorrhagic stroke.[57] Preventing this type of stroke can largely be accomplished by effective blood pressure (BP) control.[55] Four types of blood vessel abnormalities can lead to cerebral arteries rupturing: arteriovenous malformations, aneurysms, cavernomas or cavernous angiomas, and lobar hemorrhages.

The most common cause of subarachnoid hemorrhage is rupture of a saccular aneurysm at the bifurcation of a major cerebral artery.[58] Of all strokes, 87% are ischemic (either from thrombus or emboli), 10% are intracerebral hemorrhage, and 3% are subarachnoid hemorrhagic strokes.[59]

RISK FACTORS

TIAs confer a significant short-term risk for stroke, hospitalization for cardiovascular events, and death. In one study of 1707 TIA patients evaluated in the emergency room, 180 patients (10%) developed a stroke within 90 days.[60] Ninety-one patients (5%) did so within 2 days. Cigarette smoking doubles the risk for ischemic stroke compared with that of nonsmokers after adjusting for other risk factors.[61] Atrial fibrillation is an independent risk factor for stroke, increasing risk approximately fivefold.[61] Older age increases the risk for stroke. For adults older than 55, the lifetime risk is greater than one in six. Women have a higher risk than men, perhaps because of women's survival advantage. BP is a powerful determinant of stroke risk. Subjects who have BP of less than 120/80 mm Hg have approximately half the lifetime risk for stroke compared with subjects who have hypertension (higher than 120/80).[62] Diabetes increases ischemic stroke incidence at all ages but this risk is most prominent before 55 years of age in blacks and before 65 years of age in whites.[63] A study of more than 37,000 women older than 45 years of age participating in the Women's Health Study suggests that a healthy lifestyle (abstinence from smoking, low body mass index, moderate alcohol consumption, regular exercise, and a healthy diet) was associated with a significantly reduced risk for ischemic stroke but not for hemorrhagic stroke.[64] **Box 3** presents risk factors on stroke according to the ability to change, influence, or modify risk factors.

Medications can also be risk factors for strokes in several ways: by creating a tendency to form blood clots (hypercoagulable state) within the body or by increasing BP.[65] The mechanism by which some medications cause stroke remains unknown. **Table 2** lists medications and their mechanism that may lead to stroke if taken improperly or in excess.

Periodontal disease has been described as a risk factor for ischemic stroke because of the effect of inflammatory products (C-reactive protein, interleukins, and so forth) on systemic vasculature. It has been suggested that periodontal disease produces three harmful systemic responses related to strokes: inflammation in arterial walls, contributing to the build-up of atherosclerotic plaques, and increasing the risk for atheroma rupture. Studies[66–69] confirm the relationship between periodontal disease and ischemic strokes. Persons who have periodontal disease have been found to be three times as likely to have a stroke. A direct relationship has been demonstrated between

Box 3
Stroke risk factors

Stroke risk factors one can change

- Smoking
- Exercise
- Illicit drug use
- Obesity
- Physical inactivity
- Periodontal disease

Stroke risk factors one can influence (by seeking medical care)

- History of diabetes mellitus[a]
- History of high BP[a]
- Congestive heart failure[a]
- TIA or previous stroke[a]
- History of high cholesterol
- History of heart conditions (such as atrial fibrillation)
- History of narrowing of the arteries (such a carotid stenosis)

Stroke risk factors one cannot change

- Age older than 75[a]
- Race (Native Americans, Alaska Natives, multiracial persons, and blacks have higher risk)
- Sex (men have greater risk if younger than 65 and women have greater risk if older than 65)
- Family history of medical conditions related to stroke

[a] Risk for stroke increases by a factor of 1.5. Having multiple risk factors contributes to an incrementally increased risk for stroke.[4]

Data from Stein J, Silver J, Frates E. Risk factors for having a stroke. In: Life after stroke. Baltimore (MD): Johns Hopkins Press; 2006. p. 3–13, 87–90.

the thickness of the carotid artery wall and the presence of periodontal bacteria. Live periodontal bacteria have been found in atherosclerotic plaques. The conclusion from this evidence is that periodontal disease has a significant association with atheroma formation. Therefore, prevention of periodontal disease should be considered an important modifiable risk factor.

EPIDEMIOLOGY: MORTALITY, INCIDENCE, AND PREVALENCE

Stroke ranks third among all causes of death, behind diseases of the heart and cancer.[70] Mortality rates are directly related to the type of stroke, with 80% of patients dying after an intracerebral hemorrhage, 50% after a subarachnoid hemorrhage, and 30% from a thromboembolic ischemia.[58] Death from stroke may occur hours, days, or weeks after the initial stroke episode, varying by age and type of stroke. Among persons 45 to 64 years of age, approximately 10% of ischemic strokes and 38% of hemorrhagic strokes result in death within 30 days.[71] In a study of persons aged 65 and older, the 30-day fatality rate was 8% for ischemic strokes and 45% for hemorrhagic strokes.[72]

Strokes have been called a "disease of old age" because approximately half of all strokes occur in people who are older than 75. Age is considered one of the most important determinants of stroke, although 28% of people who have a stroke are younger than 65. For every 10 years after age 55, the rate of stroke more than doubles in both men and women. The prevalence of strokes increases from 35 per 100,000 people at age 35 to 1100 per 100,000 at ages 75 to 80.[56]

The 2005 Behavioral Risk Factor Surveillance System survey[70] found that many states with high stroke prevalence are concentrated in the Southeast, a region traditionally called the "stroke belt" because of its high rates of stroke mortality.[70] The overall prevalence of stroke among American Indians/Alaska natives (6%), multiracial persons (4.6%), and blacks (4%) exceeds the prevalence among whites (2.3%).[70]

On average, every 40 seconds, someone in the United States has a stroke[56] and every 3.1 minutes someone dies of one.[54] Each year in the United States, approximately 780,000 people experience a new or recurrent stroke, resulting in 253,000 deaths.[70] From 1994 to 2004, the stroke death rate fell by 24.2%, and the actual number of stroke deaths declined by 6.8%.[72] Although some of the improvement in stroke mortality may be the result of improved acute stroke care, most is thought to be the result of improved detection and treatment of hypertension.[55] Men's stroke incidence rates are greater than women's at younger ages but not at older ages. More women than men have strokes after the age of 75.

AFTERMATH OF STROKE: DISABILITY AND COST

Stroke is the leading cause of serious, long-term disability in the United States.[73] Although medical advances have reduced the mortality rate, the number of people who have strokes continues to increase every year. Approximately 50% of those who survive the acute period (the first 6 months) are alive 7 years later.[74] Of those who survive, 10% will recover with no impairment. Approximately 50% to 70% will regain functional independence but will have a mild residual disability; 15% to 30% will be permanently disabled; and 20% will require institutional care (help with daily tasks such as bathing and dressing) at 3 months after onset.[75]

The type of deficit that occurs from a stroke is directly dependent on the size and location of the infarct or hemorrhage. If many small strokes occur in the brain, a person can develop a condition called multi-infarct dementia (MID).[76] The infarcts are usually not caused by a single process but instead may result from several different ones, including ischemic and hemorrhagic processes.[77] In MID, strokes can occur on both sides of the brain and in multiple locations. Therefore, people who have MID may exhibit various symptoms because so many parts of the brain can be affected. Symptoms may include mental deterioration with memory loss (dementia), walking problems, facial muscle problems such as difficulty talking and opening the eyelids, and weakness or numbness in one or more body areas. MID is usually diagnosed through neurologic examination and brain-scanning techniques such as CT scan, although in some cases, it may not be possible to distinguish between MID and AD until after death, where autopsy findings demonstrate infarcts/hemorrhages in the brain versus beta-amyloid plaques and neurofibrillary tangles.

In a study of ischemic stroke survivors who were at least 65 years of age, the following disabilities were observed at 6 months post stroke:[78]

50% had some hemiparesis.
30% were unable to walk without some assistance.
26% were dependent in activities of daily living.

19% had aphasia.
35% had depressive symptoms.
26% were institutionalized in a nursing home.

The estimated direct and indirect cost of stroke for 2008 is $65.5 billion.[79] In 2003, $3.7 billion ($6363 per discharge) was paid to Medicare beneficiaries discharged from short-stay hospitals for stroke.[80] The mean lifetime cost of ischemic stroke in the United States is estimated at $140,048. This figure includes inpatient care, rehabilitation, and follow-up care necessary for lasting deficits.[81]

CLINICAL PRESENTATION OF STROKES: SIGNS AND SYMPTOMS

A stroke or TIA should be considered a "brain attack" and is a medical emergency that requires immediate medical attention. Because most strokes do not cause severe pain, patients often delay seeking treatment, resulting in extensive brain tissue damage. Symptoms of stroke depend on the type and area of the brain affected. Signs of ischemic stroke usually occur suddenly, and signs of hemorrhagic stroke usually develop gradually. The classic five warning signs of a TIA or a major stroke are well known[82] and include

Sudden weakness or numbness of the face, arm, or leg, especially on one side of the body
Sudden confusion, trouble speaking, or trouble understanding
Sudden trouble walking, dizziness, loss of balance or coordination
Sudden trouble seeing in one or both eyes
Sudden severe headache with no known cause

Other signs/symptoms may include sudden decrease in the level of consciousness, vision problems (blurry vision or blindness in one eye), nausea and vomiting, and seizure (rare). Even though the symptoms may disappear in minutes if the patient is having a TIA, the person still needs to seek medical attention because about 15% of strokes are preceded by a TIA.[83]

MEDICAL MANAGEMENT OF THE STROKE PATIENT

The three levels of medical management of the stroke patient are (1) prevention, (2) early diagnosis and treatment, and (3) recovery and rehabilitation.

Prevention

The best "treatment" for stroke is prevention. Although a family history of stroke plays a role in the risk, many risk factors are controllable (see **Table 2**). Controlling hypertension is the most important thing patients can do to avoid stroke. Reducing systolic pressure by 10 mm hg is associated with a documented one-third reduction in the risk for stroke.[57] The top 10 stroke-prevention guidelines published by the National Stroke Association include[77]

1. Controlling BP
2. Stopping smoking
3. Determining if you have atrial fibrillation
4. Drinking alcohol only in moderation
5. Controlling high cholesterol
6. Controlling diabetes
7. Exercising daily

8. Eating lower-sodium (salt) and low-fat diet
9. Controlling circulation problems
10. Seeking medical attention immediately if experiencing any stroke symptoms

Medications used to prevent strokes by decreasing platelet aggregation include aspirin, ticlopidine, and dipyridamole. Daily aspirin (81 mg to 325 mg) reduces the risk for stroke by about 25% among ischemic stroke patients or those who have had TIAs.[84] Similarly, cholesterol-reducing statins prescribed to control blood lipids reduce risk by about 20%. When a moderate or severe blockage in the carotid artery develops from atherosclerosis, a surgical procedure, carotid endarterectomy, can be performed to remove the inner lining of the carotid artery. As secondary stroke prevention, carotid endarterectomy reduces the risk for stroke by about 1% per year.[84]

Early Diagnosis and Treatment

If a person experiences signs or symptoms of a stroke, early diagnosis and treatment are critical. The first task is maintaining life support if the patient is not conscious and not breathing. Calling 911 and having an emergency medical technician transport to a hospital will allow for several laboratory and diagnostic imaging tests to determine if a TIA, stroke, or another condition has occurred.[58] Laboratory tests include blood glucose level, urinalysis, complete blood count and differential, blood cholesterol and lipid levels, and ECG, among others. Depending on the facility, CT is generally ordered first to determine whether the stroke is due to bleeding or a blood vessel blockage. MRI provides greater information, such as the "age" of a stroke and identifies smaller strokes but requires more time and is difficult for some patients to tolerate. Other tests used to determine the extent and location of brain injury include Doppler blood flow, MRI and CT angiograms, BP monitoring, electroencephalograms, and lumbar puncture.[85]

Early diagnosis establishes whether the stroke is due to ischemia from a thromboembolism or from a hemorrhage. Depending on what type of stroke is present, the management centers around preventing further thrombosis or hemorrhage, and to attempting to lyse the clot in the case of ischemia. Thrombolysis with intravenous administration of tissue plasminogen activator within 3 hours of ischemic stroke onset is the gold standard of early stroke management and is advocated by the American College of Emergency Physicians when time guidelines (as specified by the American College of Emergency Physicians) are followed.[83]

Anticoagulant medications, such as heparin, coumarin, aspirin, platelet receptor agonists (clopidogrel, abciximab, ticlopidine), and Aggrenox (dipyridamole combined with aspirin), are used to stabilize ischemic strokes and prevent further strokes from thromboembolism. Corticosteroids may be used in the immediate poststroke period to reduce the cerebral edema that accompanies cerebral infarction. Surgical intervention may be indicated for managing vascular obstruction or removing a superficial hematoma. Anticonvulsants such as phenytoin (Dilantin) or diazepam (Valium) are often described to manage seizures that may accompany the postoperative course of stroke.[4]

Recovery and Rehabilitation

Stroke recovery is often divided into two categories: neurologic and functional. Neurologic recovery involves the extent to which the brain is able to regain lost abilities. This recovery depends on many factors, including the extent and location of brain injury, what early treatment was done, and the individual's prestroke health and intellectual status.[86]

Functional recovery involves how much someone can improve in day-to-day activities such as bathing, dressing, walking, and talking after neurologic recovery ends. Neurologic recovery occurs in the first few months after a stroke and can possibly take up to 1 year. Functional recovery also begins immediately post stroke but usually outlasts neurologic recovery by several months. Rehabilitation works best when multidisciplinary professionals work as a team for a prolonged time, beginning immediately following a stroke and continuing until recovery is maximized. Members of a stroke rehabilitation team generally include physical, occupational, and speech therapists, nurses, social workers, and physicians, but other professionals, including dentists, may be involved, depending on the facility or community.[86]

DENTAL MANAGEMENT OF THE STROKE PATIENT

Currently, more than 5.8 million stroke survivors are living in the United States.[83] An average dental practice of 2000 adult patients will include about 31 patients who have had or will experience a stroke.[4,56]

Four main areas that dental professionals should be aware of when treating patients who have had a stroke are

1. Recognizing the patient at risk for a stroke (to prevent a stroke or recurrent stroke)
2. Preoperative modifications and approach to treatment and treatment planning
3. Intraoperative modifications for stroke patients who have residual deficits
4. Managing a patient who experiences a stroke in your office

Recognizing the Patient at Risk

The risk factors for stroke are essentially the same as those for heart disease and are seen in **Table 2**. Dentists and hygienists should assess these risk factors through standard medical history taking. As the number of risk factors increases, so does the level of risk for having a stroke, or a recurrent stroke if risk factors are not modified. Patients should be encouraged to eliminate or control risk factor through lifestyle change and medical management.

Dental professionals should take BP measurements at the initial visit, at routine visits for recalls, and before all invasive procedures (oral, periodontal, or implant surgeries). Not only is hypertension one of the most important risk factors for strokes and myocardial infarction, it is one of the most treatable conditions. According to the National Health and Nutrition Examination Survey data for the period 1999 to 2000, at least 65 million adults in the United States have high blood pressure or are taking antihypertensive medication.[87] Even more significant are the number of people who have high blood pressure who are not aware of their disease (30%) and the more than 60% of hypertensive patients who are taking medications but are not being adequately controlled.[87] **Table 3** provides the latest classification of BP in adults and recommendations for follow-up.[88]

Determining the stroke risk factors of patients may prompt postponing dental care for a period of time. In determining the risk for stroke in dental management, the American Society of Anesthesiologists (ASA) perspective can be used as a guide. ASA I is a normal healthy patient, ASA II is one who has mild systemic disease, ASA III is a patient who has severe systemic disease that limits activity but is not incapacitating, and ASA IV is a patient who has incapacitating systemic disease that is a constant

Table 3
Classification of blood pressure in adults and recommendations for follow-up

BP Classification	Systolic BP (mm Hg)	Diastolic BP (mm Hg)	Recommended Follow-Up
Normal	<120	and <80	Recheck in 2 years.
Prehypertension	120–139	or 80–89	Recheck in 1 year.
Stage 1 hypertension	140–159	or 90–99	Confirm within 2 months.
Stage 2 hypertension	or ≥160	or ≥100	Evaluate or refer to source of care within 1 month. For those who have higher pressures (eg, >180/110 mm Hg), refer for evaluation immediately or within 1 week, depending on the clinical situation and complications.

Modified from Chobanian AV, Bakris GL, Black HR, et al. Seventh report of the Joint National Committee on Prevention, Detection, Evaluation, and Treatment of High Blood Pressure. Hypertension 2003;42:1206–52; with permission.

threat to life.[89] The implication is that as the ASA class increases from I to IV, so does the risk for stroke.

Obtaining a thorough history in a patient who has had a stroke or is at risk for having a stroke is critical and may be used as a guide to dental management (**Table 4**).[90] Identifying ASA II patients who have one or more risk factors and physician referral for counseling and treatment should be performed at the initial dental visit and on recall examinations. Similarly, ASA III patients should be referred to a medical provider if their risk factors are not under medical control. If neurologic deficits are present, depending on the deficit, dental modifications should be made. For ASA IV patients,

Table 4
Risk factors and dental management of stroke patients from the perspective of the American Society of Anesthesiologists

ASA I	No Stroke Risk Factors	No Modifications Needed
ASA II	One or more stroke risk factors	Refer to physician for medical treatment of risk factors and counsel patient to quit or modify risk factors.
ASA III	History of one or more TIAs or stroke at least 6 months before dental treatment.	May or may not have some degree of residual neurologic deficit present. Refer for evaluation to medical facility if risk factors not being treated. Manage in dental office according to deficit present.
ASA IV	History of TIA or stroke within 6 months of dental treatment	TIAs or CVA with or without neurologic deficits. Deferral of dental treatment for at least 6 months because TIA/CVA recurrence is highest within the first year.

Modified from Malamed S. Medical emergencies in the dental office. 5th edition. St. Louis (MO): Mosby; 2000. p. 22; with permission.

deferral of dental treatment for at least 6 months is recommended because of the increased risk for stroke following a TIA.[91] The 90-day risk for stroke is 3% to 17%, with the highest risk within the first 30 days.[92–95] Within 1 year of a TIA, up to one fourth (25%) of patients will die.[92,96]

In addition to traditional risk factors, the finding of calcified carotid artery atheromas (CCAAs) in the region of the carotid bifurcation on a routine panoramic radiograph may indicate an increased risk for subsequent development of stroke.[97–99] Although a recent review[100] found no significant difference in the incidence of stroke between subjects who had CCAAs and subjects who did not have CCAAs, a prudent recommendation is a finding of any carotid atheromas (usually located near cervical vertebrae 3 and 4 at a 45° angle from the angle of the mandible) on a panoramic radiograph warrants referral to the patient's physician for further evaluation and treatment.[100]

Preoperative Modifications and Approach to Treatment and Treatment Planning

Oral manifestations of a stroke may include any or none of the following: slurred speech, a weak palate, difficulty swallowing, loss or difficulty in speech, unilateral paralysis of the orofacial muscles, and loss of sensory stimuli of oral tissues.[4] The tongue may be flaccid, with multiple folds, and may deviate on extrusion. Dysphagia is common and the use of rubber dams to prevent aspiration of materials should be used whenever possible. Right-sided brain damaged patients suffer more often from one-sided neglect and may be unable to clean their teeth on the affected side. Thus, food, bacteria, and debris may accumulate around the teeth, beneath the tongue, or in alveolar folds on the affected sides, resulting in pocketing of food, halitosis, risk for caries, poor oral hygiene, and the danger of aspiration. Dentists should check with the patient or the patient's therapist before treatment to determine the extent of the pocketing, and to ensure the caregiver knows how to clean the area.

Depending on the type of stroke, suggestions for dental modifications can be broken down as follows: stroke survivors who have left or right brain injuries, general communication techniques, scheduling and transferring suggestions, modifying home care practices, and other treatment issues.

Table 5
Suggestions for dental professions working with left cerebrovascular accident (brain damage)

Left Brain Damage (L-CVA) Findings	Implications for Dental Clinicians
Paralysis to right side Speech and language deficits	Because this patient has trouble communicating, it is easy to underestimate his/her abilities, which may be nonverbal.
Behavior style: slow, cautious, disorganized	Do not rush the patient in doing things.
Memory deficits: auditory	Communicate by eliminating extraneous stimuli; do not raise voice or use "baby talk;" substitute pantomime and demonstration for words; divide tasks into simple steps; give frequent, accurate, and immediate positive feedback; and ask simple and brief questions.
Anxious	Use stress-reduction techniques.

Data from American Heart Association. Strokes: how stroke affects behavior. Dallas (TX): American Heart Association National Center; 1991.

Table 6
Suggestions for dental professionals working with right cerebrovascular accident (brain damage)

Right Brain Damage (R-CVA) Findings	Implications for Dental Clinicians
Paralysis to left side Spatial and perceptual deficits	Because this patient can speak and write, it is easy to overestimate his/her abilities.
Behavior style: quick and impulsive	Do not allow the patient to do things such as transfer by him/herself unless you are there to watch and help if needed (especially transfers).
Memory deficits: visual, including visual field cuts	Move slowly around a patient's head. If moving too quickly into a patient's visual area, the risk for a patient suddenly moving is great.
Cannot monitor self (one-sided neglect)	Most patients will need assistance in brushing the left side of their mouth because they will not be able to "cross-over" to the neglected side.

Data from Fowler RS, Fordyce WE. Strokes: why they behave that way. Dallas (TX): American Heart Association; 1996.

Left and Right Brain Damaged Stroke Patients

Tables 5 and **6** summarize the differences between damage to the left and right sides of the brain and suggest some helpful modifications for dental treatment.[101]

General Communication Techniques

Effective communication techniques for the patient who has had a stroke (ASA III or IV) with deficits to speech or hearing centers include the following recommendations:[102]

Face the patient.
Use a slower, low-pitch, more deliberate, less complex pattern of speech.
Address the patient from the unimpaired side of the body.
Establish eye contact and communicate at eye level.
Be conscious of nonverbal communication to enhance messages.
Ask yes/no questions; be simple and brief.
Give frequent, accurate, and immediate feedback.
Do not raise voice or use baby talk (do not patronize).
Speak louder but do not shout.
Do not wear a mask when talking to the patient.
Be positive.
Break tasks into small steps.
Speak with the patient's significant other/personal care provider regarding important treatment planning decisions to clarify patient's wishes and desires.
For left brain injured (L-CVA) patients, use simple line drawings or write directions to explain procedures.
Especially for right brain injured (R-CVA) patients, announce to the patient what is going to be done so that he/she knows what is going to happen next. Avoid rapid, sudden movements.
If the patient can write what he/she cannot say, provide him/her with pad and pencil.
Allow more time for the patient to think or respond to questions (be patient).[102]

Scheduling and Transferring Suggestions

In general, ASA III or ASA IV stroke-prone or stroke patients should be seen during midmorning and have appointments that are stress free.[4] Reducing stress before and during dental treatment may be done by using nitrous oxide/oxygen or oral anxiolytics such as lorazepam/Ativan or triazolam/Halcion.[103] Moderate (intravenous) sedation may also be used, although only light sedation (typically using only midazolam/Versed) along with the administration of oxygen by way of nasal cannula or nasal hood during the procedure should be adhered to.[104] For extensive dental procedures, stroke patients may require airway protection through intubation in the operating room.[105]

If a stroke patient needs assistance transferring to the dental chair, ask the patient what he/she can do but be prepared to assist. Always stand in front of the patient in case he/she starts to fall. Use a transfer board for one-person transfers. For patients who cannot transfer at all from their wheelchairs, two-person transfers may be needed. In these cases, one person lifts from behind the patient, lifting the patient's crossed arms, and the other person lifts from above the patient's knees. Make sure when doing transfers that lifting is done with the legs and not the back!

All general dentistry procedures can be done on stroke patients who have residual deficits but treatment plans should incorporate the extent of disability present and the patient's and caregiver's motivation. All restorations should be placed with ease of cleaning in mind.[106] Electric toothbrushes have proved to be helpful to patients who can only use one hand, and modified toothbrushes, such as the Collis-curve (Collis Curve, Inc., Brownsville, Texas), a curved bristle brush designed to brush all three sides of the teeth are useful for caregivers for those patients who are not able to brush their own teeth. Interproximal devices such as proxybrushes (to clean in between teeth, without having to put fingers in the mouth) are more useful than floss for patients and caregivers, and work well with training.[107,108] For patients having difficulty holding their mouths open, a soft foam mouth prop, the Open-wide mouth prop (Specialized Care, Co., Hampton, New Hampshire), can help caregivers keep the mouth open to provide daily oral hygiene.

Other Treatment Planning Issues

Depression occurs in 30% to 50% of all stroke survivors and is an important determinant of functional outcome.[109] If depressed, the poststroke patient may display episodes of sadness (crying), fail their appointments, or practice no, or poor, oral hygiene. In addition, the underlying disease or conditions that caused the stroke (hypertension, diabetes, atherosclerosis, atrial fibrillation) require control, explaining why stroke patients take so many medications, including antidepressants, antihypertensives, insulin or hypoglycemics, digoxin, statins, and anticoagulants or antiplatelets. All these medications can cause dry mouth and increase the risk for caries and periodontal problems. Increasing recall frequency is one consideration for the dental team, along with educating the patient's significant other about the importance of daily care. Ideally, fluoride supplementation for stroke patients may be used; however, gels are preferable to rinses in patients at risk for aspiration due to dysphagia.

Intraoperative Modifications for Stroke Patients Who Have Residual Deficits

Intraoperative management techniques for stroke patients include monitoring BP before invasive procedures, preventing hypertensive episodes by limiting epinephrine, practicing good pain control, being aware of excessive bleeding if patients are taking anticoagulants or antiplatelet medications, and preventing aspiration through limiting ultrasonic scaling and using rubber dams. Preoperative BPs should be taken before all invasive procedures that are potentially stressful to the patient, such as oral and periodontal surgery. Not only will this establish a baseline but it will also indicate patient compliance with medical therapy, or indicate if a patient is anxious. The decision as to whether or not to proceed with dental treatment may be based on this BP finding. Delaying treatment to ensure BP is under control may prevent a hypertensive crisis, leading to a recurrent stroke or myocardial infarction.

A local anesthetic with 1:100,000 epinephrine may be used in judicious amounts (<4 mL),[110] although gingival retraction cord impregnated with epinephrine should not be used.[106] This precaution is to prevent an untoward rise in BP in stroke patients who commonly have a history of coronary artery disease. The best technique is to use intraoperative monitoring of BP following anesthetic injection to ensure BP remains within normal limits.

A stroke patient taking coumarin or antiplatelet drugs is at risk for excessive bleeding when undergoing surgical/invasive dental treatment.[4] If on coumarin, the anticoagulant effect is monitored by evaluating the international normalized ratio (INR) of the prothrombin time of a standard control versus the patient's prothrombin time. If the INR is 3.5 or less, it is considered an acceptable risk for performance of most invasive dental procedures.[4,111–113] In cases where the INR is greater than 3.5, the physician should be consulted to decrease the dose to achieve an INR less than 3.5.[111] In these cases, the anticoagulant should not be discontinued because the risk for a recurrent stroke or myocardial infarction is considered to be greater than the risk for bleeding.[111,114]

The antiplatelet effects of aspirin, clopidogrel (Plavix), and dipyridamole are monitored by the platelet function analyzer test. In general, antiplatelet agents do not lead to significant bleeding problems in oral surgical procedures and do not need to be discontinued.[115] Good surgical technique (gentle technique, removing granulation tissue, primary closure, and use of hemostatic agents as needed) prevent most postsurgical bleeding episodes.[105,113]

Postoperative pain should be managed with acetaminophen-containing products for stroke patients, with or without narcotics. Penicillins are the first choice if antibiotics are indicated. Metronidazole and tetracycline may increase the INR by inhibiting the metabolism of Coumadin; therefore, using these antibiotics should be avoided.[105,109,114]

Most strokes result in paralysis or swallowing problems on the contralateral side (ie, L-CVA, right hemiplegia). Risk for aspiration increases with the severity of the stroke and is more likely with clear liquids than solids. Aspiration may be prevented in the dental setting by using rubber dams for all restorative procedures and by avoiding the use of cavitron or air-water syringes unless absolutely necessary.[102] Primary closure for all oral surgery procedures should be done routinely to minimize the chance of aspiration of blood.

Managing a Patient Who Experiences Stroke in the Dental Office

If a patient were to develop signs and symptoms of a stroke (see **Box 3**) in the dental office, the following sequence should be followed:[116]

1. Terminate the dental procedure.
2. Position the patient in a comfortable position (if conscious, upright, and if unconscious, on back).
3. Assess the patient to determine if he/she is breathing, has an airway, or has circulation. If not breathing, open the patient's airway (basic life support) and provide two rescue breaths. Take a pulse and provide compressions if no pulse.

4. Monitor vital signs if the patient is conscious. The BP is generally elevated, whereas the heart rate may be normal or elevated. Vital signs should be recorded at least every 5 minutes during the acute episode.
5. Summon medical assistance when signs and symptoms indicate a possible stroke. Summoning early enables thrombolytic therapy to be used within the first 3 hours and helps minimize residual neurologic deficit.
6. Most TIA/CVA victims remain conscious. Patients should be allowed to remain seated upright (45° or semi-Fowler). Do not position the patient supine (flat) because this position increases blood flow to the brain, which is potentially dangerous during the time of elevated BP.
7. Oxygen may be administered through a nasal cannula or nasal hood. No central nervous system depressant should be used because using this may affect the patient's condition adversely or mask neurologic signs needed to help diagnose the condition.
8. If neurologic signs and symptoms do not resolve when emergency medical services arrive, the victim should be stabilized and transported to a hospital. Loss of consciousness is associated with a poor clinical prognosis in CVA (70%–100% initial mortality).

SUMMARY

Neurologic conditions such as AD and stroke are complex neurologic conditions and no simple description or explanation exists for their management or concomitant problems. A great deal of patience, understanding, and empathy will go a long way in the successful dental management of the patient who has AD or who has survived a stroke.

REFERENCES

1. Joynt R. Normal aging and patterns of neurologic disease. In: Berkow, R, editor. The Merck manual of geriatrics. Rahway (NJ): Merck and Co., Inc.; 1990. p. 926–44.
2. Alzheimer's disease and related disorders fact sheet. An overview of the dementias. From Alzheimer's disease and related disorders (ADRD) Association, Inc.; 2000.
3. Alzheimer's disease facts and figures. Alzheimer's association. Available at: www.alz.org. 2008.
4. Little JW, Falace DA, Miller GS, et al. Neurological disorders. In: Little JW, Falace DA, Miller GS, et al, editors. Dental management of the medically compromised patient. 7th edition. St. Louis (MO): Mosby; 2008. p. 469–87.
5. Evans D, Funkenstein H, Albert M, et al. Prevalence of Alzheimer's disease in a community population of older adults. JAMA 1989;262(18):2551–6.
6. Heyman A, Wilkenson W, Hurwitz B, et al. Alzheimer's disease. Genetic aspects and associated clinical disorders. Ann Neurol 1983;14:507.
7. Mortimer J, Hutton J. Epidemiology and etiology of Alzheimer's disease. In: Hutton J, Kennedy A, editors. Senile dementia of the Alzheimer's type. New York: Alan R. Liss; 1985. p. 177–96.
8. Bird T, Lampe T, Nemens R, et al. Familial Alzheimer's disease in American descendants of the Volga Germans: probable genetic founder effect. Ann Neurol 1988;23(1):25–31.
9. Breitner J, Silverman J, Mohs R, et al. Familial aggregation in Alzheimer's disease: comparison of risk among relatives of early- and late-onset cases, and among male and female relatives in successive generations. Neurology 1988;38(2):207–12.

10. McCarten JR, Hemmy LS, Rottunda SJ, et al. Patient age influences recognition of Alzheimer's disease. J Gerontol A Biol Sci Med Sci 2008;63:625–8.
11. Petersen R. New directions in Alzheimer's treatment. In: Mayo Clinic on Alzheimer's disease. New York: Rochester, Minn.: Kensington Publishing Corporation; 2002. p. 82–90.
12. Alzheimer's disease: unraveling the mystery. National Institute on Aging/National Institutes of Health, U.S. Dept. of Health and Human Services; Oct 2002. NIH Publication Number: 02–3782.
13. Clarfield A. The decreasing prevalence of reversible dementia: an updated meta-analysis. Arch Intern Med 2003;163:2219–29.
14. Ernst RL, Hay JW. The U.S. economic and social costs of Alzheimer's disease revisited. Am J Public Health 1994;84(8):1261–4.
15. Petersen R. Normal aging and Alzheimer's disease. In: Mayo Clinic on Alzheimer's disease. New York: Rochester, Minn.: Kensington Publishing Corporation; 2002. p. 3–9.
16. Cummings JL, Mendez MF. Alzheimer's disease and other disorders of cognition. In: Goldman L, Ausiello D, editors. Cecil textbook of medicine. 22nd edition. Philadelphia: WB Saunders; 2004. p. 2253–5.
17. Katzman R. Alzheimer's disease. N Engl J Med 1986;314(15):964–73.
18. Connelly PJ, James R. SIGN guideline for the management of patients with dementia. Int J Geriatr Psychiatry 2006;21:14–6.
19. Zimmermann M, Gardoni F, Di LLuca M. Molecular rationale for the pharmacological treatment of Alzheimer's disease. Drugs Aging 2005;22(Supp 1): 27–37.
20. Rogers SL, Farlow MR, Doody RS, et al. A 24-week, double-blind, placebo-controlled trial of donepezil in patients with Alzheimer's disease. Donepezil Study Group. Neurology 1998;50:136–45.
21. Wilkinson DG, Francis PT, Schwam E, et al. Cholinesterase inhibitors used in the treatment of Alzheimer's disease: the relationship between pharmacological effects and clinical efficacy. Drugs Aging 2004;21:453–78.
22. Petersen R. Treating the symptoms of Alzheimer's disease. In: Mayo Clinic on Alzheimer's disease. New York: Rochester, Minn.: Kensington Publishing Corporation; 2002. p. 65–76.
23. Reisberg B, Doody R, Stoffler A, et al. Memantine in moderate-to-severe Alzheimer's disease. N Engl J Med 2003;348:1333–41.
24. Doody RS. Refining treatment guidelines in Alzheimer's disease. Geriatrics 2005;(Suppl):14–20.
25. Harmann S, Mobius HJ. Tolerability of memantine in combination with cholinesterase inhibitors in dementia therapy. Int Clin Psychopharmacol 2003;18:81–5.
26. Friedlander AH, Norman DC, Mahler ME, et al. Alzheimer's disease: psychopathology, medical management and dental implications. J Am Dent Assoc 2006; 137(9):1240–51.
27. Sano M, Ernesto C, Thomas RG, et al. A controlled trial of selegiline, alpha-tocopherol, or both as treatment for Alzheimer's disease. The Alzheimer's Disease Cooperative Study. N Engl J Med 1997;336(17):1216–22.
28. Bharucha A, Pandav R, Shen C, et al. Predictors of nursing facility admission: a 12-year epidemiological study in the United States. J Am Geriatr Soc 2004; 52(3):434–9.
29. Arai K, Sumi Y, Uematsu H, et al. Association between dental health behaviors, mental/physical function and self-feeding ability among the elderly: a cross-sectional survey. Gerodontology 2003;20(2):78–83.

30. Henry R, Smith B. Treating the Alzheimer's patient: a guide for dental professionals. J Mich Dent Assoc 2004;86(10):32–6 38–40.
31. Ghezzi E, Ship J. Dementia and oral health. Oral Surg Oral Med Oral Pathol Endod 2000;89:2–5.
32. Little JW. Dental management of patients with Alzheimer's disease. Gen Dent 2005;53(4):289–96.
33. Ship JA, DeCarli C, Friedlan RP, et al. Diminished submandibular salivary flow in dementia of Alzheimer's type. J Gerontol 1990;45:61–6.
34. Ship JA. Oral health of patients with Alzheimer's disease. J Am Dent Assoc 1992; 123:53–8.
35. Screebny L, Valdini A. Xerostomia part one: relationship to other symptoms and salivary gland hypofunction. Oral Surg Oral Med Oral Pathol 1988;66:451–8.
36. Chiappelli F, Bauer J, Spackman S, et al. Dental needs of the elderly in the 21st century. Gen Dent 2002;50(4):358–63.
37. Jones JA, Lavallee N, Alman J, et al. Caries incidence in patients with dementia. Gerodontology 1993;10(2):76–82.
38. Mace N, Rabins P. The 36-hour day: a family guide to caring for persons with Alzheimer's disease. Baltimore: Johns Hopkins Press; 1991.
39. Stiefel DJ, Truelove EL, Menard TW, et al. A comparison of the oral health of persons with and without chronic mental illness in community settings. Spec Care Dentist 1990;10:6–12.
40. Friedlander AH, Jarvik LF. The dental management of the patient with dementia. Oral Surg Oral Med Oral Pathol 1987;64:549–53.
41. Henry RG, Wekstein DR. Providing dental care for patients diagnosed with Alzheimer's disease. Dent Clin North Am 1997;41(4):915–43.
42. Niessen LC, Jones JA. Alzheimer's disease: a guide for dental professionals. Spec Care Dentist 1986;6(1):6–12.
43. Niessen LC, Jones JA. Professional dental care for patients with dementia. Gerodontology 1987;6(2):67–71.
44. Kocaelli H, Yaltirik M, Yargic LI, et al. Alzheimer's disease and dental management. Oral Surg Oral Med Oral Pathol Oral Radiol Endod 2002;93(5):521–4.
45. Henry RG. Alzheimer's disease and cognitively impaired elderly: providing dental care. J Calif Dent Assoc 1999;27(9):709–17.
46. Hsu KT, Shuman SK, Hamamoto DT, et al. The application of facial assessment of orofacial pain in cognitively impaired older adults. J Am Dent Assoc 2007; 138(7):963–9.
47. Shuman S. Ethics and the patient with dementia. J Am Dent Assoc 1989;119:747–8.
48. Shuman S, Bebeau M. Ethical issues in nursing home care: practice guidelines for difficult situations. Spec Care Dentist 1996;16:170–6.
49. Wetle T. Ethical issues in geriatric dentistry. Gerondontology 1987;6:73–8.
50. Henry RG. Neurologic disorders in dentistry: managing patients with Alzheimer's disease. J Indiana Dent Assoc 1997–1998;76(4):51–7.
51. What is a stroke? National Institute of Neurological Disorders and Stroke. Office of Communications and Public Liaison. National Institute of Health. NIH publication No. 04-5517. Available at: www.ninds.nih.gov/disorders/stroke. Accessed August 15, 2008.
52. Wityk F. Foreword, Stein J, Silver F, editors. Life after stroke: the guide to recovering your health and preventing another stroke. Baltimore (MD): The John Hopkins University Press; 2006. p. xiii–xv.
53. Let's talk about stroke, TIA and warning signs. American Heart Association/ American Stroke Association. 2007 Fact Sheet.

54. Stein J, Silver J, Frates E. Understanding stroke and its consequences and Risk factors for having a stroke. In: Life after stroke: the guide to recovering your health and preventing another stroke. Baltimore (MD): The John Hopkins University Press; 2006. p. 3–13, 87–90.
55. Spence D. What is a stroke?. In: How to prevent your stroke. Nashville (TN): Vanderbilt University Press; 2006. p. 3–10.
56. American Heart Association. Heart disease and stroke statistics, 2005 update. Dallas (TX), American Heart Association, 2005. Available at: www.americanheart.org/presenter. Accessed August 18, 2008.
57. Lawes CM. Blood pressure and stroke: an overview of published reviews. Stroke 2004;35:776–85.
58. Feigin VL, Lawes CM, Bennett DA, et al. Stroke epidemiology: a review of population-based studies of incidence, prevalence, and case-fatality in the late 20th century. Lancet Neurol 2003;2:43–53.
59. Incidence and prevalence. 2006 chart book on cardiovascular and lung diseases. Bethesda (MD): National Heart, Lung, and Blood Institute; 2006.
60. Johnston SC, Gress DR, Browner WS, et al. Short-term prognosis after emergency department diagnosis of TIA. JAMA 2000;284:2901–6.
61. Wolf PA, Abbott RD, Kanel WB. Atrial fibrillation as an independent risk factor for stroke: the Framingham Study. Stroke 1991;22:983–8.
62. Seshadri S, Beiser A, Kelly-Hayes M, et al. The lifetime risk of stroke: estimates from the Framingham Study. Stroke 2006;37:345–50.
63. Kissela BM, Khoury J, Kleindorfer D, et al. Epidemiology of ischemic stroke in patients with diabetes: the greater Cincinnati/Northern Kentucky Stroke Study. Diabetes Care 2005;28:355–9.
64. Kurth T, Moore SC, Gaziano JM, et al. Healthy lifestyle and the risk of stroke in women. Arch Intern Med 2006;166:1403–19.
65. Ohira T, Shahar E, Chambless LE, et al. Risk factors for ischemic stroke subtypes: the Atherosclerosis Risk in Communities Study. Stroke 2006;37:2493–8.
66. Grau A, Becher H, Ziegler C, et al. Periodontal disease as a risk factor for ischemic stroke. Stroke 2004;35:496–501.
67. Joshipura K, Hung H, Rimm E, et al. Periodontal disease, tooth loss, and the incidence of ischemic stroke. Stroke 2003;34:47–52.
68. Elter J, Offenbacher S, Toole J, et al. Relationship of periodontal disease and edentulism to stroke/TIA. J Dent Res 2003;82:998–1001.
69. Beck J, Garcia R, Heiss G, et al. Periodontal disease and cardiovascular disease. J Periodontol 1996;67:1123–37.
70. Centers for Disease Control and Prevention. Prevalence of stroke: United States, 2005. MMWR Morb Mortal Wkly Rep 2007;56:469–74.
71. Rosamond WD, Folsom AR, Chambless LE, et al. Stroke incidence and survival among middle-aged adults: 9-year follow-up of the Atherosclerotic Risk in Communities (ARIC) cohort. Stroke 1999;30:736–43.
72. National Center for Health Statistics, Centers for Disease Control and Prevention. Compressed mortality file: underlying cause of death, 1979 to 2004. Atlanta (GA): Centers for Disease Control and Prevention. Available at: http://wonder.cdc.gov/mortSQL.html. Accessed May 29, 2007.
73. Centers for Disease Control and Prevention (CDC). Prevalence of disabilities and associated health conditions among adults: United States, 1999. MMWR Morb Mortal Wkly Rep 2001;50:120–5.
74. Wolf Pa, D'Agostino RB, Belanger AJ, et al. Probability of stroke: a risk profile from the Framingham Study. Stroke 1991;22:312–8.

75. Asplund K, Stegmayr B, Peltonen M. From the twentieth to the twenty-first century: a public health perspective on stroke. In: Ginsberg MD, Bogousslavsky J, editors, Cerebrovascular disease pathophysiology, diagnosis, and management, Vol 2. Malden (MA): Blackwell Science; 1998. chapter 64.
76. Alzheimer's disease and related disorders fact sheet: an overview of the dementias, multi-infarct dementia. Alzheimer's Association. 2008. Available at: www.alz.org. Accessed September 2, 2008.
77. Stein J, Silver J, Frates E. High blood pressure and stroke. In: Life after stroke: the guide to recovering your health and preventing another stroke. Baltimore (MD): the John Hopkins University Press; 2006. p. 131–2.
78. Kelley-Hayes M, Beiser A, Kase CS, et al. The influence of gender and age on disability following ischemic stroke: the Framingham Study. J Stroke Cerebrovasc Dis 2003;12:119–26.
79. Maron BA, Dansereau LM, Maron BJ, et al. Impact of post-graduate medical education on recognition of stroke. Cardiol Rev 2005;13:73–5.
80. Centers for Medicare and Medicaid Services. Health care financing review: Medicare and Medicaid statistical supplement. 2006 statistical supplement. Baltimore (MD): Centers for Medicare and Medicaid Services; 2006. Available at: http://www.cms.hhs.gov/apps/review/Supp/. Accessed February 7, 2007.
81. Taylor TN, Davis PH, Torner JC, et al. Lifetime cost of stroke in the United States. Stroke 1996;27:1459–66.
82. Centers of Disease Control and Prevention (CDC). Awareness of stroke warning signs: 17 states and the U.S. Virgin Islands, 2001. MMWR Morb Mortal Wkly Rep 2004;53:359–62.
83. American Heart Association and American Stroke Association. Let's talk about stroke, TIA and warning signs. American Stroke Association. 2007. Available at: www.strokeassociation.org. Accessed September 4, 2008.
84. Tonarelli SB, Hart RG. What's new in stroke? The top 10 for 2004/05. J Am Geriatr Soc 2006;54:674–9.
85. Stein J, Silver J, Frates E. Tests your doctor may order. In: Life after stroke: the guide to recovering your health and preventing another stroke. Baltimore (MD): The John Hopkins University Press; 2006. p. 24–41.
86. Stein J, Silver J, Frates E. Maximizing recovery from a stroke. In: Life after stroke: the guide to recovering your health and preventing another stroke. Baltimore (MD): The John Hopkins University Press; 2006. p. 55–69.
87. Fields L, Burt V, Cutler J, et al. The burden of adult hypertension in the United States 1999–2000: a rising tide. Hypertension 2004;44:398–404.
88. Chobanian AV, Bakris GL, Black HR, et al. Seventh report of the Joint National Committee on Prevention, Detection, Evaluation, and Treatment of High Blood Pressure. Hypertension 2003;42:1206–52.
89. McCarthy FM, Malamed SF. Physical evaluation system to determine medical risk and indicated dental therapy modifications. J Am Dent Assoc 1979;99(2):181–4.
90. Malamed SF. Prevention. In: Medical emergencies in the dental office. 5th edition. St. Louis (MO): Mosby; 2000. p. 22, 287–306.
91. Hankey GJ. Impact of treatment of people with transient ischemic attack on stroke incidence and public health. Cerebrovasc Dis 1996;6(Suppl 1):26–33.
92. Kleindorfer D, Panagos P, Pancioli A, et al. Incidence and short-term prognosis of transient ischemic attack in a population-based study. Stroke 2005;36:720–3.
93. Johnson SC, Fayad PB, Gorelick PB, et al. Prevalence and knowledge of transient ischemic attack among US adults. Neurology 2003;60:1429–34.

94. Lisabeth LD, Ireland JK, Risser JM, et al. Stroke risk after transient ischemic attack in a population-based setting. Stroke 2004;35:1842–6.
95. Coull AJ, Lovett JK, Rothwell PM. Oxford Vascular Study. Population-based study of early risk of stroke after transient ischemic attack or minor stroke: implications for public education and organization of services. Br Med J 2004;328:326.
96. Sherman DG. Reconsideration of TIA diagnostic criteria. Neurology 2004; 62(Suppl 6):S20–1.
97. Friedlander A, Lande A. Panoramic radiographic identification of carotid arterial plaques. Oral Surg Oral Med Oral Pathol 1981;52:102–4.
98. Friedlander A, Baker J. Panoramic radiography: an aid in detecting patients at risk of cerebrovascular accident. J Am Dent Assoc 1994;125:1598–603.
99. Carter LC, Haller AD, Nadarajah V, et al. Use of panoramic radiography among an ambulatory dental population to detect patients at risk of stroke. J Am Dent Assoc 1997;128:977–84.
100. Mupparapu M, Kim I. Calcified carotid artery atheroma and stroke. A systematic review. J Am Dent Assoc 2007;138:483–92.
101. American Heart Association. How stroke affects behavior. 1991. American Heart Association National Center, 7272 Greenville Ave, Dallas (TX) 75231–4596.
102. Ostuni E. Stroke and the dental patient. J Am Dent Assoc 1994;125:721–7.
103. Rose LF, Mealey B, Minsk L, et al. Oral care for patients with cardiovascular disease and stroke. J Am Dent Assoc 2002;133(Suppl):37S–44S.
104. Malamed S. Intravenous sedation: rationale. In: Sedation: a guide to patient management. 3rd edition. St Louis (MO): Mosby; 1995. p. 315.
105. Fatahzadeh M, Glick M. Stroke: epidemiology, classification, risk factors, complications, diagnosis, prevention, and medical and dental management. Oral surg Oral Med Oral Pathol Oral Radiol Endod 2006;102:180–91.
106. Sacco D, Frost D. Dental management of patients with stroke or Alzheimer's disease. Dent Clin North Am 2006;50:625–33.
107. Imm LC. Dental management of the stroke patient. Dent Hyg 1983;10:43–5.
108. Kleiman C, Zafrran J, Zayon G. Dental care for the stroke patient. Dent Hyg 1980;5:237–9.
109. Gupta A, Pansari K, Shetty H. Post-stroke depression. Int J Clin Pract 2002;56:531–7.
110. Niwa H, Satoh Y, Matsuura H. Cardiovascular responses to epinephrine-containing local anesthetics for dental use: a comparison of hemodynamic responses to infiltration anesthesia and ergometer-stress testing. Oral Surg Oral Med Oral Pathol Oral Radiol Endod 2000;90:171–81.
111. Wahl MJ. Myths of dental surgery in patients receiving anticoagulant therapy. J Am Dent Assoc 2000;131:77–81.
112. Jeske AH, Suchko GD. ADA Council on Scientific Affairs and Division of Science. Lack of a scientific basis for routine discontinuation of oral anticoagulation therapy before dental treatment. J Am Dent Assoc 2003;134(11):1492–7.
113. Blinder D, Manor Y, Martinowitz U, et al. Dental extractions in patients maintained on continued oral anticoagulants. Oral Surg Oral Med Oral Pathol Oral Radiol Endod 1999;88:137–40.
114. Rice PJ, Perry RJ, Afzal Z, et al. Antibacterial prescribing and warfarin: a review. Braz Dent J 2003;194:411–5.
115. Brennan M, Wynn R, Miller C. Aspirin and bleeding in dentistry: an update and recommendations. Oral Surg Oral Med Oral Pathol Oral Radiol Endod 2007; 104(3):316–23.
116. Malamed SF. Cerebrovascular accident. In: Medical emergencies in the dental office. 5th edition. St. Louis (MO): Mosby; 2000. p. 298–301.

Dental Management of Special Needs Patients Who Have Epilepsy

Miriam R. Robbins, DDS, MS

KEYWORDS

- Epilepsy • Seizure • Gingival hyperplasia
- Special needs patients • Developmentally disabled
- Treatment planning

The term "epilepsy" refers to a group of neurologic disorders characterized by chronic, recurrent, paroxysmal seizure activity. The word epilepsy is derived from the Greek word *epilambanein*, meaning to attack or seize. In the past, epilepsy was associated with religious experiences and even demonic possession. In ancient times, epilepsy was known as the "sacred disease" because people thought that epileptic seizures were a form of attack by demons, or that the visions experienced by persons who had epilepsy were sent by the gods. In 400 BC, Hippocrates recognized that epilepsy was a brain disorder, and he spoke out against the ideas that seizures were a curse from the gods and that people who had epilepsy held the power of prophecy.[1] The foundation of our modern understanding of the pathophysiology of epilepsy was proposed in 1873 by London neurologist John Hughlings Jackson, who proposed that seizures were the result of sudden brief electrochemical discharges in the brain. He also suggested that the character of the seizures depended on the location and function of the site of the discharges.

INCIDENCE AND PREVALENCE

Epilepsy is a common chronic neurologic disorder that is characterized by recurrent unprovoked seizures.[2] A seizure is the result of spontaneous, synchronous, inappropriate, and excessive electric discharge of cerebral neurons that interfere with the normal function of the brain and result in alterations in level of consciousness, convulsive movements or other motor activity, sensory phenomena, behavioral abnormalities, and mental impairment. Approximately 10% of Americans will experience a seizure in their lifetime.[3] Most of these seizures are attributable to a specific cause, such as a high fever or underlying metabolic disorder. Isolated seizures are most common during childhood, with as many as 4% of children having at least one seizure

Department of Oral and Maxillofacial Pathology, Radiology and Medicine, New York University College of Dentistry, 345 East 24th Street, Clinic 1B - Room 114S, NY 10010, USA
E-mail address: miriam.robbins@nyu.edu

Dent Clin N Am 53 (2009) 295–309
doi:10.1016/j.cden.2008.12.014
dental.theclinics.com
0011-8532/08/$ – see front matter

before the age of 15.[4] However, an isolated seizure does not indicate epilepsy. Epilepsy, in contrast, is a recurrent illness, and the patient must have at least two seizures before a diagnosis of epilepsy is considered.

According to the Centers for Disease Control and Prevention, epilepsy is one of the most commonly diagnosed neurologic disorders.[5] The overall incidence of epilepsy, excluding febrile convulsions and single seizures, is generally about 50 cases per 100,000 persons per year (range 40–70 per 100,000 per year)[3] in developed countries. Approximately 1% of the United States population, or 2.7 million people, have epilepsy. The incidence of this disorder is highest in patients younger than 2 years of age and rises again after 65 years of age. More than 20% of cases are discovered before a child is 5 years of age. In infants, birth injuries and congenital defects are the primary causes of epilepsy. Birth injuries, genetic factors, infections, and trauma are major contributing factors in children and adolescents from 2 to 20 years of age. For individuals between 20 and 30 years of age, brain tumors and other structural lesions are the foremost contributing causes. In those older than 50 years of age, cerebral vascular accidents and metastatic tumors are significant causes of seizure activity.[6]

DEVELOPMENTAL DISABILITIES AND EPILEPSY IN CHILDREN AND ADULTS

Epilepsy is the most common comorbid medical condition in persons who have developmental disabilities. Epilepsy occurs more frequently (25%–35%) in people who have neurologic-based disabilities. The relationship between the cause of the disability and epilepsy may be complex, although in most cases, a single underlying brain abnormality or insult to the brain causes both disorders and is another manifestation of brain injury or differences in brain development.[3] Epilepsy occurs in 15% to 55% of children and adults who have cerebral palsy, depending on the form of cerebral palsy and the severity of motor deficit.[7,8] Approximately 20% to 30% of children and adolescents who have autism develop some form of epileptic disorder.[9] The pathophysiology of epilepsy is related to the cause of the brain damage in patients who have mental retardation. The frequency and the severity of the epileptic syndrome are related more to the primary cause of mental retardation than to the severity of mental retardation. The prevalence of mental retardation is approximately 0.3% to 0.8%, but 20% to 30% of children who have mental retardation have epilepsy. Sixty-nine percent of children who have epilepsy and mental handicap have a secondary handicap such as cerebral palsy, autism, or visual impairment. Approximately 35% to 40% of children who have epilepsy also have mental retardation and up to 71% of people who have mental retardation and cerebral palsy have epilepsy.[10] The severity of intellectual disability and the frequency and severity of chronic epileptic seizures are directly related. The rate is around 20% in persons who have mild intellectual impairment and can be as high as 50% in those who have severe-to-profound intellectual disability. Epileptic seizures in adults in their late 40s who have Down syndrome are seen as an expression of Alzheimer disease, which occurs with greater frequency in individuals who have Down syndrome than in the general population.[11] The epileptic disorders in patients who have mental impairment or developmental disability are usually complex, involving more than one seizure type, and are often more severe and difficult to control than disorders in the general population.[12] Individuals who have developmental disabilities and epilepsy have higher rates of seizure recurrence after a first seizure, lower rates of "outgrowing" epilepsy, a higher degree of morbidity associated with frequent accidents and fractures, and higher rates of sudden unexpected death.[13]

CLASSIFICATION OF SEIZURES

In 1981, the International League Against Epilepsy developed an international classification of epileptic seizures based on clinical and electroencephalographic (EEG) features of the seizure.[14] All seizures are broadly divided into two major classes: partial seizures and generalized seizures. Partial seizures are further divided into simple and complex. Unclassified seizures are difficult to fit into a single class (**Box 1**). The clinical signs or symptoms of seizures depend on the location of the epileptic discharges in the cortex and the extent and pattern of the propagation of the epileptic discharge in the brain. Many patients will have more than one type of seizure and the features of each type of seizure may change from seizure to seizure or over time.

PARTIAL SEIZURES

Partial, or focal, seizures are the more common classification and occur in 75% to 80% of patients who have epilepsy. In contrast to generalized seizures, partial seizures begin focally with an abnormal electric discharge in a restricted region of the brain. Partial seizures are subclassified by their effect on consciousness, responsiveness, and memory as simple partial seizures (patient remains conscious), complex partial seizures (patient has impaired consciousness), or partial seizure evolving to secondarily generalized tonic-clonic seizures.

Simple partial seizures are the most spatially restricted of the partial seizures and are characterized by an episode of altered sensation, cognitive function, or motor activity during which consciousness and ability to interact with the external environment are not impaired. They are also known as "auras" if they precede a complex or secondarily generalized seizure. Symptoms vary, depending on the brain region involved, and can have motor signs (movement of any body part), sensory signs (visual or olfactory changes), psychic signs (fear, anxiety, déjà-vu), or autonomic signs (dizziness, tachycardia, sweating).

Box 1
Classification of seizures (adapted from International Classification of Seizures)

Partial seizures

Simple partial seizures (consciousness not impaired)

Complex partial seizures (with impairment of consciousness)

Secondarily generalized seizures

Generalized seizures

Absence seizures

Myoclonic seizures

Clonic seizures

Tonic seizures

Tonic clonic seizures

Atonic seizures

Unclassified epileptic seizures (incomplete or inadequate data)

Data from Commission on Classification and Terminology of the International League Against Epilepsy. Proposal for revised clinical and electroencephalographic classification of epileptic seizures. Epilepsia 1981;22:489–501.

Complex partial seizures are defined by an episode of impaired consciousness with altered behavior, sensation, or motor activity that can last from 30 seconds to 2 minutes. The motor activity may consist of repetitive automatic movements of the face or limbs. Partial seizures with secondary generalization occur when the seizure initially localized to one limited area spreads to involve both sides of the brain and evolves into a tonic-clonic or "grand mal" seizure.[15]

GENERALIZED SEIZURES

Generalized seizures begin with a widespread, excessive electric discharge involving most or all of the brain at the same time. They are divided into several types, including absence, myoclonic, atonic, tonic, clonic, and tonic-clonic.

The clinical signs of a generalized tonic-clonic (or grand mal) seizure are well recognized. An aura (a sensory alteration) precedes the convulsion in 35% of patients. The aura is followed by an abrupt loss of consciousness, often accompanied by an "epileptic cry" caused by air being forced out by the contraction of the diaphragm through a partially closed glottis. During the tonic phase (10–15 seconds), the whole body stiffens as the entire musculature contracts forcibly and patients may become cyanotic, tachycardic, and hypertensive. The clonic phase that follows is characterized by simultaneous rhythmic jerking of the arms and legs, usually lasting at least 1 minute. Loss of bladder control is common and patients may bite their tongues, cheeks, or lips. After this type of seizure, the patient typically enters a "postictal" state of confusion and fatigue lasting 30 minutes or longer.[15] Tonic-clonic seizures that last more than 5 minutes or recur in a series of two or more without a return to consciousness indicate a serious neurologic emergency called status epilepticus, which requires immediate medical attention because of airway impairment and aspiration. Supplemental oxygen followed by the administration of a parenteral benzodiazepine such as diazepam or midazolam should be followed by transportation to a hospital emergency department.[16]

Absence (petit mal) seizures are brief episodes of altered or impaired consciousness, unresponsiveness, and cessation of activity. No aura occurs and patients will have a brief episode of staring, usually lasting less than 10 seconds, sometimes associated with blinking or automatic movements of the hands or mouth and autonomic changes such as pallor, tachycardia, or salivation. Atypical absence seizures, which occur in patients who have symptomatic generalized epilepsies, are usually longer than typical absences and often have more gradual onset and resolution. These seizures usually occur in children who also have other types of seizure, lower than average intelligence, and more poorly controlled epilepsy.[17]

Myoclonic seizures are characterized by a brief jerk or series of jerks that may involve a small part of the body, such as a single finger, hand, or foot, or may involve both sides of the body simultaneously, most often the shoulders or upper arms. They are generally of short duration and have no postictal phase. Atonic seizures, or drop seizures, manifest as a sudden loss of muscle tone throughout most or all of the body, which may include head nodding or limb dropping, or the patient collapsing to the ground. Clonic seizures are rhythmic, jerking movements of body parts, such as the arms or legs, with impaired consciousness that occur frequently in people who have focal epilepsy. Tonic seizures are characterized by a stiffening of the body or limb, often resulting in a fall if the patient is standing. These seizures have the highest risk for traumatic injury to the head, oral, and dental structures secondary to falling and forced contraction of the jaws. Tonic seizures last 5 to 20 seconds and are followed by a postictal state.[18]

DIAGNOSIS

The diagnosis of epilepsy requires the presence of recurrent, unprovoked seizures. Patients presenting with seizures should have a general and neurologic examination, looking for other causes of loss of consciousness (eg, cardiac abnormalities, evidence of infection), contributing factors or secondary causes of epilepsy, and focal neurologic signs. Some of the important clinical findings include alterations in consciousness, sensation, motor abilities, and reflexes. Detailed accounts of the seizures from either the patient or eyewitnesses can be important in making a correct diagnosis. If seizures are due to an underlying disorder, these conditions are often discovered during the physical examination (**Box 2**).

All patients presenting with new-onset seizures should have blood taken for full blood count and biochemistry (urea and electrolytes, blood sugar, calcium, and liver function tests). They should also have an ECG to look for underlying cardiac abnormality and to exclude such conditions as long QT syndrome and other cardiac arrhythmias. Patients in whom focal neurologic signs are found in the absence of a known cause should undergo urgent neuroimaging.[19]

The EEG, combined with the clinical picture, is central to the diagnosis of epilepsy. Seizures produce characteristic spike wave patterns on EEG (**Fig. 1**). EEG changes observed in persons who have mental retardation and epilepsy are, in general, similar to the ones observed in individuals who have epilepsy without mental retardation.[20] Because the EEG is usually normal when the patient is not having a seizure, methods such as sleep deprivation, hyperventilation, or continuous monitoring using closed-circuit television videotaping and digitized EEG telemetry might be used to increase the chance of capturing abnormal activity. Other imaging and measurement technologies, such as MRI, single photon emission computed tomography, positron emission tomography, and magnetoencephalography, may be useful to discover a cause for the

Box 2
Differential diagnosis of seizures

Conditions most likely to be confused with generalized seizures

Syncope

Concussive seizures

Psychogenic nonepileptic seizures

Hypoglycemia

Breath-holding attacks

Narcolepsy

Panic attacks/hyperventilation

Toxic or metabolic disturbances

Conditions most likely to be confused with partial seizures

Transient ischemic attacks

Transient global amnesia

Vertigo

Migraine

Movement disorders (eg, tics)

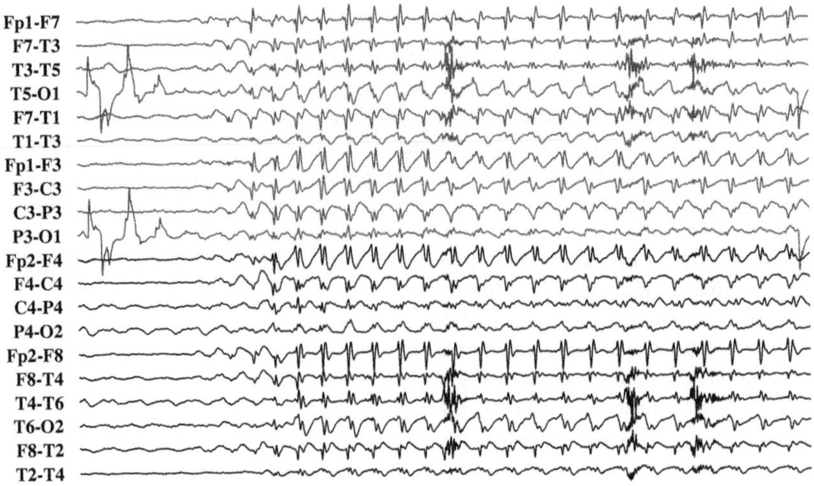

Fig. 1. EEG showing absence seizure. (*Courtesy of* the New York University Comprehensive Epilepsy Center, New York, NY; with permission.)

epilepsy, to discover the affected brain region, or to classify the epileptic syndrome, but these studies are not useful in making the initial diagnosis (**Fig. 2**).

Diagnosis of epilepsy in persons who have developmental disabilities presents unique difficulties. The patients frequently cannot describe the epileptic event and the events are infrequently observed by someone who is familiar with epileptic disorders. The patients often present with behaviors that resemble epilepsy, such as

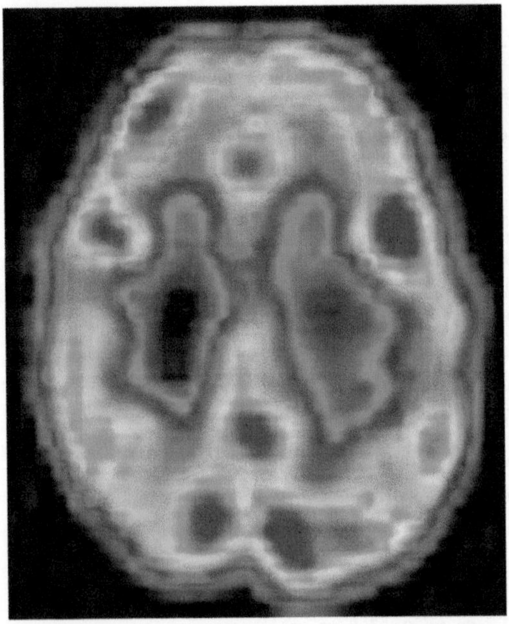

Fig. 2. Functional MRI showing generalized seizure activity. (*Courtesy of* the New York University Comprehensive Epilepsy Center, New York, NY; with permission.)

generalized tonic extension in response to stimulus in children and adults who have severe spasticity. Episodes of unresponsiveness are frequently seen in patients who have mental retardation, which can resemble absence seizures. Comorbidity with psychiatric disorders is seen in 30% to 40% of individuals who have mental retardation and some manifestations of psychiatric disorders might be confused with epileptic events. Pseudoseizures (nonepileptic seizures that are physical manifestation of a psychologic disturbance) occur in 20% to 30% of this patient population.[21] Medication-induced dystonias from psychotropic medications can be confused with epileptic events.

MANAGEMENT

Seizure disorders are generally more severe in people who have mental retardation. Patients who have developmental disabilities and epilepsy are treated for their seizure type or types and syndrome just like any other person who has epilepsy. Several options exist for the treatment of epileptic seizures, including antiseizure medications, vagal nerve stimulation, ketogenic diet, and surgery. These options are may be used concurrently in the same individual if needed.[12]

PHARMACOTHERAPY

The mainstay of treatment of epilepsy is anticonvulsant medications. Individuals who have developmental disabilities are started on an antiepileptic drug (AED) as the first-line of treatment. AEDs are a mixed blessing for patients who have developmental disabilities because they may be unusually sensitive to the adverse effects of seizures and medications. For example, the adverse-effect profiles of some older AEDs, such as phenobarbital and phenytoin, suggest that they should not be considered first-line therapies for adolescents and adults who have developmental disabilities. The newer AEDs appear to be just as effective as the older ones but are better tolerated in patients who have developmental disabilities.[20]

AEDs assist patients by stabilizing nerve cell membranes and preventing the spread of abnormal electric discharges. Many of the medications require a therapeutic level of effectiveness to provide the best seizure control with minimum side effects. Treatment with medications usually focuses on using an adequate dose of a single medication rather than smaller doses of several drugs. Monotherapy is the goal for most patients because of the benefits of improved drug compliance, reduced cost of medication and laboratory evaluations, lower risk for adverse effects, and lessened chance of drug interactions. Several AEDs can be used as the first drug in the treatment of epileptic disorders. No definitive guidelines are available to determine the first drug to use in any particular patient. AEDs are selected based on the type of seizure, age of the patient, side effects, and ability to adhere to the use of the drug. If the first AED attempted proves undesirable because of lack of efficacy or adverse effects, the first medication is tapered while a second is slowly added. After several single medications are used that are consistent with the patient's seizure type, polytherapy may be attempted. Currently, 19 medications have been approved by the Food and Drug Administration (FDA) for use in the treatment of epileptic seizures in the United States: carbamazepine (common United States brand name Tegretol), clorazepate (Tranxene), clonazepam (Klonopin), ethosuximide (Zarontin), felbamate (Felbatol), fosphenytoin (Cerebyx), gabapentin (Neurontin), lamotrigine (Lamictal), levetiracetam (Keppra), oxcarbazepine (Trileptal), phenobarbital (Luminal), phenytoin (Dilantin), pregabalin (Lyrica), primidone (Mysoline), tiagabine (Gabitril), topiramate (Topamax), valproate semisodium (Depakote), valproic acid (Depakene), and zonisamide

(Zonegran). Most of these appeared after 1990.[22] Medications commonly available outside the United States but still labeled as "investigational" within the United States are clobazam (Frisium) and vigabatrin (Sabril).

Side effects are common with many AEDs. These adverse effects include, but are not limited to, drowsiness, dizziness, nausea, visual changes, and fatigue. Intraoral symptoms can include xerostomia, soreness of the tongue, swollen or bleeding gums, and swelling of the face, lips, and tongue. Some adverse effects are related to the dose of the medications, whereas other effects, such as allergic-type reactions, occur regardless of the dose (**Table 1**).[23] Because patients who have developmental disabilities tend to have more severe seizures, it is not uncommon for these patients to be overmedicated. The evaluation of cognitive deficiencies due to the use of antiseizure drugs is difficult in persons who have intellectual disabilities. Many studies have attempted to address this issue. Unfortunately, most findings are inconclusive and even contradictory. However, no single drug causes problems in all patients taking that drug, and all the drugs can result in some form of cognitive impairment in some patients.[10]

Decreased bone mineral density has been reported with phenytoin, phenobarbital, primidone, carbamazepine, and valproic acid. This adverse effect has not been fully evaluated with the new AEDs and is particularly worrisome in individuals who have disabilities, especially if they are nonambulatory. Even though osteoporosis is present in both sexes, women who have developmental disabilities are at higher risk. For causes that are not clear, Down syndrome seems to be an independent risk factor for osteoporosis. This decrease in bone mineral density, coupled with the high fall rate in this population, results in a higher risk for osteoporotic fractures[24] and may lead to poorer bone healing following surgical procedures.

Some AEDs (carbamazepine, gabapentin, valproate, vigabatrin,) are associated with weight gain, which can have numerous health consequences, including increased risk for diabetes and cardiovascular disease. This side effect can be particularly problematic in patients who have developmental disabilities and a sedentary lifestyle.

Nonpharmacologic Treatment

Epilepsy surgery is an option for patients whose seizures remain resistant to treatment with AEDs and who have a focal abnormality that can be located and therefore removed. The goal of these procedures is total control of epileptic seizures,[25] although anticonvulsant medications may still be required. The four widely accepted surgical procedures are focal cortical resections, corpus colostomy, temporal lobectomy, and functional hemispherectomy.

The ketogenic diet was first used for the treatment of epilepsy in the 1920s. It is more effective in children than adolescents or adults and is used for those patients who have tonic-clonic, complex partial, and minor motor seizures, who do not respond or cannot tolerate the side effects of AEDs. The ketogenic diet is high in fat and low in carbohydrates and protein, and fluids are restricted. A study conducted by Johns Hopkins reported that 50% of those patients starting the ketogenic diet reported a decrease in seizures of 50% or more, with 29% of patients reporting a 90% reduction in symptoms; these patients had previously tried an average of six anticonvulsant drugs. However, the diet is nutritionally inadequate, and patients require vitamin and mineral supplementation.[26]

The vagus nerve stimulator (VNS), approved by the FDA in July 1997, was the first successful medical device for patients who have uncontrolled partial onset seizures. The current evidence suggests that VNS is a treatment option to be considered in individuals who have developmental disabilities and difficult-to-control seizures. It uses

Table 1
Adverse effects of antiepileptic drugs

Medication	Most Common Oral Side Effects and Dental Considerations
Carbamazepine (Tegretol)	Agranulocytosis, aplastic anemia, xerostomia, delayed healing, gingival bleeding (thrombocytopenia), osteoporosis
Clonazepam (Klonopin)	Drowsiness, ataxia, drug interactions
Ethosuximide (Zarontin)	Leukopenia, Stevens-Johnson syndrome, orofacial edema, dysgeusia
Felbamate (Felbatol)	Aplastic anemia, xerostomia, stomatitis, orofacial edema, dysgeusia
Gabapentin (Neurontin)	Xerostomia, stomatitis, gingivitis, glossitis, orofacial edema, dysgeusia
Lamotrigine (Lamictal)	Ataxia, Stevens-Johnson syndrome, xerostomia, stomatitis, gingivitis, glossitis, dysgeusia
Levetiracetam (Keppra)	Xerostomia, stomatitis, gingivitis, orofacial edema, dysgeusia
Oxcarbazepine (Trileptal)	Rash, xerostomia, gingivitis, stomatitis, dysgeusia
Phenobarbital (Luminal)	Drowsiness, drug interactions, xerostomia, stomatitis, osteoporosis
Phenytoin (Dilantin)	Gingival hyperplasia, delayed healing, gingival bleeding, osteoporosis
Primidone (Mysolin)	Ataxia, vertigo, stomatitis, osteoporosis
Tiagabine (Gabitril)	New-onset seizures and status epilepticus associated with unlabeled use
Topiramate (Topamax)	Impaired cognition, xerostomia, gingivitis, orofacial edema
Valproate (Depakene, Depakote)	Excessive bleeding, decreased platelet aggregation, delayed healing, osteoporosis, xerostomia, stomatitis, gingivitis, drug interactions with aspirin and nonsteroidal anti-inflammatory drugs

an implanted electric device, similar in size, shape, and implant location to a heart pacemaker, which connects to the left vagus nerve in the neck. The device can be set to emit electronic pulses, stimulating the vagus nerve at pre-set intervals and milliamp levels. Treatment studies have shown that approximately 50% of those treated in this fashion show significant seizure frequency reduction. During stimulation, patients may experience coughing, throat pain, numbness of the chin or throat, increased salivation, and dysphagia.

The responsive neurostimulator (RNS) system is currently undergoing clinical study before FDA approval. This system relies on a device implanted just under the scalp. The leads attached to the device are implanted either on the brain surface or in the brain area itself and are located close to the area where the seizures are believed to start. When a seizure begins, small amounts of electric stimulation are delivered to suppress it. This system is different from the VNS system in that the RNS relies on direct brain stimulation and the RNS is a responsive system. The VNS pulses at predetermined intervals previously set by medical personnel. The RNS system is designed to respond to detected signs that a seizure is about to begin and can record events and allow customized response patterns, which may provide a greater degree of seizure control.[27]

DENTAL MANAGEMENT

Patients who have epilepsy have been shown to have significantly worse dental condition than the general population.[28] The disease may affect the dental status and oral health of patients in several ways. Patients who have seizure disorders tend to have less than ideal oral health, with higher numbers of decayed and missing teeth. They tend to receive less dental treatment, with significantly fewer restored and replaced teeth than the general population[28] This situation can be especially true in patients who have development disabilities, who may have trouble accessing dental care anyway. The seizures themselves can cause injuries to the teeth and dental prostheses. Some of the AEDs can cause periodontal disease. Specific considerations for epileptic patients include the treatment of oral soft tissue side effects of medications and damage to the hard and soft tissue of the orofacial region secondary to seizure trauma, especially in patients who suffer from poorly controlled generalized tonic-clonic seizures.

Dentists with a thorough knowledge of seizure disorders and the medications used to treat them can provide necessary dental and oral health care for those patients. Patients who have stable seizure disorder and no associated risks can receive treatment in an outpatient setting. A thorough evaluation of a patient's seizure disorder is necessary before initiation of any dental treatment. Important aspects to evaluate include the type of seizures, any known cause, frequency, known triggers such as stress or bright lights, presence of aura before seizure activity, and history of injuries related to seizures. Drug history should be carefully reviewed and updated at each visit, and any potential drug side effects or drug interactions noted. The drug history can give some indication as to the degree of seizure severity or control. Frequent changes in medications may suggest that seizures are not optimally controlled and that it may be prudent to delay nonurgent dental care. Consultation with the patient's physician may be necessary to determine stability and the appropriate venue in which the patient should receive care (**Box 3**).

It is advisable to check that the patient has taken his/her routine medications, has eaten normally, is not excessively tired, and has not been recently ill before starting dental treatment. Stress and fatigue are factors that can trigger a seizure. If the patient is not feeling well or is overly tired, it may be prudent to reschedule the appointment. Appointments should be scheduled during a time of day when seizures are less likely to occur, if predictable, and stress and anxiety should be minimized. Explaining the dental procedures to the patient before starting, and offering assurance during the procedure may be helpful. The use of nitrous oxide or conscious sedation may be necessary to provide dental care safely and effectively. In patients whose seizure disorder is poorly controlled and whose developmental disabilities make the delivery of dental care difficult, general anesthesia may need to be considered. Light can be a trigger in inducing an epileptic seizure. Dark glasses used as eye protection and careful positioning of the dental light so that it is directed into the mouth and not flashed in the patient's eyes can minimize any problems.

AEDs can significantly impact the oral tissues and cause bleeding disorders. The most significant oral complication seen in epileptic patients is gingival hyperplasia from phenytoin, which can occur in up to 50% of patients taking the drug.[29] Valproic acid and carbamazepine have also demonstrated gingival enlargement. The anterior labial surfaces of the maxillary and mandibular gingiva are the most commonly affected (**Fig. 3**) and it is strongly correlated with poor plaque control. Evidence is lacking regarding the best treatment, but meticulous oral hygiene seems to prevent or significantly decrease the severity of the condition. In severe cases where enlarged

Box 3
Questions to ask dental patients who have epilepsy

Baseline questions as part of the medical history

1. When was the condition diagnosed?
2. What type of seizure occurs?
3. How frequent are seizures? How long do they last?
4. When was the last event?
5. What medications are taken?
6. How do the seizures begin? Do any events act as a trigger?
7. Does a warning (aura) occur before the seizure?
8. Do you lose consciousness during a seizure? Do you get confused or sleepy after a seizure?
9. Any history of seizure related injuries?

Questions asked on the day of dental appointment

1. Have you taken your medications over the last several days and today?
2. Have you had any recent seizures?
3. Are you feeling tired or stressed out today?
4. Have you had any recent illnesses?

Adapted from Jacobsen PL, Eden O. Epilepsy and the dental management of the epileptic patient. J Contemp Dent Pract 2008;9(1):54–62.

tissue interferes with function or appearance, surgical resection is necessary. AEDs can cause xerostomia, which can put patients at increased risk for developing caries, especially in the cervical region and candidiasis. In children, increased dental caries can also be seen if AEDs are delivered in a syrup form. Carbamazepine can cause ulcerations, xerostomia, glossitis, and stomatitis. Valproic acid can decrease platelet count and aggregation, resulting in bleeding problems, especially after surgical trauma.

The frequency of dental check-ups and prophylaxis appointments should be based on the patient's needs. The recall and hygiene interval may be more frequent for epileptic patients because of increased risk for gingival hyperplasia secondary to use of an AED. Patients who are xerostomic should be put on supplemental topical fluoride to prevent dental decay and monitored regularly for candidal infections. The importance of good oral hygiene should be stressed to the patient and caregivers (if appropriate). Aspirin and nonsteroidal anti-inflammatory drugs should be avoided

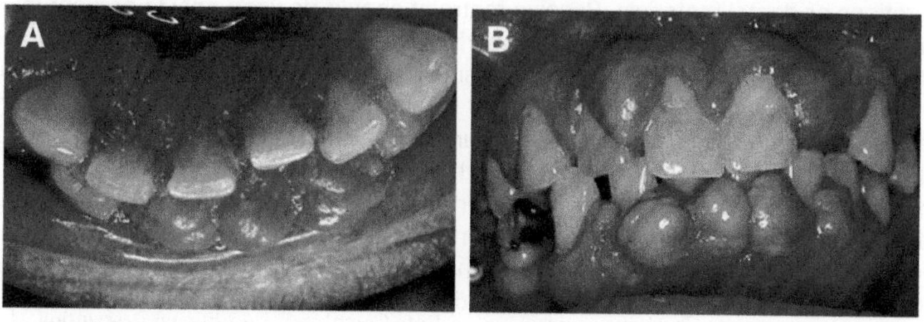

Fig. 3. (*A, B*) Gingival hyperplasia related to phenytoin.

for postoperative pain control in patients taking valproic acid because they can increase the risk for bleeding.

Generalized tonic-clonic seizures often cause minor oral injuries such as tongue biting and tooth injuries. Traumatic injury to anterior teeth should be evaluated in the standard way. Fractures of the anterior teeth can be repaired with composite restorations. A chest radiograph may be indicated if a tooth is avulsed and cannot be accounted for. Soft tissue wounds should be explored for tooth fragments when incisal fractures occur. Patients who have epilepsy can also be at increased risk for maxillofacial fractures caused by AEDs-induced osteoporosis.[30]

The presence of a seizure disorder can influence prosthodontic treatment decisions. Missing teeth should be replaced to prevent the tongue from being caught in the edentulous space and injured. Treatment planning considerations must consider fabrication of dental prostheses designed to minimize the risk for displacement of teeth or further damage. Fixed prostheses or implants are preferable to removable appliances because the latter can dislodge during a seizure and cause oral injury or airway obstruction. Large posterior restorations are prone to fracture in someone who may have jaw spasms during a tonic-clonic seizure. All-metal units should be considered whenever aesthetically possible, to minimize the chance of porcelain fracture. In the anterior, metal crowns with acrylic or composite facings can be used to facilitate repair as needed. For fixed partial dentures, the use of additional abutments may be advisable for more stability. If removable partial prostheses are unavoidable, they should be constructed with metallic palates and bases instead of acrylic and metal backings to anterior denture teeth. Acrylic should be reinforced with wire mesh[31] and more teeth should be clasped to increase retention. The base of complete dentures should also be reinforced with metal or carbon fiber because an acrylic base may fracture, increasing the risk for aspiration or dislodgement into the esophagus during a seizure.

When performing treatment in patients who have a history of generalized tonic-clonic seizures, one should schedule patients to arrive within a few hours of taking their anticonvulsive medications. If the patient can communicate, discuss with the patient the importance of mentioning any aura as soon as it is sensed. Irritability can also be a sign of an impending seizure. Minimize the risk for injury and aspiration during treatment by removing any partial or complete dentures and by using a mouth prop attached to dental floss (for easy retrievability) as a precautionary measure. A rubber dam can be used to keep the oral cavity as free from debris as possible during restorative procedures. If a seizure occurs, protect the individual from further injury by stopping treatment, removing any foreign materials from the mouth if possible, moving all instruments and equipment out of reach, and reclining the dental chair to the supine position as near to the floor as possible. Somebody should record the time the seizure began. No attempt should be made to remove the patient from the chair but, if possible, he/she should be rolled onto his/her side to prevent aspiration of secretions or dental materials. Passive restraint should be used only to prevent injury that may occur from the patient hitting nearby objects or falling out of the chair. Do not put fingers into the patient's mouth because they might be bitten if the individual clenches during a tonic clonic seizure, or attempt to force something between the teeth because this may cause further injury. Most seizures are self-limiting and do not last more than a few minutes. During the postictal state, the patient may fall into a deep sleep and be unarousable for a period of time. During this period, make sure that the patient has a patent airway. Oxygen (6–8 L/min) and suction to remove excessive secretions should be provided. Within a few minutes, the patient should regain consciousness, although he/she may be drowsy and disoriented. Once the patient is stabilized, discontinue treatment and examine the patient for any injuries. Arrange

Box 4
Dental management of the epileptic patient

1. Take a complete health history and a complete seizure history
2. List all medications, including side effects and potential drug interactions
   a. Bleeding tendencies in patients taking valproic acid
   b. Gingival hyperplasia from phenytoin
3. Treatment planning considerations
   a. Minimize risk for damaging or displacing restorations or prostheses during seizure
   b. Frequent recalls with reinforcement of good oral hygiene instructions
   c. Surgical treatment of gingival hyperplasia
4. Provision of dental care
   a. Well controlled: normal care
   b. Poorly controlled: consult with physician
      i. May require adjustment of medications
      ii. Treatment with sedation/general anesthesia
5. Careful positioning of dental light and avoidance of known precipitating factors
6. Consider use of mouth prop at beginning of procedure
7. Management of gran mal seizure
   a. Clear area, move bracket table and instruments away
   b. Chair in supported supine position
   c. If possible, remove any foreign material from mouth
   d. If possible, turn patient onto his/her side
   e. Passively restrain only to prevent patient from falling out of chair or hitting nearby objects
   f. Time duration of seizure
8. After seizure
   a. Turn patient to the side to avoid aspiration
   b. Examine for traumatic injuries
   c. Discontinue care and arrange for patient transport
9. If seizure last more than five minutes or patient become cyanotic
   a. Call 911
   b. Support airway, supplemental oxygen at 6 to 8 L/minute
   c. If equipped, administer 10 mg dose of diazepam IM/IV or 2 mg Ativan IM/IV or 5 mg midazolam IM/IV

From Malamed SF. Medical emergencies in the dental office. 5th edition. St. Louis (MO): Mosby; 2000. p. 309–32; with permission.

for the patient to be transferred to a medical facility if needed, or accompanied home with a family member or caretaker. Seizures lasting more than 5 minutes are considered medical emergencies that require immediate attention (**Box 4**). The emergency medical system should be activated and a benzodiazepine given either intramuscularly (IM) or intravenously (IV).[32]

SUMMARY

Patients who have developmental disabilities and epilepsy can be safely treated in a general dental practice. A thorough medical history should be taken and updated at every visit. A good oral examination to uncover any dental problems and possible side effects from AEDs is necessary. Stability of the seizure disorder must be taken into account when planning dental treatment. Most patients who have epilepsy can and should receive functionally and esthetically adequate dental care.

REFERENCES

1. Epilepsy: facts and myths. Available at: www.epilepsy.com. Accessed on August 20, 2008.
2. Guidelines for epidemiologic studies on epilepsy. Commission on Epidemiology and Prognosis, International League Against Epilepsy. Epilepsia 1993;34(4): 592–6.
3. Sander JW, Shorvon SD. Epidemiology of the epilepsies. J Neurol Neurosurg Psychiatr 1996;61:433–43.
4. Sander JW, Johnson AL, Shorvon SD. National general practice study of epilepsy: newly diagnosed epileptic seizures in a general population. Lancet 1990;336: 1267–71.
5. Centers for Disease Control and Prevention. Epilepsy: one of the nation's most common disabling neurological conditions. October 2005. Available at: http://www.cdc.gov/Epilepsy/index.htm. Accessed September 26, 2008.
6. Epilepsy Foundation. Epilepsy and seizure statistics. Available at: http://www.epilepsyfoundation.org/answerplace/statistics.cfm. Accessed September 26, 2008.
7. Hakijpanayis A, Hadjichrisodoulou C, Youroukos S. Epilepsy in patient with cerebral palsy. Dev Med Child Neurol 1997;39:659–63.
8. Wallace S. Epilepsy in cerebral palsy. Dev Med Child Neurol 2001;43:713–7.
9. Danielsson S, Gillberg IC, Billstedt E, et al. Epilepsy in young adults with autism: a prospective population-based follow-up study of 120 individuals diagnosed in childhood. Epilepsia 2005;46(6):918–23.
10. Sunder TR. Meeting the challenge of epilepsy in persons with multiple handicaps. J Child Neurol 1997;12:S38–43.
11. McDermott S, Moran R, Platt T, et al. Prevalence of epilepsy in adults with mental retardation and related disabilities in primary care. Am J Ment Retard 2005; 110(1):48–56.
12. Alvarez N. Epilepsy in children with mental retardation. August 2007. Available at: http://www.emedicine.com/neuro/TOPIC550.HTM. Accessed September 26, 2008.
13. McKee JR, Bodfish JW. Sudden unexpected death in epilepsy in adults with mental retardation. Am J Ment Retard 2000;105(4):229–35.
14. Proposal for revised clinical and electroencephalographic classification of epileptic seizures. The Commission for Classification and Terminology of the International League Against Epilepsy. Epilepsia 1981;22:489–501.

15. Leppick IE. Contemporary diagnosis and management of the patient with epilepsy. 5th edition. Newtown (PA): Handbooks in Health Care; 2000. p. 9–18.
16. Malamed SF. Managing medical emergencies. J Am Dent Assoc 1993;124(8): 40–51.
17. Panayiotopoulos CP. Typical absence seizures and their treatment. Arch Dis Child 1999;81(4):351–4.
18. Engel J, Pedley TA, Aicardi J. Epilepsy-a comprehensive textbook. Philadelphia: Lippincott-Raven; 1997.
19. Pohlmann-Eden B, Beghi E, Camfield C, et al. The first seizure and its management in adults and children. BMJ 2006;332:339–42.
20. Coulter DL. Comprehensive management of epilepsy in persons with mental retardation. Epilepsia 1997;38(Suppl 4):S24–31.
21. Forsgren L, Edvinsson SO, Blomquist HK, et al. Epilepsy in a population of mentally retarded children and adults. Epilepsy Res 1990;6(3):234–48.
22. Annegers JF. The epidemiology of epilepsy. The treatment of epilepsy: principles and practice. 2nd edition. Baltimore (MD): Williams & Wilkins; 1996. p. 165–72.
23. Brodie MJ, Dichter MA. Drug therapy: antiepileptic drugs. N Engl J Med 1996; 334:168–75.
24. Bryan RB, Sullivan SM. Management of dental patients with seizure disorders. Dent Clin North Am 2006;50(4):607–23.
25. Birbeck GL, Hays RD, Cui X, et al. Seizure reduction and quality of life improvements in people with epilepsy. Epilepsia 2002;43:535–8.
26. Epilepsy action. The ketogenic diet December 2005. Available at: http://www.epilepsy.org.uk/info/ketogenic.html. Accessed on September 28, 2008.
27. American Epilepsy Society – Clinical Epilepsy Education program. Available at: www.aesnet.org/go/professional-development/education/epilepsy-education-program. Accessed September 28, 2008.
28. Karolyhazy K, Kovacs E, Kivovics P, et al. Dental status and oral health of patients with epilepsy: an epidemiologic study. Epilepsia 2003;44(8):1103–8.
29. Thomason JM, Seymour RA, Rawlins MD. Incidence and severity of phenytoin induced gingival overgrowth in epileptic patients in general medical practice. Community Dent Oral Epidemiol 1992;20:288–91.
30. Turner MD, Glickman RS. Epilepsy in the oral and maxillofacial patient: current therapy. J Oral Maxillofac Surg 2005;63:996–1005.
31. Karolyhazy K, Kivovics P, Fejerdy P, et al. Prosthodontic status and recommended care of patients with epilepsy. J Prosthet Dent 2005;93:177–82.
32. Malamed SF. Medical emergencies in the dental office. 5th edition. St. Louis (MO): Mosby; 2000. p. 309–32.

HIV: Medical Milestones and Clinical Challenges

Kelly P. Halligan, DDS, RCSEd-SND[a,*], Timothy J. Halligan, DMD[b], Arthur H. Jeske, DMD, PhD[c], Sheila H. Koh, DDS[d]

KEYWORDS

• HIV • AIDS • Antiretroviral therapy • Vaccine • Dentistry • Ryan White

Since its discovery in the 1980s, HIV has infected every continent on the globe by crossing socioeconomic, racial, ethnic, and gender barriers, and continues to contribute to human morbidity and mortality. Advances in medicine and technology have lead to new combination medications for HIV-positive patients, early HIV testing methodologies, and potential for an HIV vaccine, and they have given researchers and clinicians a larger armamentarium with which to treat and prevent the disease. Even with these vast improvements in HIV prevention, detection, and treatment, scientists have been unsuccessful in developing its vaccine. Therefore, the search for a cure for HIV remains the marathon of the millennium. Dr. Berkley, President and CEO of the International AIDS Vaccine Initiative, states, "With patience and a belief in science, we expect to succeed. And when we have –and AIDS has gone the way of polio and smallpox—people will look back with gratitude on the realists who knew that the only impossible thing was giving up."[1]

Thirty-three million people are currently infected with HIV worldwide (1.1 million in the United States), and as of 2007, 26 million people worldwide have died of AIDS (566,000 in the United States, as of 2006).[2] While our military forces fight the Global War on Terror, scientists and HIV activists strive to combat the global HIV/AIDS pandemic. The demographics of the disease continue to change within and among country and world populations, with new United States cases growing fastest among

[a] Department of Restorative Dentistry, The University of Texas Health Science Center at San Antonio Dental School, Mail Code 7890, 7703 Floyd Curl Drive, San Antonio, TX 78229-3900, USA

[b] 59th Dental Group, Lackland Air Force Base, San Antonio, TX, USA

[c] Strategic Planning, The University of Texas at Houston Health Science Center Dental Branch, 6516 M.D. Anderson Boulevard, Houston, TX 77030, USA

[d] Special Patient Clinic, The University of Texas at Houston Health Science Center Dental Branch, 6516 M.D. Anderson Boulevard, Houston, TX 77030, USA

* Corresponding author.

E-mail address: petersk@uthscsa.edu (K.P. Halligan).

Dent Clin N Am 53 (2009) 311–322
doi:10.1016/j.cden.2008.12.002
0011-8532/08/$ – see front matter

minority women.[3] Because of advances in medicine, HIV-positive patients are living longer with a chronic disease, rather than succumbing to death from acute complications of AIDS. Additionally, advances in science and technology are resulting in the development of new diagnostic modalities, as well as medicines that target specific steps in the HIV lifecycle. With numbers of people living with HIV/AIDS continuing to increase, the search for eradication of this disease continues. The National Institute of Health (NIH) is currently conducting trials with multiple medications in hopes of developing a vaccine to prevent this continued global pandemic. This article reviews the current definitions and classifications of HIV and AIDS, the historical timeline from discovery of HIV until present, HIV pathogenesis, transmission of HIV and infection control issues in a clinical setting, antiretroviral therapy and potential drug interactions, rapid HIV testing, research efforts toward a vaccine, and discussion of the Ryan White Care Act.

HISTORY OF HIV AND AIDS

The history of HIV can be traced back to sub-Saharan Africa, as far back as the 1930s.[4] In 1959, scientists isolated a virus in a human male from the Democratic Republic of Congo. They believe this virus, which was genetically similar to HIV-1 and was called SIVcpz (Chimpanzee Simian Immunodeficiency Virus), migrated from the common chimpanzee to human beings when hunters were exposed to infected ape blood.[5] Using genetic sequencing, scientists later isolated HIV-1, group M, subtype B in a group of the earliest Haitian AIDS patients. According to their findings, this HIV clade originated in central Africa in the 1930s and arrived in Haiti in 1966, when a Haitian professional returned from working in the newly independent Congo.[4] After circulating in Haiti, the virus diversified before migrating to the United States around 1969.[4] It continued to diversify and cryptically circulated among United States homosexual populations until 1981, when AIDS was recognized.[4]

The 1980s and 1990s serve as the most significant historical period for HIV thus far, as this period marked the isolation and discovery of the virus that causes AIDS, the creation of guidelines to define levels of HIV infection and AIDS, and the beginning of the HIV epidemic. In 1981, the Centers for Disease Control and Prevention (CDC) reported five homosexual males in California with biopsy-confirmed *Pneumocystis carinii* pneumonia, as well as 26 cases of Kaposi's sarcoma throughout the United States.[6] By 1982, the CDC was able to link these opportunistic infections to a new blood-borne disease, which they called "Acquired Immune Deficiency Syndrome" or AIDS.[6] Multiple scientists from around the world began searching for an etiology for this disease, including Dr. Robert Gallo of the National Cancer Institute, Dr. Luc Montagnier from the Pasteur Institute in France, and Dr. Jay Levy from the University of California at San Francisco. Each of these scientists identified a retrovirus as the cause of AIDS. However, in 1983, Dr. Luc Montagnier discovered the actual virus we know today as HIV.[7] Because all three scientists had such a profound impact on the discovery of the virus, the President of the United States and the Prime Minister of France made a joint agreement in 1987 to share credit for HIV's discovery.[8] Discovery of the virus stimulated the scientific and medical communities to not only search for a cure from HIV, but also create infection-determining methodologies and epidemiologic-reporting mechanisms.

The 1990s were equally significant as the 1980s for the history of HIV. During this time period, the public became keenly aware of the virus through the efforts of Ryan White and Kimberley Bergalis. In 1990, Ryan White, a young hemophiliac patient who acquired HIV from a blood transfusion, died.[6] However, before he died, he became an HIV/AIDS activist, gaining support from such famous personalities as Elton John and Michael Jackson, and even testifying on HIV/AIDS awareness before Congress.[9] Then, in 1991, Kimberly Bergalis, a dental patient in Florida, made news headlines after acquiring the virus from her dentist. She, too, brought about public awareness of the disease, requesting Congress to mandate testing for all health care personnel.[10] With awareness came increased knowledge about the sequelae of HIV infection, opportunistic infections. Therefore, by 1993, the CDC revised the definition of AIDS to include these opportunistic infections.

Today, HIV is the leading cause of death worldwide among people ages 15 to 59.[11] Approximately 33 million people are living with HIV/AIDS, the majority of whom reside in developing countries.[11] These countries not only lack the infrastructure to combat HIV, but they still have cultural, financial, religious, and discriminatory barriers that prevent them from caring for their infected and affected populations.[11] The resultant profound effects on these populations include a reduction in their economic growth and development, a stunting of their educational systems, and a decrease in their food supply. Therefore, the HIV pandemic has been described as multiple epidemics.[12]

The onset, prevalence, and transmission of the disease remain dynamic and vary among and within countries and world populations. For example, sub-Saharan Africa remains the region with the highest prevalence of adult and childhood HIV cases.[12] The majority of these cases are transmitted through heterosexual contact or from mother to child. Women comprise over 50% of these reported infections.[12] Alternatively, the HIV epidemic was first recognized in the United States as a disease with its transmission most associated with homosexual populations. However, current data suggests the primary mode of HIV transmission in the United States has changed from homosexual to heterosexual contact, with the fastest growing numbers of AIDS cases among young African American females (49%).[12] Finally, in areas of Europe and Asia, HIV disproportionately affects intravenous drug abusers, men having sex with men, and sex workers.[13] Because of their population growth and proximity, epidemiologists predict that countries in these regions will see the next HIV epidemic.[13]

DEFINITION AND CLASSIFICATION

HIV is derived from the *Retroviridae* family of viruses and is a member of the genus, Lentivirus.[14] Two species of this retrovirus infect human beings: HIV-1 and HIV-2. These viruses are the etiology of AIDS. HIV-1 originated from the common chimpanzee, is more virulent than HIV-2, and is responsible for the majority of global HIV infections, including the majority of infections in the United States.[14] HIV-2 originated from the Sooty Mangabay, is less virulent, and is mostly confined to West Africa.[14] HIV-1 can be subdivided into three main groups: M (90% of HIV-1 infections), N (a rare group discovered in Cameroon in 1998), and O (a group restricted to West-central Africa).[15] Group M may be further divided into nine subtypes, called clades: A, B, C, D, F, G, H, J, and K.[16] HIV-1, group M, subtype B is the most widespread HIV variant.[4]

Individuals infected with the HIV virus are called "HIV-positive" and are classified according to the CDC's 1993 Revised Classification System for HIV Infection and Expanded Surveillance Case Definition for AIDS Among Adolescents and Adults or its 1994 Revised Classification System for Human Immunodeficiency Virus Infection in Children Less Than 13 Years of Age.[17] The classification system for adolescents and adults categorizes individuals based on their clinical conditions associated with HIV infection (Categories A, B, C) and their CD4 + T lymphocyte counts per microliter of blood (Categories 1, 2, 3). It is based on four criteria: (*i*) repeatedly reactive screening tests for HIV antibody, with the specific antibody identified by the use of supplemental tests (eg, Western blot, immunofluorescence assay); (*ii*) direct identification of the virus in host tissues by virus isolation; (*iii*) HIV antigen detection; or (*iv*) a positive result on any other highly-specific, licensed test for HIV.[17] Category A patients have asymptomatic HIV infection, persistent generalized lymphadenopathy, or acute (primary) HIV infection with accompanying illness or history of acute HIV infection. Category B patients display clinical conditions that are attributed to HIV infection, indicative of a defect in cell-mediated immunity or are considered by physicians to have a clinical course that is complicated by HIV infection. Common examples of conditions in clinical Category B include, but are not limited to: oropharyngeal candidiasis (thrush), fever (38.5° C), diarrhea lasting greater than 1 month, oral hairy leukoplakia, or Herpes zoster (shingles) involving at least two distinct episodes or more than one dermatome. Patients that fall into Category C have one of 26 AIDS indicator conditions. Examples of such conditions include, but are not limited to: esophageal candidiasis, extrapulmonary cryptococcosis, HIV-related encephalopathy, Human Herpes Virus I (HHV) greater than 1 month in duration, Kaposi's sarcoma, *Mycobacterium tuberculosis*, or *Pneumocystis carinii* pneumonia.[17] The three CD4+ T-lymphocyte categories are defined as follows: Category 1 patients have T cell counts greater than or equal to 500 cells/uL, Category 2 patients have T cell counts between 200 and 499 cells/uL, and Category 3 patients have T cell counts less than 200 cells/uL. Patients in clinical Category 3 are also referred to as patients with the diagnosis of AIDS. Children less than 13 years of age infected with HIV are classified into mutually exclusive categories according to three parameters: (*i*) infection status, (*ii*) clinical status, and (*iii*) immunologic status.[18] This article does not discuss the details of the HIV classification system for children under 13 years of age.

PATHOGENESIS OF HIV

HIV is a 120-nm retrovirus consisting of two copies of positive single-stranded RNA enclosed by a capsid of viral proteins and surrounded by a double-layered phospholipid envelope.[19] Each viral particle consists of 72 copies of a complex protein made up of glycoproteins 120 and 41 that traverse this phospholipid envelope and enable the virus to attach and fuse to target cells. The virus sustains itself through release of viral RNA and multiple viral enzymes into host CD4+ T cells, macrophages, and microglial cells. Its life cycle consists of six steps: binding/fusion, reverse transcription, integration, transcription, translation, and viral assembly and maturation (**Fig. 1**).[19] During binding, glycoprotein 120 (gp 120) adheres to the CD4+ T cell, macrophage, or microglial cell, causing a conformational change in the structure of gp120. While binding is crucial for viral entry, interferes with intracellular signal transduction, and promotes CD4+ apoptosis, this conformational change allows interaction of gp 120 with its coreceptor, CCR5 or CXCR4, enabling fusion.[19] Membrane fusion is dependent on coreceptor binding and is facilitated by glycoprotein 41 (gp41).[19] Once fusion occurs, the two single strands of viral RNA within the viral capsid are released into the host cell cytoplasm, leaving the viral envelope behind. The virus then releases an enzyme, reverse transcriptase, which converts the two strands of viral RNA into double stranded DNA. The viral DNA is transported to the host cell nucleus, where it is incorporated into the host DNA through the action of the viral enzyme, integrase. Once the viral DNA is integrated, the virus is called provirus. This provirus may remain dormant for years; however, once the cell is activated, the two strands of viral DNA separate and are converted into messenger RNA (transcribed) by the host enzymes. The messenger RNA is then carried outside the nucleus to the mitochondria and

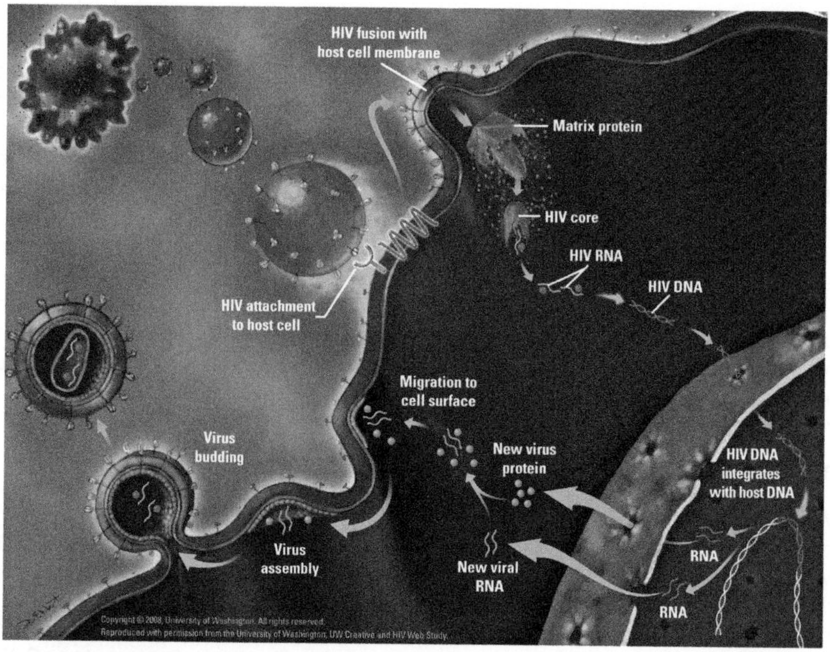

Fig. 1. The HIV lifecycle. (Copyright 2008, University of Washington, with permission.)

processed.[19] As each portion of the messenger RNA is read by the mitochondria, a complementary set of proteins is made (translation). The proteins are cut by a viral enzyme, protease, and then used to create either new viral particles or viral enzymes.[19] These new proteins and enzymes are then assembled and placed inside buds, which extrude from the cell. The buds of new immature viral proteins and enzymes break away from the infected host cell. Shortly after leaving the host cell, viral proteinases become active, cleaving the viral proteins to generate a mature form of HIV. Once mature, the virus is infective.[19]

HIV TRANSMISSION AND OCCUPATIONAL RISK

Knowledge of HIV modes of transmission and its pathogenesis are essential for the prevention of HIV infection. HIV is mainly found in blood, semen, vaginal fluids, and breast milk, and is transmitted through direct contact with these fluids via sexual contact, intravenous drug use, mother-to-child transfer, or occupational exposure.[20] The virus has also been found in small amounts in the saliva and tears of AIDS patients.[20] Oral health care personnel, in particular, are at an increased risk for occupational exposure from a percutaneous injury because of their frequent use of needles and exposure to blood and saliva. However, no cases of HIV transmission through saliva, sweat, or tears from AIDS patients have been recorded.[20]

Factors that influence occupational risk include frequency of infection among patients, type of virus, and type and frequency of blood contact.[21] Likewise, risk factors that affect transmission after a percutaneous injury include depth of the injury, amount of blood on the instrument, proximity of instrument to a vessel, and the disease status of the patient.[21] Finally, virulence of the infectious organism must also be considered. Health care personnel are more likely to acquire an infection from a Hepatitis virus, such as B or C, than HIV. The CDC reports that the risk of acquiring Hepatitis C from a needle stick injury is 1.8%, while the risk of acquiring HIV from the same injury is only 0.3%.[21] Occupational exposure to HIV through a percutaneous injury is considered a medical urgency and should be handled in a timely manner to ensure appropriate postexposure management. The CDC has developed postexposure prophylactic guidelines for health care personnel exposed to HIV-contaminated blood. These guidelines include taking a 4-week regimen of two drugs (zidovudine [ZDV] and lamivudine [3TC]; lamivudine [3TC] and stavudine [d4T]; or didanosine [ddI] and d4T) and serve to minimize the risk of seroconversion after percutaneous injury.[21] The best management of any medical urgency or emergency is prevention. Therefore, health care personnel should implement the elements of universal precautions such as hand-washing, use of personal protective equipment, care of patient equipment and environmental surfaces, and injury preventive measures when treating patients.

ANTIRETROVIRAL MEDICATIONS

HIV has a high error rate during its replication, allowing it to mutate frequently, leading to resistance in therapy. Therefore, various classes of anti-HIV medications have been developed to combat the virus at different stages of its lifecycle. Common classes of antiretroviral medications include: fusion/entry inhibitors, nucleoside, nucleotide, and non-nucleoside reverse transcriptase inhibitors, integrase inhibitors, and protease inhibitors.[22] Fusion/entry inhibitors work by either binding to the coreceptors CCR5 or CXCR4 on the CD 4 cell or by binding to glycoproteins 41 or 120 on the surface of the virus, preventing the attachment of the virus to the host cell.[22] The two Food and Drug Administration (FDA)-approved entry/fusion inhibitors are enfuvirtide (Fuzeon) and maraviroc (Selzentry). Nucleoside, nucleotide, and non-nucleoside reverse transcriptase inhibitors, otherwise known as "nukes" or "non-nukes," contain faulty building blocks used by reverse transcriptase to convert RNA to DNA. They inhibit the reverse transcription step through incorporation of these faulty DNA blocks into the newly transcribed viral DNA, preventing further elongation.[22] Examples of commonly used nucleoside, nucleotide, and non-nucleoside reverse transcriptase inhibitors include, but are not limited to: zidovudine (AZT, Retrovir); didanosine (Videx); tenofovir (Viread); and efavirenz (Sustiva).[22] Integrase inhibitors prevent the incorporation of viral DNA into the CD4 cell's DNA. Raltegravir (Isentress) is currently the only FDA-approved integrase inhibitor.[22] Finally, protease inhibitors prevent the assembly of new viruses by inhibiting the enzyme protease from cutting up the new complementary strand of viral protein from the translated messenger RNA formed during the translation step. Examples of commonly used protease inhibitors include, but are not limited to: indinavir (Crixivan); saquinavir (Invirase); and nelfinavir (Viracept).[22] Additionally, antiretrovirals may be administered in fixed-dose combinations, which combine one or more classes of drugs into one pill, reducing a patient's pill burden. Examples of commonly used fixed dose combinations include Combivir (zidovudine plus lamivudine) and Kaletra (lopinavir and ritonavir).[22]

The currently recommended treatment for HIV-positive patients, called Highly Active Antiretroviral Therapy (HAART), consists of a combination of three or more of the above antiretroviral drugs. HAART targets the virus at multiple stages of its lifecycle in hopes of halting resistant viral strains, slowing the progression of the disease, and lowering the viral load.[23] The primary goals for the initiation of antiretroviral therapy include reduction of HIV-related morbidity and prolonged survival, improved quality of life, restoration and preservation of immunologic function, maximal suppression of viral load, and prevention of vertical transmission of HIV infection.[23] Both the World Health Organization (WHO) and the United States Department of Health and Human Services (DHHS) have established guidelines for the initiation of HIV antiretroviral therapy. These guidelines are based on clinical presentation and CD4 + T cell counts. Treatment in the United States is based on the DHHS guidelines, while WHO guidelines are used in more resource-limited settings.[24] DHHS recommends the initiation of antiretroviral therapy in patients with a history of an AIDS-defining illness, a CD4 T cell count less than 350 cells/mm^3, or severe symptoms of HIV infection regardless of CD4+ T cell count.[24] Antiretroviral therapy should also be initiated in pregnant patients, patients with HIV-associated neuropathy, and patients coinfected with the Hepatitis B virus when treatment is indicated, regardless of their CD4 T cell count.[24] The preferred initial regimen of drugs is efavirenz plus zidovudine plus lamivudine. Other combinations include efavirenze plus tenofovir plus emtricitabine, lopinavir boosted with ritonavir plus zidovudine plus lamivudine, or lopinavir boosted with ritonavir plus tenofovir plus emtricitabine.[24]

The Pharmaceutical Research and Manufacturers Association of America continues to expand its database of developing drugs to treat HIV infection.[25] These new categories of drugs will exploit steps in the viral lifecycle that current medications do not target. Examples of drugs being explored or undergoing current clinical trials include maturation inhibitors, cellular metabolism modulators, immune modulators, and gene therapy, as well as more potent and less toxic protease inhibitors, and nucleoside and non-nucleoside reverse transcriptase inhibitors.[23]

DRUG INTERACTIONS AND ANTIRETROVIRAL THERAPY

A significant challenge faced by HIV-positive patients and their health care provider is the potential for adverse drug interactions. Because HIV-positive patients usually take an antiretroviral regimen of three or more drugs from at least two different classes, potential for unwanted side effects and toxicities also exists. As a matter of fact, out of the 15 approved antiretroviral drugs in 2002, Rainey reported 105 possible two-drug interactions.[26] Drug interactions can be described through their pharmacodynamic (physiologic actions on the body) and pharmacokinetic (metabolic) relationships. Common pharmacodynamic effects include additive (combined effect of two or more agents), synergistic (when the overall effect of two or more agents used together is greater than the sum of the effects the compounds would produce if used separately), and antagonistic (when one drug reduces or cancels out the effect of another drug). Successful HAART relies on additive effects.[27]

HIV antiretroviral therapy levels can also be altered by the body's pharmacokinetic properties. The majority of HIV medications on the market are metabolized through the liver via the cytochrome P450 enzyme system (CYP450). More specifically, the most abundant isoenzyme of the CYP450 system, CYP3A4, metabolizes about half of the antiretroviral drugs currently on the market.[26] Because the drugs are metabolized through the same pathway, competition exists among drugs to bind to the isoenzymes. This competition may then cause an increase in the blood plasma level of drugs, leading to drug toxicities, unwanted side effects, and potential resistant HIV strains. However, not all drug interactions have negative consequences. Some protease inhibitors, such as ritonavir, serve to boost other drug levels.[26] These protease inhibitors can be administered at lower dosages, thereby reducing the metabolism of other simultaneously administered antiretroviral drugs.[26]

Dentists should be keenly aware of potential drug interactions in their HIV-positive patients. Many of the medications dentists commonly administer or prescribe may interfere with the metabolism of the antiretroviral medications. Common examples of medications dentists may administer or prescribe that are metabolized by the cytochrome P450 enzyme system include anxiolytics, such as trizolam (Halcion), and macrolide antibiotics (such as clarithromycin, or erthromycin).[28] Because drug-drug interactions play a large role in the treatment of HIV-positive patients, oral health care personnel should take a comprehensive medical history of their patients, have a thorough understanding of potential interactions between medicines they administer or prescribe and the patient's antiretroviral medications, and consider prescribing medications from a different class to avoid these interactions.

RAPID HIV TESTING

Diagnostic methodologies to detect HIV infection have improved since the discovery of the virus. The CDC reports 40,000 new cases of HIV in the United States annually since the 1990s, with approximately 50% of patients not in treatment and approximately 25% of HIV-positive patients who do not know their HIV status.[29] Unfortunately, a disproportionate number of new cases are reported among ethnic minorities: almost one-half among African Americans, 16% among Hispanics, and 32% among Caucasians.[29] Women exhibit the fastest growth in newly diagnosed patients.[29] For those patients not in care or who do not know their status, fear seems to be the main barrier for not seeking test results or treatment. Patients state this fear as fear of rejection from family and friends, job loss and loss of benefits, and fear of needles.[30] This fear then leads to a delay in testing, continued practice of disease-transmitting behaviors, and continued progression of the disease. Because of this delay, only 40% to 50% of HIV-positive patients are diagnosed with AIDS within 1 year of first testing HIV-positive.[31]

The CDC recently announced an initiative to reduce barriers to early diagnosis and increase access to treatment and prevention. This initiative, "Advancing HIV Prevention: New Strategies for a Changing Epidemic," expands on the 1993 recommendations for testing inpatients and outpatients in acute-care hospital settings and stresses the importance of rapid HIV tests.[32] In an effort to facilitate this initiative, the FDA has approved the use of four rapid HIV tests: OraQuick/OraQuick Advance Rapid HIV-1/2 Antibody Test (OraSure Technologies, Inc., Bethlehem, Pennsylvania), Reveal/Reveal G2 Rapid HIV-1 Antibody Test (MedMira Laboratories, Inc., Halifax, Nova Scotia), Uni-Gold Recombigen HIV Test (Trinity Biotech, PLC., Bray, County Wicklow, Ireland), and Multispot HIV-1/HIV-2 Rapid Test (Bio-Rad Laboratories, Hercules, California).[32] Two of these tests, OraQuick/OraQuick Advance and Uni-Gold are CLIA-waived (Clinical Laboratory Improvements Amendment of 1988), which means that they can be performed by persons without formal laboratory training outside traditional laboratory settings.[32] However, state and local regulations and laws may still apply.[30] All four tests require whole blood samples from fingerstick or venipuncture. However, OraQuick Advance is the only test that uses saliva as a testing specimen.[32] These screening tests, which are visually interpreted, detect HIV antibodies and require confirmatory testing by Western blot or an immunofluorescent assay, if reactive. They have sensitivity levels that exceed 99%, with specificities up to 100%.[30] In 2003, the CDC, along with the FDA and the Centers for Medicare and Medicaid Services, developed guidelines for centers administering the OraQuick Rapid HIV-Antibody Test. These guidelines, called, Assurance Guidelines for Testing Using the OraQuick Rapid HIV-1 Antibody Test, allow testing centers to develop a quality-assurance program, including policies, processes, and procedures for administration of the test.[32]

All patients who take the rapid HIV test must receive before- and after-test counseling. Before-test counseling sessions should include information about HIV/AIDS, routes of transmission, sensitivities and specificities of different tests, discrimination issues, partner notification issues, and risk-reduction behaviors. After-test counseling should include assessing the client's preparedness to receive the results, the meaning of the reactive test, and the need for confirmatory testing.[30,32]

Dental offices may serve as an alternative site for HIV testing.[30] Performing rapid HIV testing in these nontraditional sites would not only decrease barriers to diagnosis and care, but would ultimately decrease the morbidity and mortality of the disease by increasing the number of people who learn their results and giving them access to early prevention and treatment measures.[32] If dental offices choose to provide HIV testing, they must comply with the Clinical Laboratory Improvements Amendment of 1988, follow the CDC/FDA-recommended quality assurance guidelines, and provide proper staff training in counseling as well as be able to direct HIV-positive patient to the appropriate social and medical support services.[32]

HIV VACCINE

Since the discovery of HIV, scientists and researchers have been unsuccessful in the search for its vaccine. Development of vaccines for diseases can take many years. For example, it took 47 years to develop the polio vaccine and 42 years to develop the measles vaccine.[31] Current viral vaccines induce humoral immunity (which uses antibodies to defend against free viruses), or cellular immunity (which uses activated immune cells to combat virus-infected cells).[33] Because HIV exists as both free virus and within infected cells, the ideal vaccine would stimulate both a humoral and cellular immunity. Additionally, because approximately 80% of HIV worldwide is transmitted sexually, scientists are looking at developing a vaccine that also produces mucosal immunity.[33] Scientists are looking at concepts including using live-attenuated virus (similar to vaccines given for measles, mumps, whooping cough), whole-killed virus (such as the influenza and Salk polio vaccines), live vectors, recombinant viral proteins, pseudovirions, DNA, peptide epitopes, or a combination of these.[33] However, the virus poses many challenges for developing a vaccine, such as its ability to continue to mutate and recombine, its ability to infect helper T cells, inhibiting the immune response, its ability to be transmitted as both free virus and in infected cells, and not having a clearly identified natural immunity to HIV.[33]

The Division of AIDS of the National Institute of Allergy and Infectious Diseases (NIAID) at the NIH continues to develop research programs focused on the discovery of an HIV vaccine.[34] Additionally, NIAID supports clinical trials currently being conducted by governmental, private, and military research programs. However, a recent human trial was unsuccessful. One of the most promising studies had been the STEP study by Merck and Co. This 3,000-patient study hypothesized that high-risk patients with a low immune response to Adenovirus 5 (a cold virus used as a vector to deliver the vaccine) would have a smaller chance of acquiring HIV when exposed to the virus or would have a decrease in their viral load if they became infected, compared with those patients who received the placebo.[35] Unfortunately, the study was halted in December 2007, as the data suggested that the vaccine did not support either hypothesis. Additionally, the initial results suggested that those study participants with preexisting immunity to Adenovirus 5 had an increased chance of acquiring HIV once exposed to the virus.[33] With this information, the scientists at NIAID have decided to rethink their goals on developing an HIV vaccine, focusing more efforts on basic research and less on human trial testing.

THE RYAN WHITE CARE ACT

In 1984, Ryan White,[36] a 13 year-old hemophiliac patient, was diagnosed with HIV after receiving a blood transfusion. Unfortunately, because of ignorance and fear, the community with which he resided responded to his diagnosis with discrimination, not allowing him to attend school. Ryan and his family gained international notoriety fighting for his right to attend school and educating others about HIV/AIDS. He was instrumental throughout the 1980s in shifting the perceptions of HIV/AIDS as a disease most associated with homosexual communities to a disease that could affect all populations. Before meeting his premature death in 1990, Ryan was invited to speak before the United States Congress and testified before the National Commission on AIDS.[36]

In 1990, the federal government created the Ryan White Comprehensive AIDS Resources Emergency (CARE) Act.[36] The Act, sponsored by Senator Edward Kennedy and administered by the U.S. Department of Human Services, Health Resources and Services Administration Bureau (HRSA), was created to improve availability of care for uninsured and under-insured HIV/AIDS patients and their families. It builds on Medicaid and is the only disease-specific discretionary grant program for care of people with HIV/AIDS. The Act is divided into different components or parts, formerly called "Titles." Funds for each part are appropriated by Congress annually and are distributed to applicants based upon meeting the defined criteria for that part. These criteria include population type (ie, state, eligible metropolitan area, and so forth), size, and prevalence of the disease within that population. A detailed description of the Act and each part can be viewed on the HRSA Web site, http://www.hrsa.gov.[37] Dental services may be reimbursed to grant recipients through parts A, B, and F by meeting the appropriate criteria. The Ryan White Care Act has been reauthorized by Congress three times: in 1996, 2000, and 2006.

HIV AND DENTISTRY

Statistically, the chances of treating a HIV-positive patient in a dental practice have increased because of a steady state of new HIV infections annually and increasing longevity from highly active antiretroviral therapy. Thus, HIV-positive patients are seeking routine dental care versus episodic treatment for the oral manifestations of HIV/AIDS, and dental clinicians should know how to appropriately care for them.[38] Controversy exists in the literature regarding the need for antibiotic coverage before performing dentistry. A small subgroup of patients with advanced HIV disease may require customized modification, such as antibiotic prophylaxis or transfusion of blood products for their care. However, no data currently exists supporting the need for routine antibiotic coverage to prevent bacteremia or septicemia arising from a dental procedure.[39] Additionally, the dental clinician should know the medications their HIV-positive patients are taking to treat their disease, understand the potential drug interactions with medications they prescribe, and be prepared to prescribe medications from a different class when interactions are possible. Finally, the practitioner should be aware of occupational risks in treating these patients, should familiarize himself or herself with the CDC's postexposure prophylactic guidelines, implement preventive measures to prevent occupational exposures, and provide occupational risk training for his or her staff.

REFERENCES

1. Berkley S. We are making progress on AIDS. Wall St J. April 25, 2008;A13. Available at: http://www.aegis.com/news/wsj/2008/WJ080406.html. Accessed June 19, 2008.

2. In search of an AIDS vaccine: rededication follows disappointment. Washington Post 2008;A14. Monday, April 21. Available at: http://www.washingtonpost.com. Accessed July 14, 2008.
3. Dietz CA, Ablah E, Reznik D, et al. Patients' attitudes about rapid oral HIV screening in an urban free clinic. AIDS Patient Care STDS 2008;22(3):205–12.
4. Gilbert MT, Rambaut A, Wlasiuk G, et al. Proceedings of the National Academy of Sciences of the United States of America. The emergence of HIV/AIDS in the Americas and beyond. Published October 31, 2007. Available at: http://www.pnas.org. Accessed August 28, 2008;104:18566–70.
5. Lears MK, Alwood K. The natural history, current status, and future trends of HIV infection. Lippincotts Prim Care Pract 2000;4(2):1–19.
6. HIV timeline. Available at: http://www.aegis.com/topics/timeline/. Accessed September 5, 2008.
7. Cichoki M, Montagnier L. Available at: http://aids.about.com/od/themindsofhivaids/p/montagnier.htm. Updated December 30, 2004. Accessed September 5, 2008.
8. Discovery of HIV. Available at: http://aidshistory.nih.gov/discovery_of_HIV/index.html. Updated June 4, 2001. Accessed August 29, 2008.
9. White Ryan. Available at: http://en.Wikipedia.org/wiki/Ryan_White#Ryan_White_and_public_perception_of_AIDS. Updated September 4, 2008. Accessed September 6, 2008.
10. Bergalis Kimberly. Available at: http://en.wikipedia.org/wiki/Kimberly_Bergalis. Updated August 28, 2008. Accessed September 3, 2008.
11. HIV Demographics. Published July, 2008, Available at: http://www.unaids.org/en/KnowledgeCentre/HIVData/Epidemiology/epidemiologySlidesAuto.asp. Accessed September 5, 2008.
12. The Henry J. Kaiser Family Foundation. The multisectoral impact of the HIV/AIDS epidemic-a primer. Published July, 2007. Available at: http://www.kff.org. Accessed September 4, 2008.
13. UNAIDS: the Joint United Nations Programme on HIV/AIDS. Published July, 2008, Available at: http://data.unaids.org/pub/GlobalReport/2008/JC1511_GR08_ExecutiveSummary_en.pdf. Accessed July 31, 2008.
14. HIV Structure. Available at: en.wikipedia.org/wiki/HIV#Structure_and_genome. Updated August 29, 2008. Accessed September 4, 2008.
15. Noble R. HIV types. Available at: http://www.avert.org/hivtypes.htm. Updated September 5, 2008. Accessed September 6, 2008.
16. Walker BD, Burton DR. Towards an AIDS vaccine. Science 2008;320:760–4.
17. Centers for Disease Control and Prevention, Morbidity and Mortality Weekly Report. HIV classification system for adults. Published December 25, 1992. Available at: http://www.cdc.gov/mmwr/preview/mmwrhtml/00018179.htm. Updated May 5, 2001. Accessed July 23, 2008.
18. Centers for Disease Control and Prevention, Morbidity and Mortality Weekly Report. HIV classification system for children. Published September 30, 1994. Available at: http://wonder.cdc.gov/wonder/prevguid/m0032890/m0032890.asp#head001000000000000. Updated August 29, 2007. Accessed July 23, 2008.
19. Noble R. HIV structure and lifecycle. Available at: http://www.avert.org/virus.htm. Updated March 14, 2008. Accessed June 28, 2008.
20. Centers for Disease Control and Prevention, HIV transmission. Available at: http://www.cdc.gov/hiv/resources/factsheets/transmission.htm. Updated March 8, 2008. Accessed July 16, 2008.

21. Centers for Disease Control and Prevention. Guidelines for infection control in dental health-care settings. Available at: http://www.cdc.gov/OralHealth/infectioncontrol/guidelines/ppt.htm. Updated November 6, 2008. Accessed July 28, 2008.
22. Aidsmeds, Antiretroviral medications. Available at: http://www.aidsmeds.com/archive/NRTIs_1082.shtml#Question. Updated May 5, 2008. Accessed July 29, 2008.
23. National Institute of Health, HIV treatment. Available at: http://www.aidsinfo.nih.gov/contentfiles/ApprovedMedstoTreatHIV_FS_en.pdf. Updated Februrary, 2008. Accessed July 16, 2008.
24. World Health Organization, HIV treatment guidelines. Published August 7, 2006. Available at: http://www.who.int/hiv/pub/guidelines/en/. Accessed July 16, 2008.
25. National Institute of Allergy and Infectious Diseases, HIV treatment. Available at: http://www.niaid.nih.gov/factsheets/treat-hiv.htm. Accessed July 16, 2008.
26. Rainey PM. HIV drug interactions: the good, the bad, and the other. Ther Drug Monit 2002;24(1):26–31.
27. HIghleyman L. HIV therapy. Published summer, 2005. Available at: http://www.thebody.com/content/art2579.html. Accessed July 30, 2008.
28. Ledirac N, de Sousa G, Fontaine F, et al. Effects of macrolide antibiotics on CYP3A expression in human and rat hepatocytes: interspecies differences in response to troleandomycin. Drug Metab Dispos 2000;28(12):1391–3.
29. Glynn M, Rhodes P. CDC. Estimated HIV prevalence in the United States at the end of 2003. Available at: http://www.cdc.gov/hiv/resources/factsheets/us.htm. Presentation at the National HIV Prevention Conference 2005. Accessed July 5, 2008.
30. Glick M. Rapid HIV testing in the dental setting. J Am Dent Assoc 2005;136:1206–7.
31. Samet JH, Freedberg KA, Savetsky JB, et al. Understanding delay to medical care for HIV infection: the long-term non-presenter. AIDS 2001;15:77–85.
32. Greenwald JL, Burstein GR, Pincus J, et al. A rapid review of rapid HIV antibody tests. Curr Infect Dis Rep 2006;8:125–31.
33. Allen MA. National Institute of Allergy and Infectious Diseases. HIV vaccine. Published November 8, 1997. Available at: http://www3.niaid.nih.gov/research/topics/HIV/vaccines/reports/forum_slides/Slide03.htm. Updated April 26, 2006. Accessed July 18, 2008.
34. Be the generation. HIV vaccine. Available at: http://www.bethegeneration.org/go/about-the-education-initiative. Updated March 13, 2007. Accessed July 23, 2008.
35. National Institute of Allergy and Infectious Diseases, HIV vaccine. Available at: http://www3.niaid.nih.gov/research/topics/HIV/vaccines/advisory/avrs/avrs.htm. Updated June 23, 2008. Accessed July 23, 2008.
36. White Ryan. Available at: www.ryanwhite.com. Accessed July 27, 2008.
37. White Ryan. U.S. Department of Health and Human Services, Health Resources and Services Administration. Available at: http://www.hrsa.gov/about. Accessed September 8, 2008.
38. Campo J, Cano J, del Romero J, et al. Oral complication risks after invasive and non-invasive dental procedures in HIV-positive patients. Oral Dis 2007;13:110–6.
39. Lyles AM. What the dentist should know about treating the patient with HIV/AIDS. J Calif Dent Assoc February, 2001. Available at: http://www.cda.org/library/cda_member/pubs/journal/jour0201/index.html. Accessed September 28, 2008.

Dental Care for Patients Who Are Unable to Open Their Mouths

Burton L. Nussbaum, DDS, RCS Ed[a,b,c,*]

KEYWORDS

- Anesthesia • Fibrodysplasia ossificans progressiva
- Mobius syndrome • Inanition • Awake fiberoptic intubation
- Buccal access • Pemphigus • Rheumatoid arthritis

There are a number of diseases and conditions that prevent the sufferer from adequately opening the mouth. These people cannot chew food, brush the lingual or palatal surfaces of the teeth, have routine dental care, or even throw up without the emesis being caught in the teeth. The danger of inanition, malnutrition, chronic periodontal disease, caries, and abscessed teeth are very real to this population. Dental treatment issues include inadequate access to the oral cavity, inability to locally anesthetize mandibular posterior teeth, inability to gain access for traditional operative dentistry, and lack of clearance for most oral surgery procedures. Even worse, these people cannot have their throats examined, their tonsils checked, or have general anesthesia by direct laryngoscopy. The purpose of this article is to provide the reader with a discussion of the various conditions and then discuss the dental and anesthesia issues for this unique population. The most extreme example of patients who cannot open their mouths is fibrodysplasia ossificans progressiva. The article presented will focus on this most extreme medical disease. The other diseases presented have problems along a continuum.

SIX DISEASES WHOSE COMMON LINK IS RESTRICTED ORAL ACCESS

Fibrodysplasia ossificans progressiva (FOP) is characterized by congenital malformation of the great toes, short thumbs, and by a progressive postnatal heterotopic ossification of the soft tissues in characteristic anatomic patterns.[1–5] It is an autosomal dominant disease that appears within the first decade of life following trauma-induced

[a] Dentistry for Special People, 1910E Marlton Pike, Suite 9, Cherry Hill, NJ 08003, USA
[b] University of Pennsylvania School of Dental Medicine, The Children's Hospital of Philadelphia, Philadelphia, PA, USA
[c] Thomas Jefferson University Medical School and Hospital, Philadelphia, PA, USA
* Dentistry for Special People, 1910E Marlton Pike, Suite 9, Cherry Hill, NJ 08003.
E-mail address: dentspecpeople@aol.com

Dent Clin N Am 53 (2009) 323–328
doi:10.1016/j.cden.2008.12.006
dental.theclinics.com

or spontaneous flare-ups.[1,4,6,7] FOP is caused by mutations in the bone morphogenetic protein type 1 receptor ACVR1.[7,8] The person is rendered immobile following progressive episodes of heterotopic ossification involving all major joints of the axial and appendicular skeletons.[5,9–11] The temperomandibular joint is not spared immobility and all joint ossifications begin within the first decade of life. In this disease, overstretching of the jaws, mandibular blocks, and surgical trauma from resecting heterotopic bone can lead to episodes of explosive bone formation around those soft tissue sights.[1,4,12] Abnormalities of the temperomandibular joint are noted early in life, even without heterotopic ossification.[10] The dental issues of patients with FOP are the same as in the general population. They can develop caries, periodontal disease, and their teeth can be impacted as well.[13]

Moebius syndrome is a rare congenital disorder primarily involving the facial (VII) and the abducent (VI) nerves. Occasionally the V, X, XI, and XII nerves are affected, causing difficulty in swallowing, chewing, and coughing. This often leads to respiratory complications. Some patients have mental retardation and autism.[14–16] Also possible in this syndrome are opthalmolplegia externa, lingual palsey, clubfoot, branchial malformation, and ptosis. From a dental point of view, multiple missing teeth in both the primary and permanent dentitions, paralysis, and hypoplasia of the tongue can be manifested.[17] A child with Moebius syndrome may not be able to close his mouth. There may be low muscle tone of the tongue, soft palate, pharynges, and the masticatory system.[18] Hypoplastic teeth are common in both the primary and permanent dentitions. The primary teeth may be slow to exfoliate.[17,18] The saliva may be thick or the patient may have dry mouth, leading to causes of tooth decay.[18]

Pemphigus describes a group of autoimmune blistering diseases of the skin and mucous membranes. The main action is caused by circulating immunoglobulin G against keratinocyte cell surfaces. Patients with active disease have circulating and tissue-bound autoantibodies og IgG1 and IgG4 subclasses. There are three subsets of the disease: pemphigus vulgaris, pemphigus foliaceus, and paraneoplastic pemphigus. Pemphigus vulgaris accounts for 70% of the cases. The incidence of the disease is 0.5 to 3.2 cases per 100,000. It is seen worldwide with a predilection to Mediterranean people and Ashkenazi Jews. The mean age of onset is at 50 to 60 years. In the mouth, intact bullae are rare, but most patients have buccal or palatal erosions that are hard to heal.[19,20] Dental management is complicated because of the oral mucosal involvement. There is increased risk of oral disease and great difficulty rendering dental care.[21] Treatment is rendered using systemic cortcosteroids.[20]

Rheumatoid arthritis (RA) is a chronic multisystem disease of autoimmune etiology. Medical complications caused by RA can affect the ability to provide oral health care. Women are three times more likely to be affected in a disease that appears between ages 35 and 50. Inflammatory disease affects small joints, leading to destruction of the cartilage and juxta-articular bone. In addition, patients feel fatigue, loss of appetite, and musculoskeketal pain. Treatment can involve physical therapy, surgery, and use of injected corticosteroids. Temperomandibular joint involvement is common. There is an increased incidence of alveolar bone involvement and teeth. There can be a decrease in salivary flow causing dental caries.[22]

Hecht-Beals syndrome (HB) is a rare condition causing congenital oral trismus. It is caused by bilateral fibrous bands on the anterior border of the masseter muscles. The condition is inoperable as the bands recur after surgery.[23,24]

Epidermolysis bullosa is a group of dermatologic diseases that are characterized by muccocutaneous fragility and blister formation. The blisters can occur spontaneously or by minimal mechanical trauma. Blistering repeatedly causes atrophy of the mucosa, causing microstomia, ankyloglossia, tongue denudation, and vestibule obliteration.[25]

The most severe form of Epidermolysis Bullosa is characterized by sub-lamina dura separation, caused by blistering below the basement membrane of the cell.[26]

To summarize, presented are six diseases and conditions that relate as having limited access to the oral cavity. Some of the problems are a result of scarring and so the limitation is that of soft tissue. Some of the limitation is a result of attack on the bone, limiting oral opening where the soft tissue is normal.

PREVENTIVE DENTISTRY

Clearly, the best way to prevent dealing with any of the six diseases of limited oral access is through a preventive dental program. It is essential in childhood that preventive measures become routine.[13,18,22,27] Fluoridated water is essential, as well as fluoridated toothpastes.[13,18,22,27] Chlorhexidine rinses are recommended, especially in places where there is disease and very little oral access. In those patients with limited access and the inability to rinse the teeth, chlorhexidine can be applied with a toothette.[13,18,22,27,28] Flossing manually or with aides is paramount.[13,18,22,27] A battery-powered dental flosser can gain access between the teeth for those unable to open their teeth. Many of these patients require a caregiver to assist in daily oral hygiene. Reduction or elimination of refined carbohydrates in the diet is essential.[13,18,22,27,28]

RESTORATIVE DENTISTRY

In patients with limited access to the oral cavity, classical restorative dentistry becomes quite difficult. It is necessary to use nontraditional approaches to caries removal and restoration. Dental materials need to be chosen to reflect the access to the cavity preparation, the oral hygiene, and the salivary flow. In patients with jaw fusion or patients with little or no vestibular access, access to caries may be accessible through a buccal approach instead of through the occlusal. Using very small round burrs on a slow speed handpiece, access to small occusal fissures can be gained. Pediatric instruments should be used, including short shank burrs.[25] For interproximal cavity preparations, metal matrix strips can be threaded between the teeth and wedged into place. Flowable dental materials allow placement in very hard-to-reach areas. For patients with poor oral hygiene, reduced salivary flow, or inability to gain complete access to the teeth, glass ionomer restorative materials offer fluoride release and protection.[27,28] In patients with vessiculo-bullous diseases, coat the mucosa with a lubricant to prevent adherence and lesion formation.[25]

ANESTHESIA: LOCAL AND GENERAL

Pain control is as important in this population as any other. When working in an area of limited access, if the patient is in pain from the procedure, accidents could happen. However, in limited access zones, how can adequate pain control be provided?

Unless the lips and anterior vestibule are so scarred that there is no access, traditional infiltration of local anesthesia can be performed on the anterior teeth. In the mandibular arch, infiltration of local anesthetic can be performed successfully through the premolar teeth. It is difficult to gain intraoseous penetration of local anesthetic in the molar regions. It may be possible to perform intraosseous anesthesia. In patients who can open their teeth, mandibular block anesthesia can be performed. In patients with RA, HB or FOP, this is not the case. None of these diseases allows opening in the advanced stages. If FOP patients have block anesthesia, they may set up a reaction that will fuse the jaw shut forever. In HB and RA, surgery on the joint is possible and temporary to gain access temporarily.

In those cases where local anesthesia is not possible, then the only answer is general anesthesia.[29] After preventive dentistry fails, if the restoration cannot be performed in the small space or periodontal disease is too great, surgical dentistry may be the only option to prevent further pain or systemic infection. The difficult part for these cases is successful intubation. Blind nasal intubations are not always successful.[30] Administration of general anesthetics can cause laryngospasms. If the patient cannot obtain oxygen during this event, death is likely to occur. In patients with slight opening, a laryngeal mask airway may be used, but the airway is not secured against fluid leakage. This may be used in nondental situations.[31,32] Another option is an "awake fiberoptic intubation." Here, a skilled anesthesiologist passes a breathing tube fiberoptically into the trachea. The patient, although sedated, can breathe spontaneously and control his secretions until general anesthesia after tube placement.[27] General anesthesia provides the pain control, relieving the need for local except for hemostasis.

ORAL SURGERY

Extraction of erupted teeth and even more in impacted teeth proves a great challenge in people who offer little access to their mouths. The really scary issue is the loss of a tooth or a piece of a tooth in a clenched mouth, with no simple way to fish out the piece. It may be possible in cases of no access or little access to use an elevator and forceps to extract anterior teeth. In the posterior dentition, no room for forceps is usually evident. For pain control these patients must be under general anesthesia.[29] A buccal approach is made to gain access to the teeth to be extracted. An incision is made along the alveolar crest and the tissue is reflected. A burr is used to remove the buccal bone, exposing the roots. A malleable neurosurgery retractor can be used to protect the palatal or lingual space. The tooth is then sectioned and removed to the buccal. Impactions are removed in a similar fashion.[33]

ACKNOWLEDGMENTS

The author thanks the surgical team at Thomas Jefferson University Hospital for their inspiration: Dr. Zvi Grunwald, Chief of Anesthesia, Dr. Robert Diecidue, Chief of Oral and Maxillofacial Surgery, and Dr. Daniel Taub, Asst Chief of Oral and Maxillofacial Surgery. Finally, the author thanks Dr. Frederick E. Kaplan, Chief of Metabolic Orthopedics, University of Pennsylvania School of Medicine, who inspired the journey into this niche of special needs dentistry.

REFERENCES

1. Connor JM, Evans DA. Fibrodysplasia ossificans progressiva (FOP): the clinical features and natural history of 34 patients. J Bone Joint Surg Br 1982;64:76–83.
2. Cohen RB, Hahn GV, Tabas J, et al. The natural history of heterotopic ossification in patients who have fibrodysplasia ossificans progressiva. J Bone Joint Surg Am 1993;75:215–9.
3. Rocke DM, Zasloff M, Peeper J, et al. Age and joint-specific risk of initial heterotopic ossification in patients who have fibrodysplasia ossificans progressiva. Clin Orthop Relat Res 1994;301:243–8.
4. Kaplan FS, Shore EM, Connor JM. Fibrodysplasia ossificans progressiva. In: Royce PM, Steinmann B, editors. Connective tissue and its heritable disorders:

molecular, genetic, and medical aspects. 2nd edition. New York: Wiley-Liss: John Wiley & Sons; 2002. p. 827–40.
5. Kaplan F, Merrer M, Glaser D, et al. Fibrodysplasia ossificans progressiva. Best Practice & Research Clinical Rheumatology 2008;22(1):191–205.
6. Lachoney TF, Cohen RB, Rocke DM, et al. Permanent heterotopic ossification at the injection site after diphtheria-tetanus-pertussis immunizations in children who have fibrodysplasia ossificans progressiva. J Pediatr 1995;126:762–4.
7. Shore E, Xu M, Feldman G, et al. A recurrent mutation in the BMP type 1 receptor ACVR1 causes inherited and sporadic fibrodysplasia ossificans progressive. Nature Genetics 2006;38(5):525–7.
8. Kaplan FS, Xu M, Seemann P, et al. Classic and atypical fibrodysplasia ossificans progressiva (FOP) phenotypes are caused by mutations in the bone morphogenetic protein (BMP) type 1 receptor ACVR1. Human Mutation 2008; e pub ahead of print.
9. Connor JM, Evans DA. Extra-articular ankylosis in fibrodysplasia ossificans progressiva. Br J Oral Surg 1982;20:117–21.
10. Renton P, Parkin SF, Stamp TV. Abnormal temperomandibular joints in fibrodysplasia ossificans progressiva. British Journal of Oral Surgery 1982;20:31–8.
11. el-Labbn NG, Hopper C, Barber P. Ultrastructural finding of vascular degeneration in fibrodysplasia ossificans progressiva. J Oral Pathol Med 1995;24:125–9.
12. Luchetti W, Cohen RB, Hahn GV, et al. Severe restriction in jaw movement after routine injection of local anesthetic in patients who have fibrodysplasia ossificans progressiva. Oral Surg Oral Med Oral Pathol Oral Radiol Endod 1996;81:21–5.
13. Nussbaum BL, O'hara I, Kaplan FS. Fibrodysplasia ossificans progressiva: report of a case with guidelines for pediatric dental and anesthetic management. J Dent Child 1996;63:448–50.
14. Sensat ML. Mobius syndrome: a dental hygiene case study and review of literature. Int J Dent Hyg 2003;1(1):62–7.
15. Gondipalli P, Tobias JD. Anesthetic implications of Mobius syndrome. J Clin Anesth 2006;18(1):55–9.
16. Ha CY, Messieha ZS. Management of a patient with Mobius syndrome: a case report. Spec Care Dentist 2003;23(3):111–6.
17. De Serpa Pinto MV, De Magalhaes MH, Nunes FD. Mobius syndrome with oral involvement. Int J Paediatr Dent 2002;123(6):446–9.
18. Osborne G. A message from a dentist and a Moebius dad. Moebius Syndrome Foundation; 1996. p. 1–3.
19. Bassam Z. Pemphigus vulgairs. Available at: EMedicine.Com. Accessed March 14, 2007. p. 1–16.
20. Scully C, Paes De Almeida O, Porter SR, et al. Pemphigus vulgaris: the manifestations and long-term management of 55 patients with oral lesions. British Journal of Dermatology 1999;140(1):84–9.
21. Fatahzadeh M, Radfar L, Sirois DA. Dental care of patients with autoimmune vesiculobullous diseases. Quintessence Int 2006;37:737–87.
22. Treister BA, Glick M. Rheumatoid arthritis: a review and suggested dental care considerations. J Am Dent Assoc 1999;130:689–98.
23. Adams C, Rees M. Congenital trismus secondasry to masseteric fibrous bands: endoscopically assisted exploration. J Craniofac Surg 1999;10(4):375–9.
24. Tveteras K, Kristensen S. The aetiology and pathogenesis of trismus. Clin Otolaryngol Allied Sci 1986;11(5):383–7.
25. Siqueira MA, de Souza Silva J, Silva FW, et al. Dental treatment in a patient with epidermolysis bullosa. Spec Care Dentist 2008;28(3):92–5.

26. Pacheco W, Marques de Sousa AR. Orthodontic treatment of a patient with recessive dystrophic epidermolysis bullosa: a case report. Spec Care Dentist 2008; 28(4):136–9.
27. Nussbaum BL, Grunwald Z, Kaplan FS. Oral and dental health care and anesthesia for persons with fibrodysplasia ossificans progressiva. Clin Rev Bone Miner Metab 2005;3(3–4):239–42.
28. Azark B, Kaevel K, Hofmann L, et al. Dystrophic epidermolysis bullosa: oral findings and problems. Spec Care Dentist 2006;26(3):111–5.
29. Akturk G, Ulusoy H, Dohman D, et al. The anesthetic management of a patient with Pemphigus vulgaris—a case report. Middle East J Anesthesiol 1997;14(2): 91–7.
30. Vaghadia H, Blackstock D. Anaesthetic implications of the trismus pseudocamptodactyly (Dutch-Kentucky or Hecht-Beals) syndrome. Can J Anaesth 1988;35(1):80–5.
31. Hung WT, Hsu SC, Kao CT. General anesthesia for developmentally disabled dental care patients: a comparison of reinforced mask laryngeal airway and endotracheal intubation anesthesia. Spec Care Dentist 2008;23(4):135–8.
32. Miyamoto E, Nagata A, Mvilao K, et al. Use of the laryngeal mask in a patient with pemphigus vulgaris. Can J Anaesth 2001;48:512.
33. Young J, Diecidue R, Nussbaum B. Oral management in a patient with fibrodysplasia ossificans progressiva. Spec Care Dentist 2007;27(3):101–4.

A Review of Cerebral Palsy for the Oral Health Professional

Nancy J. Dougherty, DMD, MPH[a,b,c,*]

KEYWORDS

- Cerebral palsy • Developmental disability
- Oral health • Dentistry • Neuromuscular disorders

Cerebral palsy (CP) is the most common form of neuromuscular disability affecting children.[1,2,3] As more and more individuals who have CP continue to live in community settings, rather than institutions, and as their life spans increase, dentists and hygienists will be responsible for providing a continuum of oral health care to this population from childhood through later life.

The definition of CP has changed through the years, as researchers have increased their knowledge of the disorder in its various permutations. In 2004, an International Workshop on the Definition and Classification of Cerebral Palsy was held, with support from United Cerebral Palsy, the Castang Foundation, and the National Institute of Neurological Disorders and Stroke.[4] Attendees at this meeting agreed on an updated definition of CP as follows:

> *Cerebral palsy (CP) describes a group of disorders of the development of movement and posture, causing activity limitation, that are attributed to non-progressive disturbances that occurred in the developing fetal or infant brain. The motor disorders of cerebral palsy are often accompanied by disturbances of sensation, cognition, communication, perception, and/or behavior, and/or by a seizure disorder.*

This definition differs from earlier ones that focused solely on motor impairments and did not include mention of the additional developmental disorders that often are observed in individuals who have CP. This definition excludes discussions of what constitutes an immature brain and levels of functioning. These exclusions were

[a] Department of Pediatric Dentistry, New York University College of Dentistry, 345 East 24th Street, 967W, New York, NY 10010, USA
[b] Departments of Dentistry and Pediatrics, Albert Einstein College of Medicine, 1300 Morris Park Avenue, Bronx, NY 10461, USA
[c] Postgraduate Program in Pediatric Dentistry, Department of Dentistry, North Bronx Healthcare Network, Jacobi Medical Center, 1400 Pelham Parkway South, Bronx, NY 10461, USA
* Department of Pediatric Dentistry, New York University College of Dentistry, 345 East 24th Street, 967W, New York, NY 10010.
E-mail address: nid201@nyu.edu

Dent Clin N Am 53 (2009) 329–338
doi:10.1016/j.cden.2008.12.001
0011-8532/08/$ – see front matter

intentional, with the belief that more precise definitions might result in limitations of services for many individuals who have CP.[4]

RISK FACTORS

"Cerebral paresis" first was described in 1861 in an article by William Little, an English surgeon. Little noted that most of the children who developed CP had histories of difficult births, and he theorized that the condition was the result of hypoxia during the birth process.[1] Until recently, this belief remained widespread among the public and the medical profession. Biomedical research done in the past 20 years has shown that, in reality, birth complications are responsible for only a small fraction of cases of CP. It has been estimated that up to 70% to 80% of CP cases can be attributed to prenatal factors, with birth asphyxia responsible for a small number (approximately 10%) and the remainder due to identifiable postnatal conditions.[5]

As stated in the definition of CP, the disorder develops subsequent to some type of insult to the immature brain. This insult can occur, however, anytime from during the prenatal period through the first few years of life. A wide range of risk factors have been implicated in the development of CP. **Table 1** provides a list of conditions shown to place a child at risk for developing CP.[1,2]

It is not always possible to determine an exact cause in individual cases. Approximately 30% of cases have none of the known risk factors.[1,6] Premature birth, especially associated with extreme low birth weight (<1000 g), places infants at significant risk for subsequent CP. The rate of CP in this population of infants is approximately 8% to 10%. Improved fetal monitoring during birth and higher rates of cesarean section have not had an impact on the rates of CP, however, and some

Table 1
Risk factors associated with cerebral palsy

Prenatal	Perinatal	Postnatal
Hypoxia	Premature birth <32 wk or <2500 g	Asphyxia
Genetic disorders	Asphyxia	Seizures in postnatal period
Metabolic disorders	Blood incompatibility	Cerebral infarction
Multiple gestation	Infection	Hyperbilirubinemia
Intrauterine infection	Abnormal fetal presentation	Sepsis
Thrombophilic disorders	Placental abruption	Respiratory distress syndrome
Teratogenic exposure	Instrument delivery	Chronic lung disease
Chorioamnionitis	—	Meningitis
Maternal fever	—	Postnatal steroids
Exposure to toxins	—	Intraventricular hemorrhage
Malformation of brain structures	—	Periventricular leukomalacia
Intrauterine growth restriction	—	Shaken baby syndrome
Abdominal trauma	—	Head injury
Vascular insults	—	—

From Jones MW, Morgan E, Shelton J.E. Cerebral palsy: introduction and diagnosis (Part 1). J Pediatr Health Care 2007;21(3):147; with permission.

investigators question whether or not many of these infants have pre-existing conditions that precipitate preterm birth and subsequent development of CP.[7]

PREVALENCE

Birth prevalence rates for CP have not decreased in the United States or Europe over the past 30 years. One European study showed a slight increase in CP from the 1970s to the 1990s. The rate has remained approximately 2 to 3 per 1000 live births during that time. Rates in underdeveloped countries are similar or, in some cases, even lower than in developed countries.[7,8] Some researchers have theorized that a greater incidence of multiple births and increased survival rates for extreme low birth weight infants in recent years may account for some of this inability to lower CP rates.[5,7,9] United Cerebral Palsy has estimated that currently there are more than 500,000 individuals who have CP living in the United States.[10] An estimated 87% to 93% of children who have CP are now living into adulthood, which increases prevalence in the adult population.[11]

SUBCLASSIFICATION OF CEREBRAL PALSY

One method of classifying types of CP is according to the nature of the motor disorder observed.[1,2] Three major types of motor disorders are encountered:

- Spastic CP, which accounts for 70% to 80% of cases. Its predominant characteristic is increased muscle tone. This type of CP results from pyramidal (upper motor neuron) damage.
- Dyskinetic CP, which is observed in 10% to 15% of cases. Motor characteristics include hypotonia, athetotic (slow, writhing) movements, abnormal postural control, and overall problems with coordination. Oromotor difficulties, including speech and swallowing difficulties, commonly are seen. Damage to basal ganglia or deep motor neurons is responsible for this type of CP.
- Ataxic CP, which accounts for only approximately 5% of cases. These individuals have problems with voluntary movement, balance, and depth perception. It is caused by damage to cerebellar neurons.

Many individuals exhibit mixed motor involvement and cannot be categorized exclusively in any one of these groups.

Spastic CP can be subclassified further according to topography, that is, depending on which extremities are involved:[2]

- Quadriplegia: All four extremities, the trunk, and oromotor musculature are involved. This accounts for 10% to 15% of cases of spastic CP. Most of these individuals exhibit some degree of intellectual disability in addition to the motor disorder. These patients also are at high risk for seizures and sensory impairments. This type of CP has been associated with asphyxia in all infants and severe intraventricular hemorrhage in preterm infants.
- Diplegia: 30% to 40% of cases of spastic CP, characterized by spasticity in the legs. Arms also can be affected but to a lesser extent. Approximately 30% of these individuals have intellectual disabilities or learning difficulties. Most are able to ambulate independently or with assistance. Approximately 50% of these cases are associated with preterm birth.
- Hemiplegia: 20% to 30% of cases of spastic CP. One side of the body is involved. Usually, the arm is more involved than the leg. More than 60% of these individuals have normal intellectual development and are able to ambulate with or

without assistance. They are at high risk for development of partial seizures. This type of CP is associated with vascular malformations in the brain and limited intraventricular hemorrhage in early childhood.
- Monoplegia: This condition is extremely rare. Only one limb is involved, an arm or leg. Patients who have this subtype as an initial clinical diagnosis often are shown to have an underlying etiology other than CP.

DIAGNOSIS

The diagnosis of CP not always is straightforward, but an early diagnosis is important in terms of optimizing therapeutic interventions. Clinical observation and parental report are the initial stages in formulating this diagnosis. Children who are severely affected, or who have a known risk factor, often are diagnosed at an earlier age than those who are affected more mildly.

Parents may report concerns in early infancy, such as difficulty with feeding, excessive crying, jitteriness, "stiff" posturing, or limpness (indicative of hypotonia). As children age, motor milestones, such as the ability to sit up unassisted or learning to walk, may be delayed. Physicians may note a persistence of primitive reflexes that normally are lost in the first few months of life. In a toddler who has learned to walk, abnormal gait patterns may be observed.[1]

Part of the diagnostic process involves the exclusion of other etiologies, such as neurodegenerative, metabolic, or genetic disorders that have clinical presentations similar to CP. Neuroimaging studies, electroencephalography, chromosomal studies, and an array of blood tests all may be useful in making a definitive diagnosis.[2]

MEDICAL ISSUES

Although the encephalopathy responsible for CP may be static, the physical and medical status seen in individuals who have CP is anything but static. CP is a lifelong disorder that requires a range of long-term therapies and acute interventions. Several physical complications are commonly associated with CP (**Box 1**).[2,6] Early predictions of future neuromuscular and intellectual deficits can be difficult or impossible to make, and the course of complications varies greatly from person to another.[1]

Box 1
Medical complications associated with cerebral palsy

Spasticity

Joint contractures, misalignment secondary to muscle spasticity

Hip dislocation

Spinal disorders (scoliosis or kyphosis)

Osteoporosis

Intellectual disability (seen in 30%–50% of individuals)

Seizures

Gastroesophageal reflux

Dysphagia or aphagia

Failure to thrive/malnutrition

Hearing loss

A team of health care professionals is required to help individuals who have CP achieve and maintain their own optimal functioning. Physical, occupational, and speech therapies may be necessary over the long-term. Surgical interventions also may be required at various times for procedures that address the secondary complications of CP. These can include scoliosis repair, hip relocation, tendon lengthening, gastric tube placement, and insertion of baclofen pumps (to relieve spasticity).[2]

Gastrointestinal problems are common in individuals who have CP.[2,12,13,14,15,16,17] Several reports place the prevalence of various gastrointestinal disorders as high as 90% in populations of children who have CP.[14,16] These disorders can include dysphagia, gastroesophageal reflux, gastritis, chronic pulmonary aspiration, and constipation.

Dysphagia is defined as difficulty with eating resulting from some type of disorder in the process of swallowing.[15] Aphagia refers to the complete inability to swallow. Individuals who have aphagia or a history of chronic aspiration secondary to feeding may require feedings through a type of tube—nasogastric, oroesophageal, or gastric.[14,15]

Gastroesophageal reflux disease (GERD) refers to pathologic reflux of gastric juices into the esophagus. Similarly to dysphagia, GERD has an increased prevalence in individuals who have neuromuscular disorders.[13,16,18] Untreated GERD can lead to erosive esophagitis, increased bronchial aspiration, and malnutrition.[13,16]

INTELLECTUAL DISABILITY

Although intellectual disability is not a diagnostic feature of CP, it is present in a significant number of individuals.[1,2,4] Prevalence is variable, depending on the subtype of CP. The highest rate of intellectual impairment is seen in individuals who have spastic quadriplegia. It is estimated that more than 50% of these individuals have some level of intellectual disability. Much lower rates are observed in individuals who have ataxic and dyskinetic forms of CP. Prevalence rates of intellectual disability in these groups are estimated in the range of 20% to 30%.[1,2]

DENTAL TREATMENT CONCERNS

The neuromuscular problems inherent in CP can affect oral health significantly in several ways. These can include changes in structure to the orofacial region, development of parafunctional habits, feeding problems, difficulties with maintaining oral hygiene, and encountering barriers to oral care access.

Malocclusions

Several articles have reported an increased rate of malocclusion in individuals who have CP compared with the general public. Prevalence rates are reported between 59% and 92%, with the vast majority of malocclusions classified as Angle Class II.[19,20,21,22] The frequent occurrence of anterior open bite, with prominent maxillary incisors, also is reported. At least one study reported an increase in overjet as individuals age.[20] It has been suggested that the high rate of Class II malocclusion and anterior open bite can be attributed to hypotonia of the orofacial musculature, with resultant forward tongue posturing, a poor swallow reflex, and frequent mouth breathing.[19,20]

Traumatic Dental Injuries

Theoretically, it could be assumed that individuals who have CP may be at increased risk for dental trauma as a result of several factors. These considerations include the high prevalence of Class II malocclusion with prominent maxillary incisors and difficulties with ambulation and an increased incidence of seizures. Few studies, however, actually have studied the incidence of dental trauma in people who have CP. Holan and colleagues[23] found greatly increased incidence of dental trauma in a CP population when compared with reports in general populations (57% of children who had CP versus 18% to 22% in studies of general populations). Two other studies found that the incidence of dental trauma in children who had CP was only slightly or not significantly higher than that of the general population (18% and 28.8%).[24,25] This small number of studies makes it difficult to draw conclusions concerning the prevalence of dental trauma in individuals who have CP. It is possible that children who have CP are unable to participate in as many unrestricted physical activities as children who do not have disabilities, and this could act as a mitigating factor in the incidence of dental trauma.

Bruxism

A high prevalence of bruxism in individuals who have CP has been reported in several articles.[19,20,26,27,28] Ortega and colleagues[26] found the prevalence of bruxism in a group of children and young adults who had CP to be 36.9%. An age-comparable group of nondisabled individuals had a rate of only 15.3%. dos Santos and colleagues[20] found similarly high rates of bruxism in a population of children who had CP in Brazil. Several studies have noted that the prevalence of bruxism is increased in individuals who had severe to profound intellectual disability (not necessarily with a diagnosis of CP) and in institutionalized populations.[28,29] Lobbezoo and Naije have hypothesized that bruxism habits in these populations are related to problems with dopamine function and not regulated by local factors, such as malocclusion.[30] Few studies have been published that report success with treatment of bruxism in populations who have intellectual disability. The studies that do exist have reported success with aversive behavioral techniques.[29] This is an area that requires further research into techniques that may be effective in extinguishing a habit that potentially is of great detriment to the dentition.

Sialorrhea

Sialorrhea (drooling) can be a significant problem for individuals who have neuromotor disorders, such as CP. Prevalence rates of sialorrhea in children who have CP are reported range from 10% to 58%.[31,32,33,34] Drooling is normal in infants and young children. Past age 4, however, it is considered pathologic. The majority of individuals who have CP who experience sialorrhea are not producing excess saliva; rather, they are unable to swallow normal outputs of saliva because of oromotor dysfunction. Perioral chapping, infection, and dehydration are physical complications that can result from sialorrhea. The psychosocial ramifications of drooling, however, may be more serious than the physical ones. The disorder can be stigmatizing, causing social isolation and a reluctance for close contact by caregivers, therapists, and others who normally may interact closely with individuals who have disabilities.[34,35]

Several therapeutic modalities exist to treat sialorrhea. These include anticholinergic medications (which often have too many side effects to be considered a long-term therapy), speech therapy, intraoral appliance therapy, biofeedback, and various surgical procedures that involve the salivary glands. A recent treatment that has had success is the injection of botulinum toxin A into the salivary glands (primarily the parotid glands).[33,34,35] A team approach is most appropriate for treatment of sialorrhea, and therapeutic decisions depend on various factors, such as the severity of the problem, patient's medical status, and patient's ability to cooperate and benefit from modalities, such as speech, behavioral, and appliance therapy.[31]

Oral Hygiene

Poor oral hygiene frequently is cited as a problem affecting the oral health status of individuals who have CP.[19,20,25,36,37] The ability to maintain adequate oral hygiene is complicated by many factors, including dyskinetic movements, the presence of pathologic oral reflexes (biting and vomiting), and the inability to manipulate a toothbrush. Many individuals who have CP, even those who do not have intellectual impairment, are dependent on another person to help with activities of daily living, such as toothbrushing. In such cases, it is imperative that caregivers are given instructions in the maintenance of daily oral hygiene for the individuals who have CP. Ideally, an individual hygiene plan should be designed for each patient. This plan may include alternative positioning techniques during hygiene and the use of assistive devices, such as mouth props, floss holders, toothbrushes with large handles, or electric toothbrushes.

Individuals who experience chronic pooling of saliva tend to build up extensive calculus deposits. These same patients often are at risk for pneumonia secondary to aspiration. Increased colonization of the oral cavity by respiratory pathogens can be a serious concern, and maintenance of adequate oral hygiene to minimize bacteria levels and gingival inflammation is important.[2] In any patient for whom aspiration is a concern, use of rigorous high-speed suction during hygiene procedures is a must.

Dental Caries

Several studies have examined caries rates in individuals who have CP.[19,20,38] Results from these studies make it impossible to generalize about caries rates in individuals who have CP. Pope and Curzon[19] did not find significant differences in the levels of decayed, missing, and filled teeth between children who had CP and a control group of children who did not have disabilities. They did find, however, that the children who had CP had more untreated decay than the nondisabled children, indicative of difficulties people who have disabilities often have in accessing care. Nielsen, in Denmark, found lower decayed, missing, and filled tooth surfaces scores in adolescents who had CP than in a control group.[38] A Brazilian study found significantly higher decayed, missing, and filled tooth surfaces scores in children who had CP when compared with a control group of children who did not have disabilities. The investigators of this study also note, however, that the children who had CP had higher plaque indexes, food residue, and rates of mouth breathing than the control group. This could help account for the higher caries rate.[20]

BEHAVIORAL CONSIDERATIONS

The definition of CP (discussed previously) includes "disturbances of sensation, cognition, communication, perception, and/or behavior" that often accompany the central neuromotor disability.[4]

All of these must be taken into consideration when providing dental treatment to patients who have CP. The goal should be to provide optimal oral health care in the least restrictive environment, with patient safety and comfort as primary concerns.

Little research has been done that examines the effectiveness of various behavior management techniques in the provision of dental treatment to individuals who have CP. One Brazilian study compared various management techniques in an institutionalized population with CP. The researchers concluded that the use of assistive stabilization and postural maintenance reduced the number of patients requiring referral to a hospital for treatment under general anesthesia.[39] Stabilization and postural maintenance can be achieved through a combination of cushions and physical restraint, adapted for individuals. Oral stability can be accomplished with the use of a mouth prop.

A rehabilitation professional, such as a physical or occupational therapist, can be invaluable in determining appropriate positioning and stabilization techniques.

Outpatient sedation also may be useful in the treatment of patients who have CP. There are, however, several features of CP that can complicate sedation in these individuals:[40]

- Scoliosis can affect a patient's ventilatory capacity.
- A compromised gag reflex can put a patient at more risk for aspiration.
- A patient who has compromised communication ability may be unable to express breathing difficulties.
- Joint contractures may make patient positioning difficult.
- Poorly controlled seizures can complicate sedation.

As this list makes clear, a thorough medical history must be elicited along with a careful consideration of risks and benefits before appropriate management decisions can be made in the provision of dental treatment for patients who have CP.

SUMMARY

Individuals who have CP face many physical challenges throughout their lifetimes in addition to societal barriers that can have an impact on quality of life. The ability to readily access appropriate dental care has long been an issue for people who have disabilities. Dentists should be considered integral members of teams of professionals involved in optimizing the health of individuals who have CP. As with all other members of this interdisciplinary team, oral health care providers should have a thorough knowledge of the medical, cognitive, and rehabilitative issues associated with CP. It is with this knowledge that the best possible health care can be provided.

REFERENCES

1. Jones MW, Morgan E, Shelton JE. Cerebral palsy: introduction and diagnosis (part 1). J Pediatr Health Care 2007;21(3):146–52.
2. Thorogood C, Alexander MA. Cerebral palsy. eMedicine. Available at: www.emedicine.com/pmr/topic24.htm. Accessed December 12, 2007.
3. Yeargin-Allsopp M, Van Naarden Braun K, Doernberg NS, et al. Prevalence of cerebral palsy in 8-year-old children in three areas of the United States in 2002: a multisite collaboration. Pediatrics 2008;121(3):547–54.
4. Bax M, Goldstein M, Rosenbaum P, et al. Proposed definition and classification of cerebral palsy. Dev Med Child Neurol 2005;47:571–6.
5. Jacobsson B, Hagberg G. Antenatal risk factors for cerebral palsy. Best Pract Res Clin Obstet Gynaecol 2004;18(3):425–36.
6. Rosenbaum P. Cerebral palsy: what parents and doctors want to know. BMJ 2003;326:970–4.
7. Clark SL, Hankins GDV. Temporal and demographic trends in cerebral pals—fact and fiction. Am J Obstet Gynecol 2003;188(3):628–33.
8. Odding E, Roebroeck ME, Stam HJ. The epidemiology of cerebral palsy: incidence, impairments and risk factors. Disabil Rehabil 2006;28(4):183–91.
9. Platt MJ, Cans C, Johnson A, et al. Trends in cerebral palsy among infants of very low birthweight (<1500g) or born prematurely (<32 weeks) in 16 European centres: a database study. Lancet 2007;369:43–50.
10. Cerebral palsy. Medical College of Wisconsin Healthlink. Available at: http://healthlink.mcw.edu/article/931225858.html. Accessed May 8, 2008.

11. Hutton JL, Cooke T, Pharoah PO. Life expectancy in children with cerebral palsy. BMJ 1994;309(6952):431–5.
12. Jones MW, Morgan E, Shelton JE. Primary care of the child with cerebral palsy: a review of systems (part II). J Pediatr Health Care 2007;21(4):226–37.
13. Bohmer CJM, Klinkenberg-Knol EC, Niezen-de Boer MC, et al. Gastroesophageal reflux disease in intellectually disabled individuals: how often, how serious, how manageable? Am J Gastroenterol 2000;95(8):1868–72.
14. Reilly S, Skuse D, Poblete X. Prevalence of feeding problems and oral motor dysfunction in children with cerebral palsy: a community survey. J Pediatr 1996;129(6):877–82.
15. Paik NJ. Dysphagia. eMedicine. Available at: www.emedicine.com/pmr/topic194.htm. Accessed May 11, 2008.
16. Chong SKF. Gastrointestinal problems in the handicapped child. Curr Opin Pediatr 2001;13:441–6.
17. Kozma C, Mason S. Survey of nursing and medical profile prior to deinstitutionalization of a population with profound mental retardation. Clin Nurs Res 2003;12(8):8–22.
18. Fisichella PM, Patti MG. Gastroesophageal reflux disease. eMedicine. Available at: www.emedicine.com/med/topic857.htm. Accessed July 20, 2008.
19. Pope JEC, Curzon MEJ. The dental status of cerebral palsied children. Pediatr Dent 1991;13(3):156–62.
20. dos Santos MTBR, Masiero D, Novo NF, et al. Oral conditions in children with cerebral palsy. J Dent Child 2003;70:40–6.
21. Winter K, Baccaglini L, Tomar S. A review of malocclusion among individuals with mental and physical disabilities. Spec Care Dentist 2008;28(1):19–26.
22. Franklin DC, Luther F, Curzon ME. The prevalence of malocclusion in children with cerebral palsy. Eur J Orthod 1996;18:637–43.
23. Holan G, Peretz B, Jacob E, et al. Traumatic injuries to the teeth in young individuals with cerebral palsy. Dent Traumatol 2005;21:65–9.
24. Ohito FA, Opinya GN, Wangombe J. Traumatic dental injuries in normal and handicapped children in Nairobi, Kenya. East Afr Med J 1992;69:680–2.
25. Nunn JH, Murray JJ. The dental health of handicapped children in Newcastle and Northumberland. Br Dent J 1987;62:9–14.
26. Ortega AOL, Guimaraes AS, Ciamponi AL, et al. Frequency of parafunctional oral habits in patients with cerebral palsy. J Oral Rehabil 2007;34:323–8.
27. Dura JR, Torsell E, Heinzerling RA, et al. Special oral concerns in people with severe and profound mental retardation. Spec Care Dentist 1988;8:265–7.
28. Lindqvist B, Heijbel J. Bruxism in children with brain damage. Acta Odontol Scand 1974;32:313–9.
29. Long ES, Miltenberger RG. A review of behavioral and pharmacological treatments for habit disorders in individuals with mental retardation. J Behav Ther Exp Psychiatry 1998;29:143–56.
30. Lobbezoo F, Naije M. Bruxism is mainly regulated centrally, not peripherally. J Oral Rehabil 2001;28:1085–91.
31. Mathur NN, Vaughn TL. Drooling. eMedicine. Available at: www.emedicine.com/ent/topic629.htm. Accessed August 1, 2008.
32. Tahmassebi JF, Curzon MEJ. Prevalence of drooling in children with cerebral palsy attending special schools. Dev Med Child Neurol 2003;45:613–7.
33. Jongerius PH, van den Hoogen FJA, et al. Effect of botulinum toxin in the treatment of drooling: a controlled clinical trial. Pediatrics 2004;114:L620–7.
34. Bothwell JE, Clarke K, et al. Botulinum toxin A as a treatment for excessive drooling in children. Pediatr Neurol 2002;27(1):18–22.

35. Hockstein NG, Samadi DS, Gendron K, et al. Sialorrhea: a management challenge. Am Fam Physician 2004;69(11):2628–34.
36. Subasi F, Mumcu G, et al. Factors affecting oral health habits among children with cerebral palsy: pilot study. Pediatr Int 2007;49:853–7.
37. dos Santos MTBR, Nogueira MLG. Infantile reflexes and their effects on dental caries and oral hygiene in cerebral palsy individuals. J Oral Rehabil 2005;32: 880–5.
38. Nielsen LA. Caries among children with cerebral palsy. Proceedings of the 9th Congress of the International Association of Dentistry for the Handicapped. Philadelphia, PA, August 7–10, 1988.
39. Santos MTBR, Manzano FS. Assistive stabilization based on the neurodevelopmental treatment approach for dental care in individuals with cerebral palsy. Quintessence Int 2007;38(8):681–7.
40. Wongprasartsuk P, Stevens J. Cerebral palsy and anaesthesia. Paediatr Anaesth 2002;12:296–303.

Oral Self-Injurious Behaviors in Patients with Developmental Disabilities

Maureen Romer, DDS, MPA[a,*], Nancy J. Dougherty, DMD, MPH[b,c,d]

KEYWORDS

- Self-injurious behavior • Self-injurious behaviors
- Factitial injury • Intellectual disabilities
- Developmental disabilities • Autism • Mental retardation
- Lesch-Nyhan syndrome • Familial dysautonomia

Behaviors that result in self-induced wounds stem from a wide range of etiologies including those of an organic nature, those that seem to serve a function, or those that are habitual.[1,2] Although some self-injurious behaviors (SIB) may be unintentional, when the term is used in the medical and psychiatric literature, it usually refers to *intentional* acts that result in organ or tissue damage.[3]

SIB encompasses a wide range of behaviors, some resulting in relatively minor tissue damage, others with very severe consequences (**Fig. 1**).[3,4] The medical sequelae of these behaviors can include soft tissue infection, loss of vision, injury to the dentition, bone fracture, as well as scarring and disfigurement.[5] Additionally, side effects of psychotropic medications that are used to manage SIB can have long-term, unintended health consequences. SIB may also interfere indirectly with an individual's social and educational opportunities.[6]

Diverse populations have been known to exhibit SIB. These include individuals with psychiatric diagnoses such as bipolar disorder and depression, those with conditions that result in indifference to pain, such as familial dysautonomia, and others with a variety of developmental disabilities.[3,4,7]

[a] Arizona School of Dentistry and Oral Health, A.T. Still University, 5855 E. Still Circle, Mesa, AZ 85206, USA
[b] Department of Pediatric Dentistry, New York University College of Dentistry, 345 East 24th Street, 967W, New York, NY 10010, USA
[c] Departments of Dentistry and Pediatrics, Albert Einstein College of Medicine, 1300 Morris Park Avenue, Bronx, NY 10461, USA
[d] Postgraduate Program in Pediatric Dentistry, Department of Dentistry, North Bronx Healthcare Network, Jacobi Medical Center, 1400 Pelham Parkway South, Bronx, NY 10461, USA
* Corresponding author.
E-mail address: mromer@atsu.edu (M. Romer).

Dent Clin N Am 53 (2009) 339–350
doi:10.1016/j.cden.2008.12.015
dental.theclinics.com
0011-8532/08/$ – see front matter

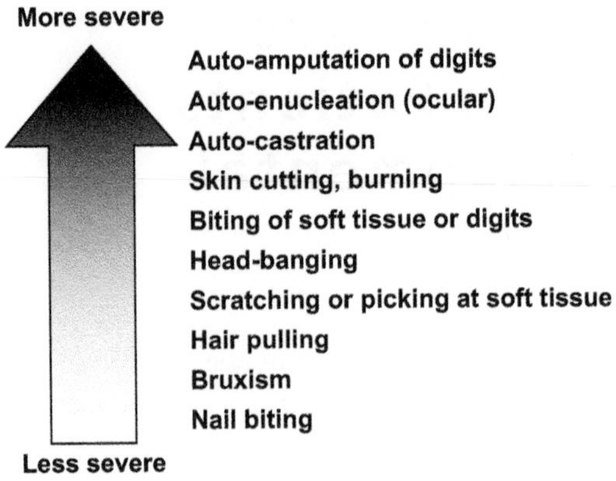

Fig. 1. Range of self-injurious behaviors.[3,4]

There is some variation in the behaviors engaged in by these different groups. Individuals with psychiatric disorders tend to engage more in non-oral forms of SIB, such as auto-amputation, cutting and burning of skin, or picking and scratching of soft tissue. SIB in this group also tends to be sporadic, rather than a chronic behavior.[4] Oral SIB is seen more frequently in patients with intellectual disabilities, autism, and specific genetic disorders, most notably, Lesch-Nyhan syndrome.[1] Although SIB in this group may be sporadic, in response to specific stimuli, the pattern more often tends to be chronic and/or stereotypic.[4] Patients with disorders of decreased pain sensation may experience oral soft tissue self-inflicted wounds, but this is often not intentional in nature. This type of injury is related to an impaired ability to perceive and/or react to painful stimuli.[8,9] Comatose or decerebrate patients may also experience severe oral soft tissue mutilation, but this, too, is unintentional and can be attributed to neuropathologic chewing that is associated with injury to the cerebral cortex and pyramidal system.[10]

The focus of this article is oral SIB as manifested by individuals with developmental disabilities. Prevalence estimates of SIB in this group have ranged from 3.5% to 40%.[2–4,11] In 1989, the National Institutes of Health estimated that approximately 25,000 people with developmental disabilities in the United States exhibit some type of SIB.[12] In addition to the physical and psychologic hardships brought on by SIB, the behavior brings with it financial burdens. It is a significant factor in hospitalizations, decisions to use psychotropic medications, and institutional placement for people with developmental disabilities.[5]

RISK FACTORS FOR SELF-INJURIOUS BEHAVIOR

The literature is replete with reports on SIB in patients with normal intellect and psychiatric disorders such as bipolar disorder,[13] obsessive compulsive disorder,[14] schizophrenia,[13–15] borderline personality disorder,[13] severe depression,[13–15] eating disorders,[3,16,17] and self-mutilation disorders.[18] For the psychiatric population with SIB, the behavior is often described as a "relief" from psychic pain or tension.[16,17] Yates[19] proposed a psychopathology framework for SIB that is a result of childhood trauma such as sexual abuse. The psychopathology of SIB in patients with psychiatric diagnosis (but normal range of intelligence) most likely serves a different function than for individuals with intellectual disability (ID).

An increased incidence of SIB is noted in individuals with severe-to- profound intellectual disability and those with additional sensory impairments.[11,20–23] Blindness in particular has been associated with increased risk of SIB.[24] It is postulated that eye poking serves a self-stimulatory function in those with visual impairment.[24] Presence of stereotypies (purposeless repetitive movements), movement disorders, and sleep disturbances are associated with the occurrence of SIB in patients with ID.[13] As mentioned previously, individuals with a diagnosis of autism are also at increased risk for SIB.[3,11,20,25–27]In McClintock and colleagues'[11] meta-analysis of studies of SIB in ID populations over the last 30 years, the top risk factors for SIB are listed as severe or profound ID, diagnosis of autism, and deficits in receptive or expressive communication. SIB has also been reported in patients with altered states of consciousness[28,29] due to brain injury[30] or infection.[31,32] The lip or cheek may act as a bolus that initiates the chewing cycle[29] in a patient without cerebral control of the masticatory muscles.

There have been several case reports of patients with cerebral palsy (CP)[33,34] exhibiting SIB as a result of involuntary movement. Patients with seizure disorders,[24,35] as well as Chiari type II malformation[36] have also been reported to exhibit SIB.

GENETIC SYNDROMES ASSOCIATED WITH SELF-INJURIOUS BEHAVIOR

Genetic disorders associated with SIB include: Lesch-Nyhan syndrome,[37] Tourette-syndrome,[38–42] Cornelia de Lange syndrome,[43,44] familial dysautonomia,[45–47] Fragile X,[48] Leigh disease,[49] Hallervorden-Spatz disease,[50] Prader-Willi syndrome,[51,52] Rett syndrome,[52,53] and Richner-Hanhart syndrome.[54] Several of the more commonly reported syndromes are detailed below.

Lesch-Nyhan syndrome (LNS) is an X-linked disorder of purine metabolism (specifically the lack of hypoxanthine-guanine phosphoribosyltransferase) that is perhaps the most notable genetic condition associated with SIB.[37,53,55,56] Patients present with ID, choreoathetosis, hyperuricemia, uricosuria, and SIB.[53,56] Biting of the lips, tongue, fingers, and hands is the predominant form of SIB in LNS patients and thus these patients are often referred to the dentist for treatment. The dental literature contains numerous reports of patients with LNS who have undergone a range of treatments with varying degrees of success.[53,55,57–61]

Tourette syndrome (TS) is characterized by tics, both motor and vocal, as well as compulsions and attention deficits.[38,39] The method of inheritance is unclear; however, familial history is implicated in nearly 50% of cases.[40,42] Up to 60% of patients with TS exhibit SIB.[38,40,41] Behavior such as lip and hand biting, head banging, and skin picking have been reported.[38] Mathews and colleagues[41] have correlated SIB with impulsivity, compulsivity, and affect disregulation, suggesting that in mild cases, SIB in TS may be closer to the SIB symptoms in psychiatric patients rather than patients with ID and other genetic syndromes.

Familial dysautonomia (also known as Riley-Day syndrome or hereditary sensory and autonomic neuropathy type III) is an autosomal recessive disorder. It is most often seen in patients of Ashkenazi Jewish descent.[46] Patients have a progressive loss of small myelinated fibers and neurons in the autonomic and sensory ganglion.[46] This inability to feel pain (eg, loss of pain as a protective mechanism) can result in accidental tissue damage such as biting, burns, and lacerations.[47] Interestingly, these patients lack fungiform papillae and this unique finding can be diagnostically significant.

Individuals with Cornelia de Lange (CDL) syndrome have a characteristic appearance consisting of microbrachycephaly, micrognathia, low hairline, coarse hair, synophrys, and long eyelashes. Intellectual disability and foreshortened hands and feet are also features of this syndrome.[44] Hyman and Oliver[43] reported SIB in 62% of patients studied with CDL. Another report of two patients with CDL documented finger sucking, biting of digits and lips, and skin picking.[44] It can be theorized that because these patients have many of the risk factors for SIB, including ID, "autistic tendencies," lack of communication skills, and physical impairments, it is logical that there would be reports of SIB in this population.[43]

ETIOLOGIES

Underlying etiologies for SIB are poorly understood. As research in this area progresses, it is quite possible that multiple neuropathologic mechanisms will be uncovered, all with the final outcome of self-injurious behavior.[3,4,21,22]

Physicians and psychologists have been shown to differ in their approaches to research in the area of SIB etiologies.[5] Many physicians, who tend to be biologically oriented, have theorized that SIB has a primary *biologic* basis. This theory implicates organic processes such as abnormalities in neurotransmitter pathways, hormone fluctuations; or SIB as a response to underlying pain (primarily in patients who have deficient communication skills).[3,5,21,22,61] In support of this theory, painful stimulation has been shown to increase the release of endorphins, resulting in a pleasurable response.[4] The fact that certain genetic syndromes, especially Lesch-Nyhan and Cornelia de Lange, have SIB as a prominent feature would also appear to support this biologic basis.[22,61,62] In fact, imaging studies of patients with Lesch-Nyhan have demonstrated elevated numbers of dopamine receptors, accompanied by reductions in dopamine transporters and overall dopamine levels.[62–65] Other papers have reported increased incidence of SIB associated with menstrual cycles.[61,66] A study of 25 individuals who had been admitted to an in-patient unit for treatment of SIB showed that 28% had undiagnosed underlying medical problems that could be a source of discomfort. Conditions such as constipation, otitis media, gastroesophageal reflux, abscessed teeth, and pneumonia have been associated with periods of SIB in individuals with ID.[2,22,61]

Psychologists, on the other hand, have investigated SIB as an *operant* phenomenon. This theory posits that SIB is a learned behavior, that it serves a specific function in the patient's life, and that it can be modified by environmental changes and behavioral therapy.[3,4,21,22,67] Behaviorists hypothesize that individuals may be motivated to use SIB in various situations:[4,5,67]

- as an attention-getting device (positive reinforcement of behavior)
- as a means of obtaining materials or activities that may otherwise be inaccessible (positive reinforcement of behavior)
- as a way of avoiding stressful situations or undesirable tasks (negative reinforcement)

These situations are especially relevant to individuals who have limited cognitive abilities and/or compromised communication skills. The SIB acts, effectively, as a means of communication.

Patients with intellectual disability accompanied by severe sensory deficits, especially visual and auditory, receive little stimulation from the surrounding environment. It is possible that the increased incidence of SIB in this population may be interpreted as serving a pleasurable, self-stimulatory function.[5]

FUNCTIONAL ANALYSIS

The ability to make appropriate treatment decisions is dependent on accurate diagnosis. Unfortunately, it can be very difficult to pinpoint underlying causes for SIB. Functional analysis provides a methodical system that can help interpret what environmental conditions are responsible for triggering episodes of SIB. It can also be useful in distinguishing when an underlying medical condition, rather than environment, might be responsible for a person's SIB.

Briefly, during a functional analysis, a patient will be placed in several experimental conditions. During each of these controlled sessions, various behavioral reinforcers are presented to the patient. Observations will determine, which, of any, of these reinforcers results in SIB.[4,5,22,67,68] An example of this is the "escape" condition, in which the patient is requested to perform a task (ie, putting away toys, helping to clean a kitchen). If the request provokes SIB, a break is provided, and the patient is ignored. The observer will then determine if escape from the demand results in a lessening of the SIB. Increased incidence of SIB in this type of situation would indicated that the patient has "learned" that SIB is a technique for avoiding undesirable demands.[22] Other contingencies that might be tested are social interaction (attempting to attract attention via SIB), and using SIB in an attempt to obtain items such as toys or food.[5,22]

The control situation is observation of the patient alone, without any demands and without the ability to interact with another person. In other words, the patient receives no reinforcement, either positive or negative, in response to an incident of SIB. Persistence of SIB during this "alone" contingency is an indication that the behavior may have a biologic, or internal, reinforcer rather than an environmental, or external, one. This type of automatic SIB warrants investigation into underlying medical conditions as a cause for the behavior.[22]

Frequently, the results of a functional analysis may not be clear-cut. Many individuals have mixed bio-behavioral etiologies for SIB, a complication that makes definitive therapeutic interventions difficult.[5]

MANAGEMENT OF SELF-INJURIOUS BEHAVIOR

A review of the medical, psychiatric, and dental literature reveals several common themes regarding the treatment of SIB. It is clear that the underlying mechanism of the patient's behavior must be understood (ie, what purpose does the SIB serve?). Because many such patients lack communication skills, it may be a "cry for help." A thorough medical assessment is needed to rule out undiagnosed medical reasons for SIB such as otitis media, infection, and pneumonia.[14,69] Should no physical cause be found, and the patient is determined to be in good physical health, then a psychiatric evaluation may be advisable to determine the existence of comorbid psychiatric conditions that may respond to pharmacotherapy.[70]

The dental literature consists largely of individual case reports. Most of these focus on appliance therapy to manage SIB. Management with soft resin bite guards (ie, sports guards),[50,71] acrylic mouth guards,[39,55] lip bumpers or plumpers,[36,60] oral screens or tongue shields,[28,33] appliances attached to head gear or helmets,[15,34,72] acrylic splints attached with brass ligatures,[31] and acrylic appliances designed with blocks to maintain an open bite[73] have all met with varying degrees of success.

Patients with LNS are particularly refractory to appliance therapy and several authors have ultimately opted for extraction as treatment[57,59,61] Cusamano,[58] in his review of LNS, points out that appliance therapy should be tried first and extraction should be a last resort. However, in a study by Anderson and Ernst,[74] 60% of parents of children with LNS would prefer extraction over appliance therapy. A report of crown amputation and pulpotomies in an LNS patient offers a treatment alternative to extraction.[53]

Patients with familial dysautonomia may require extraction of primary teeth to prevent SIB to the lips and cheeks. These patients can later be taught not to bite.[45,47]

Alternative therapies such as botulinum toxin injections in the orofacial musculature[75] and orthognathic surgery to create an open bite[76] have been reported to be successful in extinguishing SIB.

Dental therapy has focused on symptomatic treatment rather than attempts to treat the underlying mechanism of SIB. It should be noted, however, that although this type of therapy may extinguish oral SIB, the failure to address underlying reasons for the behavior may result in the emergence of other forms of SIB (**Fig. 2**A–C).

BEHAVIORAL TREATMENT

A bio-behavioral approach including functional analysis may lead to better outcomes than oral appliance therapy alone.[5] Potential intervention strategies include positive reinforcement (by attention or tangible items), negative reinforcement by escape/avoidance of task demands and sensory reinforcement.[5,13,77,78]

It has also been theorized that SIB may be a form of self stimulation that is used to compensate for limited sensory input or for sensory "overload."[24,79] Sensory integration has been suggested as a treatment modality that may decrease self-stimulating activities and allow for more functional ones to replace them.[80] Extinction, systematic desensitization, and play therapy together have been reported to decrease SIB in patients with LNS.[81] Aversive therapy such as shock,[62,69,82] lemon juice,[83] and aromatic ammonia[84] have also been reported.

Richman and Lindauer[85] advise an early intervention (EI) program for children at high risk for SIB, theorizing that non-socially mediated SIB may become sensitive to social consequences and then be maintained.

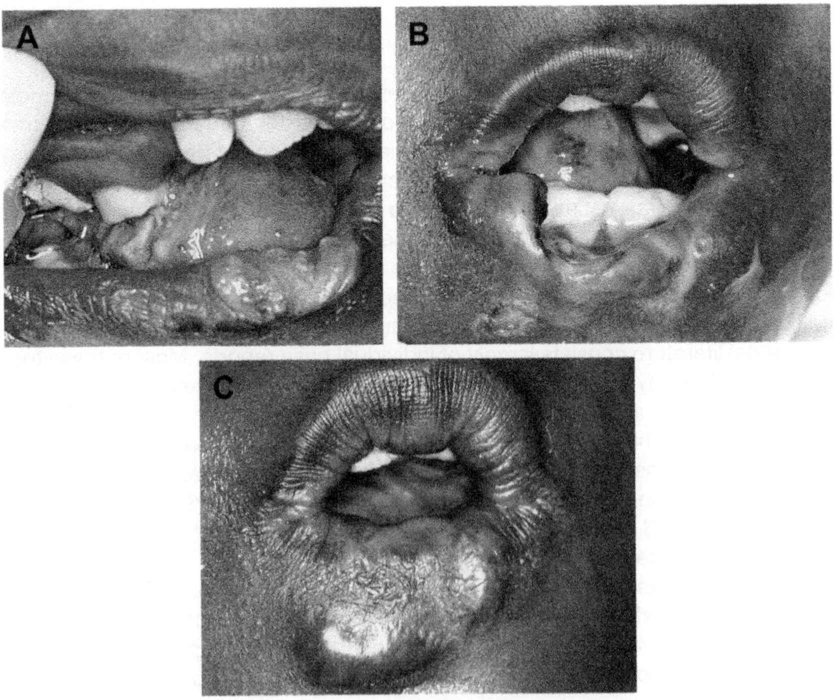

Fig. 2. Six- year-old child with severe intellectual disability, treated by authors. Patient was refractory to symptomatic treatment of oral SIB, but responded well to behavioral therapy. (*A*) and (*B*) show mutilation of lower lip and tongue. (*C*) shows healing of lower lip 4 mos. after initiation of behavioral therapy. (*From* Romer M, Dougherty N, Fruchter M. Alternative therapies in the treatment of oral self-injurious behavior: a case report. J Spec Care Dentist 1998;18(2):66–9; with permission).

PHARMACOLOGIC TREATMENT

The seratonergic, dopaminergic, and opioid neurotransmitter systems have all been implicated in the mechanism of SIB.[3,13,86,87] Seratonergic agents such as fluoxetine, sertraline, trazodone, clomipramine, and fenfluramine have been used with variable success in patients with SIB.[3,13,41,86] Buspirone (BuSpar) has had some effect on SIB and agitation and is not associated with unwanted sedation.[3,86] Lithium has also had some effect in reducing SIB, but is unclear if this is due to treatment of an underlying affective disorder.[3,86]

Beta blockers can be effective in treating agitation and have been tried as a treatment for SIB.[86] Clonidine, an α-adrenergic blocker, was reported to decrease SIB in a young girl with pervasive developmental disorder.[88]

Dopamine agonists (neuroleptics) have been used for treatment of SIB in patients with LNS,[89] TS,[38,42] and ID.[52,90] However, side effects such as tardive dyskinesia, impaired cognition, and motor skills may make neuroleptics a less desirable choice than other medications.[86]

Increased levels of endogenous opiates and opioid disregulation have been reported in patients with autism.[91] At the National Institute of Child Health and Human Development Conference on SIB, Sandman[13] reported that 30%–70% of patients with SIB have opioid disregulation. It stands to reason that opioid agonists such as naltrexone would be effective in treating patients with SIB. Interestingly, some authors report failure of naltrexone in patients with SIB.[92,93] Medications such as benzodiapines and other GABA agonists have been reported with conflicting success in the literature.[3] In a study of 31 patients, Ruedrich and colleagues[94] found atypical antipsychotics to decrease aggression but not SIB in institutionalized adults with ID.

NEUROSURGERY

Fountas and colleagues[18] reported a case of a young woman with severe SIB and psychiatric disorder refractory to behavioral and pharmacologic intervention who was successfully treated with bilateral stereotactic amygdalotomy. Deep brain stimulation of the hypothalamus[30] and bilateral chronic stimulation of the globus pallidus internus[95] were also reported to be successful in extinguishing SIB.

SUMMARY

It should be clear to the reader at this point that SIB in patients with developmental disabilities is a complex disorder without a universally successful course of treatment.

While oral appliance therapy may be indicated to minimize tissue damage caused by SIB, addressing the underlying impetus for the behavior is essential for successful treatment. The dentist may be the first professional called upon to evaluate a patient with oral SIB. However, the probability of a favorable outcome is likely to increase with the incorporation of a team approach that includes medical and behavioral specialists.

REFERENCES

1. Johnson CD, Matt MK, Dennison D, et al. Preventing factitious gingival injury in an autistic patient. J Am Dent Assoc 1996;127:244–7.
2. Romer M, Dougherty N, Fruchter M. Alternative therapies in the treatment of oral self-injurious behavior: a case report. Spec Care Dentist 1998;18(2):66–9.
3. Pies R, Popli A. Self-injurious behavior: pathophysiology and implications for treatment. J Clin Psychiatry 1995;56(12):580–8.

4. Winchel RM, Stanley M. Self-injurious behavior: a review of the behavior and biology of self-mutilation. Am J Psychiatry 1991;148(3):306–17.
5. Mace FC, Mauk JE. Bio-behavioral diagnosis and treatment of self-injury. MRDD Res Rev 1995;1:104–10.
6. Kahng SW, Iwata BA, Lewin AB. Behavioral treatment of self-injury, 1964 to 2000. Am J Ment Retard 2002;107(3):212–21.
7. Chen LR, Liu JF. Successful treatment of self-inflicted oral mutilation using an acrylic splint retained by a head gear. Pediatr Dentistry 1996;18(5):408–10.
8. Eichenfield LF, Honig PJ, Nelson L. Traumatic granuloma of the tongue (Riga-Fede disease): association with familial dysautonomia. J Pediatr 1990;116(5): 742–4.
9. D'Amico RA, Axelrod FB. Familial dysautonomia. eMedicine. Available at. www.emedicine.com/oph/topic678.htm. Accessed September 10, 2008.
10. Hanson GE, Ogle RG, Giron L. A tongue stent for prevention of oral trauma in the comatose patient. Crit Care Med 1975;3(5):200–3.
11. McClintock K, Hall S, Oliver C. Risk markers associated with challenging behaviors in people with disabilities: a meta-analysis study. J Intellect Disabil Res 2001; 47:405–16.
12. National Institutes of Health. NIH consensus development conference on the treatment of destructive behaviors in persons with developmental disabilities. Bethesda (MD): U.S. Department of Health and Human Services; 1989.
13. Schroeder S, Oster-Granite M, Berkson G, et al. Self-injurious behavior: gene-brain-behavior relationships. MRDD Res Rev 2001;7:3–12.
14. Loschen EL, Osman OT. Self-injurious behavior in the developmentally disabled: assessment techniques. Psychopharmacol Bull 1992;28:433–8.
15. Davila J, Aslani M, Wentworth E. Oral appliance attached to a bubble helmet for prevention of self-inflicted injury. J Dent Child 1996;63(2):131–4.
16. Cordás TA, et al. Oxcarbazepine for self-mutilating bulimic patients. Int J Neuropsychopharmacol 2006;9:769–71.
17. Herpertz S. Self-injurious behavior psychopathological and nosological characteristics in subtypes of self-injurers. Acta Psychiatr Scand 1995;91: 57–68.
18. Fountas K, Smith J, Lee G. Bilateral stereotactic amygdalotomy for self-mutilation disorder: a case report. Stereotact Funct Neurosurg 2007;85:121–8.
19. Yates T. The developmental psychopathology of self-injurious behavior: Compensatory regulation in posttraumatic adaptation. Clin Psychol Rev 2004;24:35–74.
20. Hall S, Oliver C, Murphy G. Early development of self-injurious behavior: an empirical study. Am J Ment Retard 2001;106(2):189–99.
21. Aman MG. Efficacy of psychotropic drugs for reducing self-injurious behavior in the developmental disabilities. Ann Clin Psychiatry 1993;5:171–88.
22. Bosch JJ, Ringdahl J. Functional analysis of problem behavior in children with mental retardation. MCN Am J Maternal Child Nurs 2001;26(6):307–11.
23. Oliver C. Self-injurious behavior in children with learning disabilities: recent advances in assessment and intervention. J Child Psychol Psychiatry 1995;30: 909–27.
24. Hyman S, Fisher W, Mercugliano M, et al. Children with self-injurious behavior. Pediatrics 1990;85:437–41.
25. ElChaar GM, Maisch NM, Augusto LMG, et al. Efficacy and safety of naltrexone use in pediatric patients with autistic disorder. Ann Pharmacother 2006;40: 1086–94.

26. Canitano R. Self injurious behavior in autism: clinical aspects and treatment with risperidone. J Neural Transm 2006;113:425–31.
27. Klein U, Nowak AJ. Autistic disorder: a review for the pediatric dentist. Pediatr Dent 1998;20(5):312–7.
28. Wood AJ. A tongue shield appliance: design, fabrication, and case report. Spec Care Dentist 1991;11(1):12–4, 9.
29. Kobayashi T, Ghanem H, Umexawa K, et al. Treatment of self-inflicted oral trauma in a comatose patient: a case report. J Can Dent Assoc 2005;71(9):661–4.
30. Kuhn J, Lenartz D, Mai J, et al. Disappearance of self-aggressive behavior in a brain-injured patient after deep brain stimulation of the hypothalamus: a technical case report. Neurosurgery 2008;62(5):E1182.
31. Finger S, Duperon D. The management of self-inflicted oral trauma secondary to encephalitis: a clinical report. J Dent Child 1991;58(1):60–3.
32. Coyne B, Montague T. Teeth grinding, tongue and lip biting in a 24-month-old boy with meningococcal septicaemia: a case report. Int J Paediatr Dent 2002;12:277–80.
33. Yasui E, Kimura R, Kawamura A, et al. A modified oral screen appliance to prevent self-inflicted oral trauma in an infant with cerebral palsy: a case report. Oral Surg Oral Med Oral Pathol Oral Radiol Endod 2004;97:471–5.
34. Sonnenberg E. Treatment of self-induced trauma in a patient with cerebral palsy. Spec Care Dentist 1990;10(3):89–90.
35. Geyde A. Extreme self-injury attributed to frontal lobe seizures. Am J Ment Retard 1989;1:20–6.
36. Nurko C, Errington B, Taylor W, et al. Lip biting in a patient with Chiari type II malformation: case report. Pediatr Dent 1999;21(3):209–12.
37. Lesch M, Nyhan WL. A familiar disorder of uric acid metabolism and central nervous system function. Am J Med 1964;36:561–70.
38. Robertson M. Tourette syndrome, associated conditions and the complexities of treatment: invited review. Brain 2000;123:425–62.
39. Lowe O. Tourette's syndrome: management of oral complications. J Dent Child 1986;53(6):456–60.
40. Freeman R, Fast D, Burd L, et al. An international perspective on Tourette syndrome: selected findings from 3500 individuals in 22 countries. Dev Med Child Neurol 2000;42:436–47.
41. Mathews CA, Waller J, Glidden DV, et al. Self injurious behavior in Tourette syndrome: correlates with impulsivity and impulse control. J Neurol Neurosurg Psychiatry 2004;75:1149–55.
42. Janik P, Kalbarczyk A, Sitek M. Clinical analysis of Gilles de la Tourette syndrome based on 126 cases. Neurol Neurochir Pol 2007;41(5):381–7.
43. Hyman P, Oliver C. Causal explanations, concern and optimism regarding self-injurious behavior displayed by individuals with Cornelia de Lange syndrome: the parents' perspective. J Intellect Disabil Res 2001;45(4):326–34.
44. Shear C, Nyhan W, Kirman B, et al. Self-mutilative behavior as a feature of the de Lange syndrome. J Pediatr 1971;78(3):506–9.
45. Amano A, Akyiama S, Ikeda M, et al. Oral manifestations of hereditary sensory and autonomic neuropathy type IV: congenital insensitivity to pain with anhidrosis. Oral Surg Oral Med Oral Pathol 1998;86(4):425–31.
46. Mass E, Gadoth N. Oro-dental self-mutilation in familial dysautonomia. J Oral Pathol Med 1994;23:273–6.
47. Butler J, Fleming P, Webb D. Congenital insensitivity to pain – review and report of a case with dental implication. Oral Surg Oral Med Oral Pathol Oral Radiol Endod 2006;101:58–62.

48. Hall S, Lightbody A, Reiss A. Compulsive, self-injurious, and autistic behavior in children and adolescents with Fragile X syndrome. Am J Ment Retard 2008; 113(1):44–53.
49. Diab M. Self-inflicted orodental injury in a child with Leigh disease. Int J Paediatr Dent 2004;14:73–7.
50. Sheehy E, Longhurst P, Pool D, et al. Self-inflicted injury in a case of Hallervorden-Spatz disease. Int J Paediatr Dent 1999;9:299–302.
51. Hiraiwa R, Maegaki Y, Oka A, et al. Behavioral and psychiatric disorders in Prader-Willi syndrome: a population study in Japan. Brain Dev 2007;29:535–42.
52. Schroeder S, Hammock R, Mulick J, et al. Clinical trials of D_1 and D_2 dopamine modulating drugs and self-injury in mental retardation and developmental disabilities. MRD Res Rev 1995;1:120–9.
53. Lee J, Berkowitz R, Choi B. Oral self-mutilation in the Lesch-Nyhan syndrome. J Dent Child 2002;69(1):66–9.
54. Madan V, Gupta U. Tyrosinaemia type II with diffuse plantar keratoderma and self-mutilation. Clin Exp Dermatol 2005;31:54–6.
55. Shapira J, Zilberman Y, Becker A. Lesch-Nyhan syndrome: a nonextracting approach to prevent mutilation. Spec Care Dentist 1985;5(5):210–2.
56. Torres R, Puig J. Hypoxanthine-guanine phosophoribosyltransferase (HPRT) deficiency: Lesch-Nyhan syndrome. Orphanet J Rare Dis 2007;2(48):1–10.
57. LaBanc J, Epker B. Lesch-Nyhan Syndrome: surgical treatment in a case with lip chewing: a case report. J Maxillofac Surg 1981;9:64–7.
58. Cusumano F, Penna K, Panossian G. Prevention of self-mutilation in patients with Lesch-Nyhan syndrome: review of literature. J Dent Child 2001;68(3):175–8.
59. Dicks J. Lesch-Nyhan syndrome: a treatment planning dilemma: a case review. Pediatr Dent 1982;4(2):127–30.
60. Benz C, Reeka-Bartschmid A, Agostini F. The Lesch-Nyhan syndrome: a case report. Eur J Pediatr Dent 2004;5(2):110–4.
61. Bosch J, Van Dyke DC, Smith SM, et al. Role of medical conditions in the exacerbation of self-injurious behavior: an exploratory study. Ment Retard 1997;35(2):124–9.
62. Zilli E, Hasselmo M. A model of behavioral treatment for self-mutilation behavior in Lesch-Nyhan syndrome. Neuroreport 2008;19(4):459–62.
63. Lloyd KG, Hornykiewicz O, Davidson L, et al. Biochemical evidence of dysfunction of brain neurotransmitters in the Lesch-Nyhan syndrome. N Engl J Med 1981; 305:1106–11.
64. Ernst M, Zametkin AJ, Matochik Ja, et al. Presynaptic dopaminergic deficits in Lesch-Nyhan disease. N Engl J Med 1996;334:1568–72.
65. Wong DF, Harris JC, Naidu S, et al. Dopamine transporters are markedly reduced in Lesch-Nyhan disease in vivo. Proc Natl Acad Sci U S A 1996;93:5539–43.
66. Lee DO. Menstrually related self-injurious behavior in adolescents with autism [letter to editor]. J Am Acad Child Adolesc Psychiatry 2004;43(10):1193.
67. Mace FC, Blum NJ, Sierp BJ, et al. Differential response of operant self-injury to pharmacologic versus behavioral treatment. J Dev Behav Pediatr 2001;22(2):85–91.
68. Rooker GW, Roscoe EM. Functional analysis of self-injurious behavior and its relation to self-restraint. J Appl Behav Anal 2005;38(4):537–42.
69. Frey L, Szalda-Petree A, Seekins M, et al. Prevention of secondary health conditions in adults with developmental disabilities: a review of literature. Disabil Rehabil 2001;23(9):361–9.
70. Tsiouris J, Cohen I, Patti P, et al. Treatment of previously undiagnosed psychiatric disorders in persons with developmental disabilities decreased or eliminated self-injurious behavior. J Clin Psychiatry 2003;64:1081–90.

71. Sugahara T, Mishima K, Mori Y. Lesch-Nyhan syndrome: successful prevention of lower lip ulceration caused by self-mutilation by use of mouth guard. Int J Oral Maxillofac Surg 1994;23:37–8.
72. Evans J, Sirikumara M, Gregory M. Lesch-Nyhan syndrome and the lower lip guard. Oral Surg Oral Med Oral Pathol 1993;76:437–40.
73. Fardi K, Topouzelis N, Kotsanos N. Lesch-Nyhan syndrome: a preventive approach to self-mutilation. Int J Paediatr Dent 2003;13:51–6.
74. Anderson L, Ernst M. Self-injury in Lesch-Nyhan disease. J Autism Dev Disord 1994;24(1):67–81.
75. Santos M, Manzano F, Genovese W. Different approaches to dental management of self-inflicted oral trauma: oral shield, botulinum toxin type A neuromuscular block, and oral surgery. Quintessence Int 2008;38(2):e63–9.
76. Macpherson DW, Wolford LM, Kortebein MJ. Orthognathic surgery for the treatment of chronic self-mutilation of the lips. Int J Oral Maxillofac Surg. 1992;21:133–6.
77. Saemundsson S, Odont C, Roberts M. Oral self-injurious behavior in the developmentally disabled: review and a case. J Dent Child 1997;64(3):205–9, 228.
78. Thompson T, Symons F, Delaney D, et al. Self-injurious behavior as endogenous neurochemical self-administration. MRDD Res Rev 1995;1:137–48.
79. Smith S, Press B, Koening K, et al. Effects of sensory integration intervention on self-stimulating and self-injurious behaviors. Am J Occup Ther 2005;59(4):418–25.
80. Richman DM. Early intervention and prevention of self-injurious behavior exhibited by young children with developmental disabilities. J Intellect Disabil Res 2008;52(1):3–17.
81. Olson L, Houlihan D. A review of behavioral treatments used for Lesch-Nyhan syndrome. Behav Modif 2000;24(2):202–22.
82. Lovass IO. Building social behavior in autistic children by use of electric shock. J Exp Res Personality. 1965;1:99–109.
83. Rapoff ME, Altman K, Christopher ER. Suppression of self-injurious behavior: determination of the least restrictive alternative. J Ment Defic Res 1980;24:37–46.
84. Altaman K, Haavik S, Cook JW. Punishment of self-injurious behavior in natural settings using contingent aromatic ammonia. J Behav Res Ther 1978;16(2):85–96.
85. Richman D, Lindauer S. Longitudinal assessment of stereotypic proto-injurious, and self-injurious behavior exhibited by young children with developmental delays. Am J Ment Retard 2005;110(6):439–50.
86. Osman O, Loschen E. Self-injurious behavior in the developmentally disabled: pharmacologic treatment. Psychopharmacol Bull 1992;28(4):439–49.
87. Symons F, Thompson A, Rodriguez M. Self-injurious behavior and the efficacy of naltrexone treatment: a quantitative synthesis. MRDDD Res Rev 2004;10:193–200.
88. Blew P, Luiselli J, Thibadeau S. Beneficial effects of clonidine on severe self-injurious behavior in a 9-year-old girl with pervasive developmental disorder: a case report. J Child Adolesc Psychopharmacol 1999;9(4):285–91.
89. Jinnah HA, Visser J, Harris J, et al. Delineation of the motor disorder of Lesch-Nyhan disease. Brain 2006;129:1201–17.
90. Mikkelsen E. Low-dose haloperidol for stereotypic self-injurious behavior in the mentally retarded. N Engl J Med 1986;315(6):398–9.
91. Parksepp J, Vilberg T, Bean NJ. Reduction of distress vocalization in chicks by opiate peptides. Brain Res Bull 1978;3:633–67.

92. Willemsen-Swinkels S, Buitelaar J, Nijhof G, et al. Failure of naltrexone hydrochloride to reduce self-injurious and autistic behavior in mentally retarded adults. Arch Gen Psychiatry 1995;52:766–73.
93. McDougle CJ. Psychopharmacology. In: Cohen DJ, Volkmar FR, editors. Handbook of autism and pervasive developmental disorders. 2nd edition. New York: John Wiley & Sons, Inc; 1997. p. 707–29.
94. Ruedrich SL, Swales TP, Rossvanes C, et al. Atypical antipsychotic medication improves aggression, but not self-injurious behavior, in adults with intellectual disabilities. J Intellect Disabil Res 2008;52(2):132–40.
95. Taira T, Kobayashi T, Hori T. Disappearance of self-mutilating behavior in a patient with Lesch-Nyhan syndrome after bilateral chronic stimulation of the globus pallidus internus. J Neurosurg 2003;98:414–6.

Oral Health Burden in Children with Systemic Diseases

S. Thikkurissy, DDS, MS[a], Shantanu Lal, DDS[b,*]

KEYWORDS

• Special needs • Pediatric • Burden of oral disease

Children with special health care needs (CSHCN) comprise nearly 13% of all children in the United States, approximately 9.3 million children in all.[1] The National Survey of Children with Special Health Care Needs (NS-CHSCN) defined this population as those with "a chronic physical, developmental, behavioral or emotional condition and who also require health and related services of a type or amount beyond that required by children generally."[1] The very carefully worded definition employed by this survey, which evaluated variables for 373,055 children under the age of 18 from 196,888 households, describes how these children face a "burden of disease" distinctly greater than their healthy counterparts. Neglect or delay of addressing this burden cannot only lead to significant morbidity for the child but to family dysfunction as well. These children are generally at a higher risk for mental or behavioral problems, such as developmental delay, school absences, unscheduled intensive care unit admissions, and related health care costs.[2–4] All of the aforementioned issues put a considerable strain on the family unit. Van Dyck and colleagues[4] noted that "having a child with an SCHN can result in considerable financial challenges, substantial demands on time and lost parental employment opportunities." Within these intricately overlapping issues rests associated oral health morbidities.

While every illness carries its own oral health burden and space precludes an in-depth discussion, this article addresses issues salient to the understanding of oral health burden in children and families living with systemic disease. A list of conditions in **Table 1** demonstrates, by example, how oral physiology and treatment considerations are directly impacted by systemic illness.

A CHILD'S LIFE AT HOME

Children (both healthy and those with systemic illness) are more likely to have some form of medical insurance than dental coverage. While 6 million children lack medical

[a] Pediatric Dentistry, The Ohio State University College of Dentistry, Nationwide Children's Hospital, Columbus, OH, USA
[b] Division of Pediatric Dentistry, Columbia University College of Dental Medicine, 630 West 168th Street, P&S 3-454C, New York, NY 10032, USA
* Corresponding author.
E-mail address: sl784@columbia.edu (S. Lal).

Dent Clin N Am 53 (2009) 351–357
doi:10.1016/j.cden.2008.12.004

Table 1
Oral impacts of systemic illness

Systemic Condition	Oral Health Burden
Diabetes mellitus	Periodontal disease/gingival bleeding
Hemophilia	Increased oral and mucosal bleeding
Cancer	Infection, impaired healing, eruption disturbances, mucositis, xerostomia, caries
Gastrostomy	Increased calculus formation, sialorrhea
Cerebral palsy	Reduced oral clearance of foods; inability to maintain oral hygiene and associated complications.
HIV/AIDS	Opportunistic infections, periodontal disease, oral malignancies
Craniofacial anomalies and syndromes	Abberrations in dental development, craniofacial defects, loss of function

insurance, 16.3 million lack dental coverage.[5] Children with special health care needs are more likely to have access to a physician than they are to a dentist. When the NS-CHCSN was evaluated for unmet health care needs, it was determined that dental needs were second in frequency of need behind mental health needs. Dental needs were also the number one unmet health care need.[6] It has been estimated that in some populations of CSHCN, as many as one child in seven lack dental insurance.[7] The incorporation of oral health into the medical home, particularly for CSHCN, has been fraught with issues in training physicians and service-delivery concerns. This is especially true for facilities providing alternate living arrangements for patients with systemic illness.

Many such children, particularly those that are older, live in group facilities. In many cases, requirements for periodic oral health examinations are marginal and pursuance of actual dental care minimal, at best. While many case managers can identify the importance of dental care, to what extent they bear responsibility remains unclear.[8] Even for those CSHCN who are deinstitutionalized, as is the growing trend, finding a local dentist to provide routine care poses a challenge.[9]

One of the aims of the Dental Home concept relies on the recruitment of dentists to assume care for CSHCN into their practices.[10] Progress has been slow. From a legislative standpoint, a key to improving access to dental care for this vulnerable population is understanding that incorporation into a medical and dental home is vital to overall health and a sustained quality of life.

MY CHILD, MY PATIENT

An increasingly common phenomenon is the assumption of some aspects of preventive medical care—typically those performed by nursing staff —by parents of CSHCN. Parents who assume a nursing role change the dynamic of their relationship with their child.[11] This additional responsibility on the caregiver-parent-nurse can cause social isolation, greater anxiety, and stress in a marriage or relationship.[12–14]

In a 2008 study of parents of children requiring complex medical care, MacDonald and Callery related one mother's feelings as her daughter with a neurodevelopmental delay transitioned from infancy and toddler to school age:

> *I can't imagine giving up caring for her, although I'm sure a time will come as she gets older, I mean she's a lot heavier now, she's quite a big girl, she weighs about eight stone and I do find that moving around, even changing a nappy, is getting*

more and more difficult. It's not like lifting a baby's legs up anymore. She's heavy physically; she's become more of a problem.[15]

The above parent's concern is emblematic of the dilemma that a child with systemic illness can place on a parent who also functions as a caregiver. There is no doubt in this mother's words of her devotion to her child's care, yet there is the reality that the child is getting heavier and living with a static condition that will likely not improve. This underscores the idea that, perhaps when anticipatory guidance is provided in a dental setting, it must be done as speaking to a caregiver who has cognition of how oral health can impact the child's systemic disease, not simply to a parent who may find the thought of wrestling a large child to the ground to brush their teeth an insurmountable obstacle. Instructions and recommendations must be framed within the context of the child's systemic condition.

ORAL HEALTH AND CHRONIC PHYSICAL ILLNESS

Children with chronic physical illness that limit movement or motor function face a daily obstacle in maintaining optimal oral health. The oral health burden in children goes far beyond caries. An emblematic example of a chronic physical illness is cerebral palsy (CP). CP is a relatively common (1 to 2 per 1,000 live births) static encephalopathy in which many of the challenges of oral health can be seen. Despite the reduction of neonatal and perinatal mortality rates, CP rates have continued to rise, and as a result more children are surviving with severe CP that would not have survived 20 years ago.[16] Children with CP often present with poorly coordinated/pathologic oral reflexes. Dysfunctional swallow and chew mechanisms impact the diet that a child with CP can tolerate. Diet impacts plaque composition and the plaque composition impacts the balance of remineralization/demineralization that can lead to hard tissue dental disease.[17] Children with CP have been shown to have significant food residue present on their teeth. Removal of this food residue can be a challenge to the patient and caregiver.

Another systemic illness that often presents with physical disability that impacts oral health is juvenile arthritis, including juvenile rheumatoid arthritis (JRA) and juvenille idiopathic arthritis (JIA). JIA represents the most common arthritis of childhood, has a reported prevalence of 1 in 1,000 births, and can result in significant orthopedic and psychologic morbidities.[18] Children with upper limb JRA/JIA have been shown to have limited oral hygiene reach and poorer plaque removal.[19] Children with JRA/JIA are often treated with low-dose chemotherapeutic agents, such as methotrexate, and our understanding on the long-term effect of these agents is limited. Methotrexate has been reported to have interactions with inflammatory cytokines, such as tumor necrosis factor.[20] There is very limited understanding, if any, on how such interactions may affect oral development (eruption/exfolitation) and even response of pulpal and periradicular tissues to dental trauma.

Over time, the picture of caries prevalence in children with physical disabilities has changed. Historical studies demonstrated lower or equivalent decayed, missing or filled teeth or surface (DMFT/S) values in children with CP and those without.[21,22] Dos-Santos and colleagues[23] demonstrated children with CP were significantly more likely to be affected by caries than those without.

Caution must be exercised when interpreting how DMFT/DMFS relates the complete oral health picture of a child with systemic illness as CP and JIA/JRA. According to the World Health Organization, "DMFT and DMFS are means to numerically express the caries prevalence and are obtained by calculating the number of Decayed (D), Missing (M) and Filled (F) teeth (T) or surfaces (S). It is thus used to get an estimation illustrating how much the dentition until the day of examination has become affected by dental caries."[24] While DMFS and DMFT may give us the prevalence of caries, it represents a fragment of the overall oral health burden, as described in the opening section. In a 2008 study, Tickle and colleagues discussed surveillance methods used to assess the impact of dental pain on 3- to 6-year-old healthy children. The point is made that "person-level outcome measures are more important than tooth-level measures."[25] This speaks to the notion that our methods of assessing morbidity of the true impact of dental disease on a child are still in their infancy.

ORAL HEALTH AND NEUROBEHAVIORAL ILLNESS

If we go back to The National Survey of Children with Special Health Care Needs definition, those with "a chronic physical, developmental, behavioral or emotional condition and who also require health and related services of a type or amount beyond that required by children generally," neurobehavioral illness encompass those children with developmental, behavioral, and emotional conditions.

Children with developmental delay (DD) comprise 2% to 10% of the pediatric population.[26] Studies have shown this population twice as likely to have one or more chronic health conditions, with only 32% having isolated DD. In fact, 16.5% of children with DD had three or more chronic health conditions, compared with 1.5% for a cohort without DD. In many cases, accompanying these multiple medical conditions are polypharmacy and increased health care use, particularly during early childhood.

One hypothetical consideration is whether, as the number of medical-based visits increase and costs increase, a prioritization of care might occur, with an asymptomatic oral cavity potentially left without adequate attention. This supposition is not that far off when considering recent struggles with the dental applications of medically necessary care in operating room and hospital settings.[27] Furthermore, as Edelstein notes, while dentistry should ideally occupy a place as a specialty of medicine, it instead occupies a separate locus, both in terms of funding and case coordination. Children with neurobehavioral illness face these challenges, as exemplified by the fact that during the first 3 years of life, children with DD had significantly more physician and emergency department visits.[26] For some neurobehavioral illness however, we lack a clear picture of what the true oral health burden may be. Examples of this are the Autism Spectrum Disorders (ASD).

ASD is an umbrella term, encompassing a wide range of neurobehavioral illnesses including; autism, pervasive developmental delay not otherwise specified (PDD-NOS), and Asperger Syndrome. The overall prevalence has been reported to range from 5.2 to 7.6 per 1,000 children.[28] Specific oral health issues include oral aversions and dietary hypersensitivities to color, texture, and taste, as well as pouching of food.[29] The pouching of food, particularly cariogenic food, pushes the balance of oral health toward demineralization and possible cavitations. While existing studies have provided snapshot DMFT scores for autistic patients, currently we have no examination of these patients longitudinally. As with any child, an autistic child's diet and taste will develop but we have a poor understanding why certain foods might be favored over others, and how or if this can contribute to poor oral health. Finally, another burden in these patients that can impact oral health is the notion that many of the patients exist in a "diagnosis limbo," with no actual *Diagnostic and Statistical Manual of Mental Disorders* (DSM IV) diagnosis. This directly impacts medical (and dental coverage), particularly for general anesthesia, a forum in which many of these patients are ultimately treated, and quite often on repeated occasions.

Aside from the neurobehavioral impact of DD and ASD, children are also susceptible to emotional disturbances, and the therapies can have oral health implications as well.

Treatment-resistant clinical depression (TRCD) is a DSM-IV diagnosis that affects 1% of children, up to 8% of adolescents, and nearly 4 million people diagnosed with depression.[30] An increasingly popular treatment for TRCD is the use of a Vagus nerve stimulator (VNS). Though not fully understood, the theory behind the mechanism of the VNS is alteration of blood flow to the thalamus. VNS are also used to treat intractable epilepsy, in which at least two medications have failed to reduce seizure frequencies. An interesting side note relevant to the burden of these diseases: some state Medicaid agencies will only fund a VNS for intractable epilepsy when conventional medication therapy has failed for 12 months, thus forcing a family to live with a child with systemic illness for an additional year before approving VNS therapy, which has proved overwhelmingly effective in the treatment of intractable epilepsy. In children with VNS, there is an overall 3% to 5% infection rate, and there are potential oral health comorbidities as well. Dysphagia, Sialorrhea, vocal cord paralysis, and alteration of pain thresholds are possible adverse effects. This underscores a point for many of these children, for many of these families living with systemic illness: the main outcome is not eliminating disease or morbidity, but rather minimizing it. Implanted devices all have failures, polypharmacy can lead to untoward physiologic side effects, and the issue becomes: what choices will maximize the child's quality of life?

ORAL HEALTH AND ORGAN DISEASE

Aside from chronic physical illness and neurobehavioral illness, organ disease encompasses a large and particularly varied group of systemic illness. Children account for approximately 7% of all renal and liver transplants in the United States.[31] When parents were surveyed regarding the oral health of their children, 59% reported their child's oral health as "fair" or "poor." A high proportion of these parents reported being unable to find a dentist who felt comfortable treating their child during the various phases of the solid organ-transplant process.[32] Another disease characterized by treatment-phase specific oral health concerns is childhood cancer.

Current 5-year survivorship rates for children diagnosed with cancer exceed 75%. The 3-year survivorship rate exceeds 80%.[33] With medical advances aimed at evidence-based rather than empiric combinations of radiation and chemotherapy, there is every reason to expect these survival rates to increase in the future. Even as survival rates increase, the specter of the disease remains in the minds of the families it has affected. Kinahan and colleagues[34] surveyed adult childhood-cancer survivors and their parents, and found that 45% of surveyed parents reported thinking about the cancer experience more often than their child. The oral health burden of childhood cancer has been established in the literature, citing increased caries susceptibility, xerostomia associated with treatment regimens, mucositis, and abberations in dento-facial development.[35,36] In both solid organ transplant and cancer patients, the burden of oral disease can be acutely felt by adverse effects, such as graft-versus-host disease. Approximately 20% of patients who receive matched sibling transplants and 40% of matched unrelated donor recipients will develop chronic graft-versus-host disease.[25]

SUMMARY

Our picture of the oral health burden in children with systemic illness is incomplete. Limited tooth-based surveillance tools, an oral-systemic connection research base still relatively in its infancy, a continually diminishing number of dental providers comfortable in treating populations of children with systemic illness, and the fact that children are living longer with more serious illness all contribute to a considerable burden of oral health. In light of the last point mentioned, our attentions must also be focused on the long-term impact of systemic illness on family function. Moreso in children, systemic diseases have far reaching oral health implications (perhaps beyond periodontal disease-atheroscelrosis) that warrants our attention as a first priority. More efforts and resources need to be directed toward advocacy, policy, legislation, education, research, and clinical care, ultimately leading to a much deserved and enhanced quality of life for our very special population.

REFERENCES

1. McPherson M, Arango P, Fox H. A new definition of children with special health care needs. Pediatrics 1998;102:137–40.
2. Newacheck PW, Strickland B, Shonkoff JP, et al. An epidemiological profile of children with special health care needs. Pediatrics 1998;102:117–23.
3. Dosa NP, Boeing MM, Kanter RK. Excess risk of severe acute illness in children with chronic health conditions. Pediatrics 2001;107:499–504.
4. Van Dyck P, Kogan MD, McPherson MG, et al. Prevalence and characteristics of children with special health care needs. Arch Pediatr Adolesc Med 2004;158:884–90.
5. Lewis C, Mouradian W, Slayton R, et al. Dental Insurance and its impact on preventive dental care visits for U.S. children. J Am Dent Assoc 2007;138:369–80.
6. Lewis C, Robertson AS, Phelps S. Unmet dental care needs among children with special health care needs: Implications for the medical home. Pediatrics 2005;116:e426–31.
7. Ngui EM, Flores G. Unmet needs for speciality, dental, mental and allied health care among children with special health care needs: are there racial/ethnic disparities? J Health Care Poor Underserved 2007;18:931–49.
8. Hagman-Gustafsson ML, Holmen A, Stromberg E, et al. Who cares for the oral health of dependent elderly and disabled persons living at home? A qualitative study of case managers' knowledge, attitudes and initatives. Swed Dent J 2008;32:95–104.
9. Waldman HB, Perlman SP. Deinstitutionalization of children with mental retardation: what of dental services? ASDC J Dent Child 2000;67:413–7.
10. Nowak AJ, Casamassimo PS. The dental home: a primary oral health concept. J Am Dent Assoc 2002;133:93–104.
11. Kirk S, Glendinning C, Callery P. Parent or nurse? The experience of being the parent of a technologically-dependant child. J Adv Nurs 2005;51:456–64.
12. Diehl S, Moffitt K, Wade SM. Focus group interviews with parents of children with medically complex needs: an intimate look at their perceptions and feelings. Child Health Care 1991;20:170–8.
13. McKeever P. Mothering chronically-ill technology dependant children: an analysis using critical theory. 1991. PhD These. York University. Toronto.
14. Petr CG, Murdock B, Chapin R. Home care for children dependant on medical technology: the family perspective. Soc Work Health Care 1995;21:5–22.
15. MacDonald H, Callery P. Parenting children requiring complex care: a journey through time. Child Care Health Dev 2008;34:207–13.
16. Colver AF, Gibson M, Hey EN, et al. Increasing rates of cerebral palsy across the severity spectrum in northeast New England: collaborative cerebral palsy survey. Arch Dis Child Fetal Neonatal Ed 2000;83:F7–12.
17. Brown J, Schodel B. A review of controlled surveys of dental disease in handicapped persons. J Dent Child 1976;83:313–20.

18. Walton AG, Welbury RR, Thomason JM, et al. Oral health and juvenile idiopathic arthritis: a review. Rheumatology 2000;39:550–5.
19. Welbury RR, Thomason JM, Fitzgerald JL, et al. Increased prevalence of dental caries and poor oral hygiene in juvenile idiopathic arthritis. Rheumatology 2003; 42:1445–51.
20. Feldmann M, Maini SR. Role of cytokines in rheumatoid arthritis: an education in pathophysiology and therepeutics. Immunol Rev 2008;223:7–19.
21. Magnusson B, Deval R. Oral conditions in a group of children with cerebral palsy. Odontol Revy 1963;14:385–402.
22. Swallow J. The dental problems of handicapped children. J R Soc Health 1968; 85:152–7.
23. dos Santos MT, Masiero D, Novo NF, et al. Oral conditions in children with cerebral palsy. J Dent Child 2003;70:40–6.
24. WHO Oral Health Country/Area Profile Programme. Caries prevalence: DMFT and DMFS. WHO Collaborating Centre, Malmo University, Sweden. Available at: http://www.whocollab.od.mah.se/expl/orhdmft.html.
25. Tickle M, Blinkhorn AS, Milsom KM. The occurrence of dental pain and extractions over a 3-year period in a cohort of children aged 3-6 years. J Public Health Dent 2008;68:63–9.
26. Gallaher MM, Christakis DA, Connell FA. Health care use by children diagnosed as having developmental delay. Arch Pediatr Adolesc Med 2002;156:246–51.
27. Edelstein BL. Conceptual frameworks for understanding system capacity in the care of people with special health care needs. Pediatr Dent 2007;29:108–16.
28. Kopychka-Kedzierawski DT, Auigner P. Dental needs and status of autistic children: results from the National Survey of Children's Health. Pediatr Dent 2008; 30:54–8.
29. Herndon AC, DiGuiseppi C, Johnson SL. Does nutritional intake differ between children with autism spectrum disorders and children with typical development. J Autism Dev Disord 2008 [Epub ahead of print].
30. National Institutes of Health. Depression. U.S. Department of Health and human Services. NIH Publication 2008;083561.
31. The Organ procurement and transplantation network [Web site]. Transplants in the US by recepients age, 2006. Available at: http://www.optn.org/latestdata/rptData.asp. Accessed September 11, 2008.
32. Shiboski CH, Kawada P, Golinveaux M, et al. Oral disease burden and utilization of dental care patterns among pediatric solid organ transplant recepients. J Public Health Dent 2008; epub ahead of print.
33. Smith MA, Ries LAG. Childhood cancer: incidence, survival, and mortality. In: Pizzo PA, Poplack DG, editors. Principles and practice of pediatric oncology. 4th edition. Philadelphia: Lippincott Williams & Wilkins; 2002. p. 1–12.
34. Kinahan KE, Sharp LK, Arnston P, et al. Adult survivors of childhood cancer and their parents: experiences with survivorship and long-term follow up. J Pediatr Hematol Oncol 2008;30:651–8.
35. Schubert MM, Epstein JB, Peterson DE. Oral complications of cancer therapy. In: Yagiela JA, Neidle EA, Dowd FJ, editors. Pharmacology and therapeutics for dentistry. 4th edition. St. Louis (MO): Mosby-Year Book Inc; 1998. p. 644–55.
36. Dahllof G. Craniofacial growth in children treated for malignant diseases. Acta Odontol Scand 1998;56:378–82.

Behavioral Management for Patients with Intellectual and Developmental Disorders

Karen A. Raposa, RDH, MBA

KEYWORDS

- Autism spectrum disorders • Sensory modulation
- Pica • Receptive language Expressive language
- Applied behavior analysis • Dyspraxia
- Individualized education plan

Intellectual and developmental disorders (I&DDs) can severely impair a patient's ability to communicate and socialize. Individuals with such disorders tend to have unusual ways of learning, paying attention, and reacting to different sensations.[1] Symptoms can range from very mild to very severe. To properly treat these patients and, if necessary, refer them for appropriate medical care, dental professionals must be able to recognize the signs and symptoms of each patient's specific disability. Treating patients with I&DDs can be both challenging and rewarding.

As a parent of a child with autism–pervasive development delay, which is one type of I&DD, I can offer a personal as well as a professional perspective. Living with an individual with an I&DD involves ongoing challenges that dental professionals are unlikely to face in the short time the patient spends in the dental office. This article gives details about behaviors associated with I&DDs—behaviors that caregivers come to understand through constant care and supervision—and provides specific techniques that may be used routinely at home and carried into the dental setting. Researchers have not sufficiently studied the effectiveness of many suggested treatment accommodations for this patient population. So, to effectively provide good dental care to such patients, dental professionals must learn through interviews with caregivers about which behavior management techniques are most effective for each individual patient.

Colgate Oral Pharmaceuticals, Inc., 300 Park Avenue, New York, NY 10022, USA
E-mail address: Karen_raposa@colpal.com

Dent Clin N Am 53 (2009) 359–373
doi:10.1016/j.cden.2008.12.013
dental.theclinics.com

Today, dental and dental hygiene programs offer little formal education specific to the care of patients with I&DDs. To make up for this virtual absence of educational preparation for the care of patients with special needs, Special Olympics initiated an effort that brought about a modification in the Standards of Accreditation of all dental and dental hygiene schools in the United States. Beginning in 2006, all schools considered for accreditation by the Commission on Dental Accreditation must offer didactic and clinical opportunities to better prepare dental professionals for the care of persons with intellectual and other developmental disabilities.[2] While these standards are in place, many schools still struggle to meet all of the clinical requirements to include significant experiences with this patient population. In fact, in a recent study conducted at the University of Iowa, graduating dental students reported that their comfort level in treating patients who are mentally compromised was equal to their comfort level for treating patients who are drug users, who are jailed, or who have HIV.[3] In addition, a Special Olympics study conducted by Reuters Health found that "more than half of medical school deans and dental school deans, respectively, said that their graduates were 'not competent' to treat patients with intellectual disabilities."

For patients with I&DDs, it is crucial to introduce the patient to the dental environment and provide patient-appropriate care in a slow and gentle manner that builds trust and cooperation. Caries risk must be part of the initial assessment, and it is important that both the parent/caregiver and patient be introduced to a viable home care regimen that is tailored to the patient's abilities and not focused on the disabilities.

WHAT ARE INTELLECTUAL AND DEVELOPMENTAL DISORDERS?

I&DDs are classified as a complex group of neurobiological disorders that are caused by unusual brain development and that usually last throughout a lifetime. I&DDs include autism spectrum disorders (ASDs), which are associated with rigid routines and repetitive behaviors. Those afflicted have unusual ways of learning, paying attention, and reacting to different sensations.

Autism was first described in 1943 by American psychiatrist Leo Kanner of Johns Hopkins University. At the same time in Germany, Dr. Hans Asperger described a milder form of ASD, which eventually became known as Asperger's syndrome. These disorders, along with several others, including but not limited to Rett syndrome, pervasive developmental disorder, and childhood disintegrative disorder, are seen in children with varying degrees of communication disorders or delays. For children experiencing developmental delays, skills develop at a slower rate than normal (based on age appropriateness, whether it be a communication or motor skill). The skills of a delayed child are present but are slow to emerge. Meanwhile, a child who presents with a disorder, such as an ASD, either has skills that develop abnormally (eg, the child once possessed a skill and then regressed, losing the skill) or does not develop skills at all at age-appropriate intervals. These developmental delays result in such symptoms as speech difficulties, lack of eye contact, isolation, and no fear of danger.[4] I&DDs, including autism, can inhibit a person's ability to communicate and develop social relationships and are often accompanied by extreme behavioral challenges.

INTELLECTUAL AND DEVELOPMENTAL DISORDERS AND THE DENTAL PROFESSIONAL

Dental professionals must be knowledgeable and comfortable treating patients who have these disorders. In the past, many dental professionals were not exposed in an educational setting to the challenges and rewards associated with treating this patient population. Based on the prevalence of these types of disorders, including ASDs, a dental professional will likely meet at least seven or eight patients this year who have been diagnosed with some form of an I&DD.

To provide the most appropriate treatment for each patient and to be successful in providing that care, the dental professional must take time to learn about each patient's abilities prior to the initial dental visit. Dental professionals must request written information, which can be acquired in the form of a questionnaire prior to the visit. Furthermore, professionals must provide time during the initial visit to get to know the patient through interview and behavior assessment. These assessments should include inquiries about each patient's situation at home and that patient' specific abilities. Knowledge of the patient's home environment and specific capabilities gives the dental professional a basis for tailoring dental care to the patient's needs and capacities.

PREVALENCE OF INTELLECTUAL AND DEVELOPMENTAL DISORDERS

Because autism is the most common form of I&DD, the following statistics are specific to ASDs to help put into perspective the significant size of this patient population. ASDs usually develop between ages 2 and 3, although recent research is beginning to look at diagnosis as early as 6 months of age. Autism is seen across all racial, ethnic, and social groups, with a male predominance of four to one. Symptoms can be very mild to very severe. Today 1 in 150 individuals is diagnosed with autism, making it more common than pediatric cancer, diabetes, and AIDS combined.[5] It is seen in greater numbers than cerebral palsy, Down syndrome, and hearing and vision impairment (**Table 1**).[1] Three children per hour are diagnosed with ASDs, and the rate of diagnosis has increased 10-fold in the last decade, with 24,000 children currently diagnosed every year. Three million United States citizens have autism and the annual cost in the United States for caring for these individuals is estimated at $35 billion.[6]

AUTISM-SPECIFIC ETIOLOGIES

The etiology of autism is multifaceted, and no one particular factor has been proven to be "the" cause. The Centers for Disease Control and Prevention has called autism a national public health crisis whose cause and cure remain unknown. In May 2008, the International Meeting for Autism Research held its seventh annual meeting, with more than 850 presentations on various subjects related to autism, including etiology, biology, diagnosis, and treatment. Several of the presentations focused on the role of the environment as a risk factor for autism. Some discussion centered on the possibility that environmental factors may affect genetic risk factors.[7]

Table 1
Prevalence of childhood conditions

Condition	Prevalence
Autism	1 in 150 individuals
Cerebral palsy	1 in 357 individuals
Juvenile diabetes	1 in 450 individuals
Down syndrome	1 in 800 individuals
Deafness/hearing loss	1 in 909 individuals
Blindness/vision impairment	1 in 1111 individuals

Additionally, research is beginning to show that there is a familial pattern to symptoms of autism: If one child presents with symptoms, the parents are encouraged to be diligent in watching for signs/symptoms in other siblings, especially males. Other mechanisms being researched include nerve synapse connectivity and neuropathology of various structures of the brain.[8] Preliminary research also indicates that a high percentage of patients with autism exhibit autoimmune disorders, such as food allergies or rhinitis. It has been demonstrated that maternal infections can result in the elevation of cytokines in the fetal environment, which in turn may be a risk factor for developmental disorders.[1] Other hypotheses on the etiology of autism have been circulating for years, with no real definitive answers having been found. Some have speculated that autism might be a psychiatric disorder and have implicated the roles of amino acids, stress, prenatal aspartame exposure, vitamin A deficiencies, air pollution, and vaccinations. But the bottom line is that there is no answer yet and further research is needed in all areas of autism.

SIGNS AND SYMPTOMS OF AUTISM

Autism is diagnosed according to a pattern of symptoms rather than one single symptom. The main characteristics involve difficulties with social interaction and communication, limited interests, and repetitive behavior. Early signs and symptoms of ASDs include:

- No big smiles or other warm, joyful expressions by 6 months of age or thereafter
- No back-and-forth sharing of sounds, smiles, or other facial expressions by 9 months of age (communication skills)
- No babbling by 12 months of age
- No back-and-forth gestures, such as pointing, showing, reaching, or waving by 12 months of age (motor skills)
- No words by 16 months of age
- No two-word meaningful phrases, without modeling or repeating, by 24 months of age
- Any loss of speech or babbling or social skills at any age
- Underdeveloped play skills for a particular age
- Oversensitivity to textures

As there is no medical test or biomarker for autism, diagnosis is based on observation of the child's behavior, educational and psychological testing, and parent reporting. Several diagnostic tools are used in assessing for ASDs. The Autism Diagnostic Interview–Revised (ADI-R) and the Autism Diagnostic Observation Schedule (ADOS) are two of the most widely used. ADI-R can be used for both children and adults with a mental age of 18 months or above and contains 93 items. It focuses on behavior in three main areas: reciprocal social interaction, communication and language, and restrictive/repetitive stereotyped interests and behaviors. The ADOS is a semistructured assessment of communication, social interaction, and play or imaginative use of materials for individuals suspected of having autism or other ASDs. It enables the examiner to observe over a 30- to 45-minute period the occurrence or nonoccurrence of behaviors that have been linked to ASDs, and is appropriate for all age levels and developmental abilities. A team of specialists is usually involved in the diagnosis and evaluation. The team may include a neurologist, a psychiatrist, a developmental pediatrician, a psychologist, a gastroenterologist, an audiologist, a speech therapist, and an occupational therapist, as well as other professionals.

PREPARATION FOR TREATMENT OF PATIENTS WITH INTELLECTUAL AND DEVELOPMENTAL DISORDERS

To treat patients with I&DDs, one needs an open mind and heart. Emotional skills may be more useful than intellectual and clinical skills. The ability to get close to the patient both physically and emotionally, and the ability to be guided by instinct and creativity, rather than by strict reasoning, are important. This is a very different and sometimes challenging way of practicing dentistry and dental hygiene, but it is often a rewarding experience. Much understanding of the patient's condition can be obtained from the patient or parent/caregiver through documentation and interviews; however, because each patient is unique, most of the details are learned from one-on-one experience with the patient.

Documentation of the specific characteristics and abilities of the patient prior to the initial appointment is important for both the parent/caregiver and the dental professional. This provides an opportunity for the parent/caregiver to share with the dental professional all aspects of the patient's life and abilities. Ultimately the family will recognize that the professional cares and understands that these disorders present differently in all cases. For the dental professional, a patient information form with questions about crucial aspects of the patient's abilities is necessary to determine the proper skills and techniques required to provide successful dental treatment. This form should include sections for personal and medical information, dental experiences, oral habits, physical function, sensations, communication, vision, hearing, and behavior/emotions. A basic medical history form should be completed in its entirety and the additional information provided in this patient information form should be considered supplemental.

Personal and Medical Information

This first section of the form should include basic contact information as well as emergency names and phone numbers. A section should be included to provide the names and contact information of the general physician, as well as those of any developmental specialist or other specialists who routinely care for the individual. The nature and diagnosis of the condition needs to be addressed and a list of all medications should be provided. Allergies and sensitivities can be common in patients with I&DDs and should be discussed. In addition, the dental professional needs to be aware of any bowel or bladder adaptations necessary prior to performing dental treatment.

Dental Experiences

Information requested in the section on dental experiences should include those that have occurred in previous dental settings, as well as those that occur on a daily basis in the home. A discussion is necessary to explore the history of these experiences, as well as details about the daily at-home dental care routine, including products being used. Families/caregivers should be asked to provide information about the tolerance level of dental treatment both in-office and at-home daily. Finally, this section must include a statement of dental goals and expectations, both short term as it relates to the upcoming dental visit, as well as long-term expected care and realized benefits.

Oral Habits

Individuals with I&DDs can have any number of oral habits that should be discovered prior to the first dental appointment. Many of these individuals snack routinely through the course of the day as part of their need to satisfy oral sensory issues. In addition, because of food sensitivities or aversions, individuals may tend to always choose foods of a specific texture. Some patients may routinely choose a soft diet, while others may require hard crunchy foods to satisfy their sensory needs.

It is also important to ask about the type and frequency of nonnutritive behaviors. For some, sensory chewing involves chewing on rubber tubing or other materials as a stress release or to increase the muscular and sensing abilities of the masticatory muscles. Nonnutritive behaviors range from thumb/finger/pacifier sucking to pica, the ingestion of nonedible materials, including dirt, clay, paint, plaster, chalk, cigarette butts/ashes, glue, paper, buttons, toothpaste, or soap. While parents may think toothpaste is the lesser of the evils in this list, they should be instructed about the danger of toothpaste ingestion and provided with clear instructions on the proper amount of toothpaste to be used during brushing.

For teaching purposes, many therapists may choose caries-prone foods as a consistent reward for appropriate behaviors. Also, speech therapists may tend to choose foods that are sour or tart to help stimulate the mouth to entice language. Some of these choices, such as sour tarts, carbonated products, or lemons, can be erosive in nature and parents/caregivers need to provide therapists with more appropriate options (**Fig. 1**).

Finally, clenching and grinding habits are common in individuals with I&DDs. Such habits can be exacerbated by the use of inappropriate oral stimulation or sensory chewing devices. Appropriate devices for these purposes can be found at www.sensorycomfort.com.

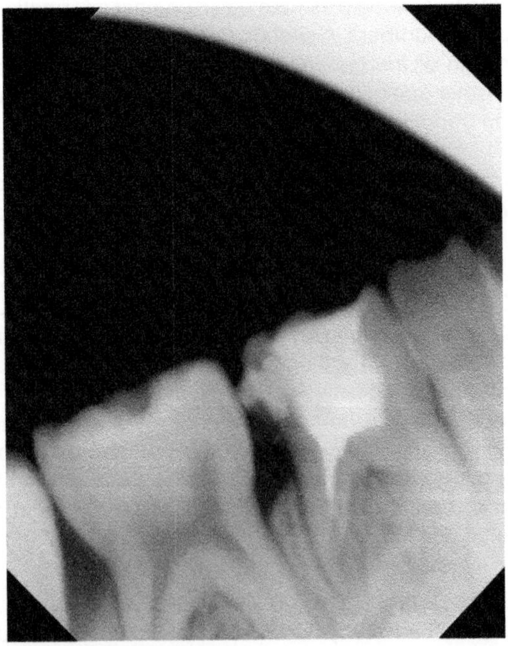

Fig. 1. Root canal–treated deciduous tooth as a result of being consistently rewarded with caries-prone foods for proper behavior.

Physical Function

It is important to learn the patient's daily habits and routines. Understanding whether the individual attends school or works and for what length of time can help gauge stamina and tolerability of procedures. Details about respiratory functioning, range of motion, and upper body strength are necessary in determining appropriate in-office treatment, as well as home care recommendations.

Sensations

Sensory issues involve visual, auditory, olfactory, gustatory (taste and texture), and tactile cues. Many I&DD patients exhibit sensory modulation processing disorders that manifest as underresponsivity (when stronger input is needed to register sensations), overresponsivity (when slight input causes extreme reactions), or sensory seeking (hypo- and hypersensitivities comingling with the same sense).

Within the dental environment, a sensory modulation processing disorder may be affected by the patient's olfactory sense of the operatory; auditory response to the high-speed handpiece; visual response to the lights; proximity to people and water; vestibular reactions to the chair movements; proprioceptive reactions to gagging and the lead apron; touch and temperature reactions to gloves, cotton rolls, and air/water; texture reactions to radiographic film or sensors, cotton rolls, or metal instruments; or taste sensations to gloves or medicaments (**Table 2**).

Every I&DD patient reacts differently according to each sense, and even the same patient may react differently to the same sensation at different times. A patient may experience a positive sensation on one visit, but the next time the same stimuli could produce a negative reaction. Understanding how a patient reacts to various sensory issues takes time, patience, and repeated work with the individual. The interview process is the beginning of this understanding.

Communication

Understanding how an I&DD patient communicates is an important goal of the interview process. Many patients may exhibit hearing or speech/language difficulties. Receptive language (what is heard/received) and expressive language (what is said) are often areas within the speech/language arena that present issues. The ability to follow directions, learn new things, and articulate wants and needs may be difficult for some patients with an I&DD. Many rely on verbal and nonverbal cues; others do

Table 2
Factors in the dental environment that may affect sensory modulation disorder

Environmental Factors	Affected Senses
Operatory smells	Smell
High-speed handpiece, among other noises	Hearing
Operatory light	Vision
Close proximity of people	Touch, smell, hearing
Water usage	Taste, touch, hearing
Operatory chair	Sense of motion
Gloves, cotton gauze, instruments, air/water syringe, textures of all other intraoral objects	Touch; sense of different temperatures, textures
Medicaments, gloves, dental materials	Taste

not understand nonverbal language. Therefore it is essential for the dental professional to be aware of the patient's manner of communication. Some require assistive communicative devices, such as an AlphaSmart (portable word processor), an augmentative communication device (**Fig. 2**), or a Picture Exchange Communication System (PECS).

PECS is an alternative communication technique for those who have little or no verbal skills. The PECS consists of a book of pictures to express desires, observations, and feelings (**Fig. 3**). The book grows as the patient grows, with more words and pictures, and is very helpful for those who are nonverbal.

Vision and Hearing

Elements to consider as they relate to vision include whether the patient routinely wears glasses or contacts, complains of double vision, has dominant peripheral vision, or can see effectively in both or only one eye. Patients who are hearing impaired may have auditory processing issues or wear hearing aides. Understanding all of these details helps with both effective communication and treatment.

Behavior/Emotions

Patients with I&DDs can exhibit a wide range of behavioral and emotional issues. Impulsiveness and a low threshold for frustration are common. These individuals often verbally or physically lose control and may have physical/verbal cues that set them off or calm them down. Verbally, they may use inappropriate language or speak at inappropriate times. Physically, they may pinch themselves or others; head bang or bite themselves or others; or self-induce vomiting. Information gained during the initial

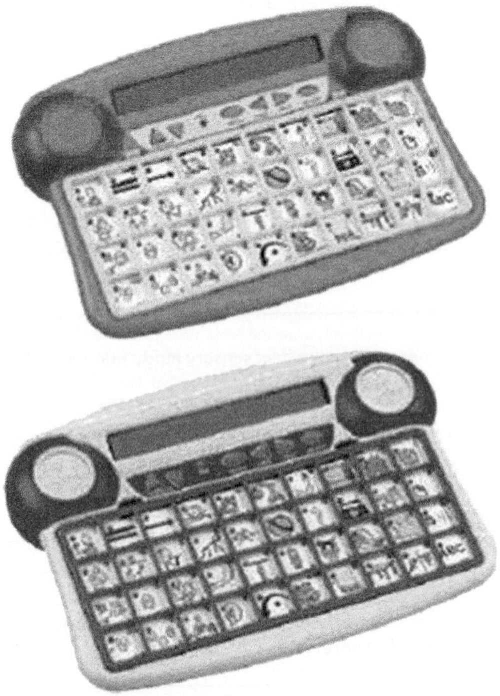

Fig. 2. Augmentative communication devices.

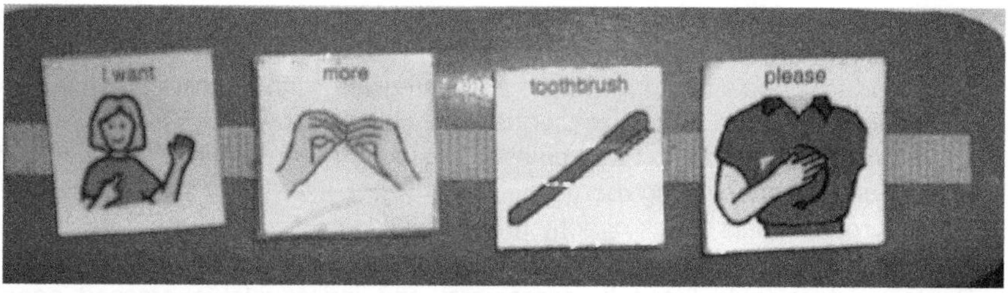

Fig. 3. PECS. (*Courtesy of* Woodlake Technologies, Inc., Chicago, IL. Available at: http://www.woodlaketechnologies.com; with permission.)

interview as to what may frustrate or calm the patient is important in providing dental care. Some parents/caregivers rely on applied behavior analysis techniques, based on B. F. Skinner's model of positive reinforcements, to enhance the patients' cooperation. Others may use a variety of other techniques and modalities to calm or soothe the individual. Behavior for patients with I&DDs is, in some cases, their only mode of communication. As this relates to dental pain, it is critical to ask parents/caregivers if they have noted any changes in behavior or prolonged episodes of behavioral abnormalities, as this could be an indicator of pain in the mouth.

THE INITIAL APPOINTMENT

The initial appointment for patients with I&DDs should include an interview. If possible, this should be conducted by telephone prior to the first visit to the dental office. Caregivers of patients with I&DDs have expressed a desire to speak with the dental care provider prior to the first appointment so that the needs of the patient can be discussed without the added stress of having the patient sitting in the office waiting for the interview to be completed. It would be ideal to have the patient return the completed patient information form prior to the call so it can be reviewed and discussed during the phone interview. Dental care goals and expectations should be agreed upon prior to scheduling the first appointment.

When scheduling the initial appointment, the front office personnel should inquire as to the best time of day for the appointment and should find out how the patient relates to having several people in a room at one time. In addition, it should be suggested that the parent/caregiver bring a comfort object or other coping device for the child as well as a second adult or friend who may stay with the child while the appropriate forms are reviewed with the parent. Prior to the initial appointment (and reinforced as necessary at subsequent appointments), photos of the office or a dental story can be sent to the parent/caregiver to familiarize the patient with the office. Finally, it should be suggested to the parent/caregiver that they bring an appropriate reward (sometimes wrapped gifts work well), as the rewards that may be available in the practice may not be appropriate or valuable to the individual.

The goal of the initial appointment is to establish trust and develop a relationship so the family gets to know that the dental professional is interested in the patient's well-being. It is important to learn what the patient is capable of doing versus learning what the patient is not able to do.

In a survey conducted on August 1, 2008, by the New York State Developmental Disabilities Planning Council, parents and caregivers stated what they need from dental care providers:

- Dental office staff have an understanding of the disability and the anxiety that individuals may have about dental visits
- Dental professionals treat individuals and caregivers with the same respect and dignity as others and recognize unique family strengths
- The dental office have short wait times and a low-stress, quiet environment, with special or separate waiting rooms
- Dental professionals speak directly to the individual
- The dental office allows extra time for the appointment
- Dental professionals listen to caregivers' and individuals' expressed needs (verbal and nonverbal)
- Dental professionals share complete and unbiased information with families
- Dental professionals allow caregivers to be present during the visit and give caregivers ample opportunities to ask questions
- The dental professional sees the individual as a person with unique needs, not as a "disabled person"
- The dental professional make appropriate referrals and timely follow through with paperwork

In turn, these individuals in the same study provided a list of items they felt they should do themselves to prepare their family member with an I&DD for the first dental visit:

- Prepare the individual for dental visit through role-play, books, and pictures
- Bring distractions for waiting and examination rooms (eg, books, music, video, games) and offer rewards (eg, prizes, outings)
- Ask for a "get acquainted" visit
- Schedule appointment at a time that is best for the individual (first or last appointment of the day)
- Keep a dental journal of copayments, medications, treatments, prior visits, and referrals
- Make sure the parking lot, building, and office are accessible
- Talk to the dentist and staff before the visit; prepare staff ahead of time and remind them of the individual's needs; mail or fax a summary letter (ie. patient information form)
- Bring a support person to listen to the dentist/hygienist/assistant, write things down, and help with other children
- Research dental issues in books, journals, and online, and ask lots of questions
- Ask for the same staff each time

This first trust-building appointment may be only 20 minutes in length and can be considered an orientation to the dental practice, including staff and facility, as warranted. The appointment should begin on time so there is very little wait time for the patient. In addition, the patient should be allowed to determine where the visit takes place (ie, reception area, operatory, business office, staff lunch area) and the parent/caregiver should be present during the appointment. This allows a trust-building relationship to begin between the patient and the dental professional. If possible, a brief examination could be conducted without dental instruments at first. Then, instruments could be introduced gradually later on, possibly at a rate of only one new instrument at each subsequent appointment. This introduction should involve the "tell-show-do" method of communication and engagement.

Dr. David Tesini, a pediatric dentist in Sudbury, Massachusetts, developed the D-Termined Program of Repetitive Tasking and Familiarization in Dentistry, in which the dental professional presents one new step to the patient at each visit and the patient must master it before moving on to the next step. Parents/caregivers must practice a given routine at home so that visiting the dental office becomes a "game" with rewards. This game can include the use of plastic mirrors or dental films, which the dental office can supply, to simulate dental procedures at home. Dividing the skill into small parts, demonstrating the skill, drilling of the skill, delighting the learner (individualized reward), and delegating the repetition (reinforcement of the skill) are components of the D-Termined program. Additionally, three factors are important for success from a dental standpoint: maintenance of eye contact ("look at me" statements), educational modeling (clear, understandable directions), and the use of a counting framework ("Let me do this for a count of 10").

The dental professional should "reward" the patient at the end of the appointment immediately following an appropriate behavior, even if the behavior is only a handshake that was given when asked. I&DD patients enjoy receiving rewards and will look forward to seeing the dental professional at a future date if the first experience has been rewarding.

FOLLOW-UP AND THE SECOND APPOINTMENT

Dental professionals should follow up with a phone call to the family a day or two after the procedure and then at regular intervals (2, 5, and 12 weeks following). This conveys a sense of concern to the parent/caregiver and reminds the parent/caregiver to keep working on all recommendation recommendationss for practice dental stimulation routines and home care. It also provides an opportunity for coaching on home care strategies and techniques. Appropriate reinforcement recommendations should be sent home with the patient for practicing the dental office visit and proper home care. A recare/reevaluation appointment 3 to 6 months in the future should be arranged before the patient leaves the office.

The next appointment should be based on what was learned during the initial visit. The second and subsequent appointments should be kept short with treatment being provided in a timely manner. A smile and a sense of playfulness, while understanding the patient's developmental age, helps in the treatment process. It is also important to continue to build on the trust relationship.

To determine what will work during treatment, dental professionals should focus on the patient's abilities rather than disabilities. Information gleaned from the initial interview can answer such questions as:

- How much time will be needed for a procedure?
- What do the dental professional, parent/caregiver, and patient want to accomplish in the visit?
- What accommodations will be necessary?
- How will "success" be measured?

TREATMENT CONSIDERATIONS AND ACCOMMODATIONS

When initially approaching a patient with an I&DD, a request for a "high five" can be very effective. This approach is generally used by therapists, teachers, and caregivers, so it is familiar to patients in this population. In addition, it allows the patient to approach the dental professional and help avoid the hesitation that can occur when a dental professional walks toward the individual for the first time.

Since many patients with autism act out for a reason and many cannot communicate if they are uncomfortable, these individuals can become aggressive. Therefore, planning for success is crucial to maintaining control of the dental situation. Developing relationships, reducing anxiety, and understanding and using the patient's strengths all increase the control the dental professional has with this patient population. Many patients may also exhibit levels of dyspraxia (developmental coordination disorder). Patients who present with dyspraxia may not be able to perform basic tasks asked by dental professionals, including opening the mouth wide, closing the mouth a little, and turning the head. The dental professional must be aware of this and must adjust treatment modalities as necessary. With any modification in treatment protocols for the patients, the dental professional must remember that all of it means nothing unless that patient is handled with a "special touch."[9]

Keeping instruments out of sight until needed, keeping lights out of the patient's eyes, and keeping distracting noises to a minimum add to the confidence and trust factor. The use of a headlamp allows for both the overhead lights and dental lights to remain turned off, which can be very effective in calming a patient with an I&DD. Dental professionals should also consider noise-aversion devices, which make "white noise" or musical sounds, as well as headphones that drown out surrounding sounds.

Simple, creative tools can smooth the way to complete success in many cases. Calming devices, such as weighted vests, warm moist pillows for under the neck, or even the use of the lead apron can be very effective. Fidget toys and chew tubes can help to keep the appointment moving forward. A fidget toy can be an effective distraction and a chew tube that is allowed in the mouth as a reward for each 10 seconds of allowed treatment can provide great success. In addition, while bite blocks are necessary in most cases, they are difficult to maintain in the mouth and patients may tend to reject them. Since the handles on children's toothbrushes in today's market are very large, they can serve very well as a bite block if held on the opposite side of the proposed treatment. The end result is less rejection because a toothbrush is something that a patient is accustomed to having in his or her mouth.

While body wraps and joint stabilizers are available and some dental professionals have found them to be beneficial, in most states they are categorized as restraining devices and should only be used if the specific state laws are researched and understood and then only when a dental professional has been properly trained in their use. In most cases, if dental care begins early in the patient's life and the techniques discussed in this article are provided routinely and consistently, the use of stabilizing restraint devices will most likely not be necessary.

Constant sincere reinforcement and consistent praise or high fives help improve trust. Involving the same dental team members in the patient's care each time helps avoid unnecessary anxiety and frustration for the patient. In addition, patients with I&DDs crave consistency, and seeing the same faces at each visit helps build trust and confidence. Use of the tell-show-do technique of treatment allows familiarization and confidence and familiarizing the parent/caregiver with the procedure via a telephone conversation prior to the office visit can also improve outcomes. Individuals with I&DDs can be very cooperative with dental treatment if an approach based on trust, tailored communication, and appropriate appointment length is developed.

HOME CARE FOR PATIENTS WITH INTELLECTUAL AND DEVELOPMENTAL DISORDERS

Beyond treatment modality concerns, patients and parents/caregivers need to be educated about the importance of home care therapies. It is crucial that the parent/caregiver be provided with hands-on training, and issues of accountability should be discussed. An appropriate special-needs health history form should include the question: "Who will be responsible for the success or failure of the patient's oral health?" This question should be addressed and signed by the parent/caregiver.

When basic toothbrushing is discussed, it is critical that its importance be reinforced. One method of doing this is by changing the terminology so the parents/caregivers do not feel they are hearing the same information they have heard about their own mouths for many years. Instructing the parent/caregiver in daily full-mouth disinfection rather than toothbrushing can help. Also, talking about toothpaste as medication and the toothbrush as the device used to deliver the medication can elevate the importance of this daily regimen. An antibacterial toothpaste that does not cause tooth staining is recommended for this patient population. Consider altering conversations to include the use of the terms *debridement* and *medication* rather than *brushing with toothpaste*. Finally, offering the parent/caregiver the information in writing also reinforces the concepts discussed.

Parents/caregivers need the dental professional to show them several options for positioning their loved one during home care. Depending on the size of the individual with an I&DD, positioning can be demonstrated in several ways. One way is to have the parent/caregiver sit down with the individual sitting on the floor between the parent's or caregiver's knees. Another way is to have the individual lay down on a beanbag on the floor to allow homecare. It is important to remind the parent/caregiver that brushing does not have to be performed in the bathroom.

Begin educating the parent/caregiver and the patient in baby steps. Recommend that a timer be set for 5 to 10 seconds for the first brushing session and that this be conducted several times during the course of the day. At 2- to 3-day intervals, the brushing time can be increased and the frequency decreased until the patient is allowed at least a full minute of brushing three times a day (note that it would be ideal to extend this to a 2-minute brushing, but it may not be realistic to expect this in all cases). Allowing the patient to brush alone at each session, even if it is only for a second or two, will help build confidence in the skill. In addition, it is important to provide a reward at the end of every session to encourage cooperation from session to session. The use of a power toothbrush is recommended as it is not only more effective in removing plaque, but it also works to desensitize patients to similar types of oral sensations when they have their dental visits. This may require a slow build similar to the conditioning to allow manual brushing, but with time and persistence, the long-term advantages are significant.

Fluoride is critical in this patient population because these patients are all at high risk for caries due to any number of factors (diet, constant snacking, xerostomia, poor oral hygiene). Many prescription fluoride gels and rinses may not be safe for use if the individual is unable to effectively expectorate. However, over-the-counter toothpaste, which contains approximately 1100-ppm fluoride, can be very beneficial if left on the teeth after brushing and not rinsed out of the mouth. Parents/caregivers must be instructed to place only a smear of paste on the brushhead because most patients in this population will swallow all of the paste placed on the brush. The in-office fluoride of choice for patients with I&DDs is fluoride varnish. At approximately 22,500 ppm, fluoride varnish provides the highest concentration of fluoride with the lowest risk of ingestion. It works effectively in a wet environment and is quick and easy to apply, no trays necessary. For dental professionals concerned with the color of fluoride varnishes, several available today are white or clear and such varnishes need to be applied only in areas of the mouth most at risk, so it is not necessary to apply varnish to the buccal surfaces of maxillary lateral and central incisors.

In addition, discuss with the parent/caregiver the roles of saliva substitutes, sealants, and xylitol. For patients taking medications that may cause xerostomia, parents/caregivers need to understand the role of saliva in order to elevate the need for additional homecare strategies. In cases where increased saliva is necessary or where constant snacking is an issue, a nice alternative to fluoride when it is not available is the use of xylitol containing candy and gum. These products can help stimulate salivary flow and they provide an effective substitute for other less-appropriate food snacks.

Finally, understanding the individualized education plan (IEP) developed for the overall education of your patient with an I&DD helps you build bridges with the patient and provide oral health care and education at an appropriate pace and level of complexity. It is also important to look at the IEP to see if oral hygiene education has been included and, if not, to recommend that the parent call the school to request that this be incorporated into the IEP.

MEASURING SUCCESS

Success in treating patients with I&DDs is measured exactly the same way as it is for the general patient population:

- Determine how the patient and parent/caregiver feel about visiting the dental practice.
- Measure how the patient responds to treatment.
- Evaluate actual home care routines.
- Look for presence of any new disease.
- Document successes and failures.

Thomas A. Edison once said: "Many of life's failures are people who did not realize how close they were to success when they gave up." This is an important thought when considering whether to refer a patient with an I&DD to a specialist outside of your practice. The Academy of General Dentistry notes that, while all dental professionals are encouraged to treat individuals with special needs, the law does not require professionals to accept these patients into their practice. However, practitioners should try to provide some guidance by knowing who in their community does have the experience and education to treat patients with special needs.[10] Recognize that parents/caregivers know the patient very well, so plan to use their insights to help make this decision. If a referral is best, then help educate the family about alternatives, which can include but are not limited to an educational setting, hospital setting, or pediatric dental office.

In addition to treating patients with I&DDs, dental professionals should consider evaluating all children for signs and symptoms of developmental delays/disorders. For dental professionals, it is beyond the scope of practice to "diagnose" a child with a delay/disorder, but the recognition and referral to the appropriate resources is invaluable to those parents/caregivers who may not otherwise seek out such services. The earlier delays are recognized and treatment implemented, the better the outcome for the child and family. One effective way of providing referral information without an implied "diagnosis" is to contact such organizations as Autism Speaks and request brochures that list the signs and symptoms of developmental delays. This brochure can be placed in a home care packet provided to parents at the child's first dental visit.

Dental professionals should build relationships with pediatricians, early intervention specialists, and special education therapists in their area to provide a network of resources for families. The American Academy of Pediatric Dentistry and the American Academy of Pediatrics recommend initial dental visits for all children by age 1. This initial visit serves a number of purposes but is primarily educational for the parent/caregiver.

SUMMARY

Dental care for the I&DD patient population makes a long-term impact that affects the patient, family, and dental professional in ways that are often overlooked. For patients with I&DDs receiving treatment, they have an opportunity to experience lifelong dental health from a team of caring dental professionals they know and trust. In the hands of such sensitive and qualified professionals, these individuals have one less event in their lives to be anxious about. For the families and caregivers of these individuals, they experience a feeling of acceptance and trust not typically found in many environments they encounter and they will tell others about it. For dental professionals and the dental practice, they will receive referrals from the patients' families and friends and these same parents/caregivers will be discussing the positive experience of a caring, thoughtful, and kind staff with all of their friends. In addition, working with these individuals provides an opportunity to meet and work with some exceptional families. Dr. Gregory Folse described it best in his article for *Access* in January 2006: "It is hard to describe the elation one can feel when a patient who doesn't speak to anyone speaks to you."

REFERENCES

1. Centers for Disease Control and Prevention. Commission on Dental Accreditation – 2006. Available at: www.cdc.gov. Accessed February 17, 2006.
2. Folse G, Glassman P, Miller C. Serving the patient with special needs. Access 2006;20(1):8–13.
3. Kathy R, McQuistan M, Riniker K, et al. Students' comfort level in treating vulnerable opulations and future willingness to treat: results prior to extramural participation. J Dent Educ 2005;69(12):1307–14.
4. The Healing Center. Available at: www.healing-arts.org. Accessed March 4, 2006.
5. Autism Speaks. Available at: www.autismspeaks.org. Accessed March 4, 2006.
6. Harvard School of Public Health. Available at: www.hsph.harvard.edu. Accessed March 11, 2008.
7. International Meeting for Autism Research—Final Recap. London, United Kingdom, May 15–17, 2008.
8. Ramachandran V, Oberman L. "Broken mirrors: a theory of autism." Sci Am November 2006;295(5):63–9.
9. Elliott-Smith S. Special products for patients with special needs. Access 2006; 20(1):18–20.
10. Asa R. Special care: treating patients with special needs requires both training and compassion. AGD Impact 2007;35(10):34–6, 38,40.

Home Oral Health Practice: The Foundation for Desensitization and Dental Care for Special Needs

Fred S. Ferguson, DDS[a,*], Debra Cinotti, DDS[b]

KEYWORDS

• Home • Oral health • Desensitization • Special needs
• Dental care • Risk assessment

Obstacles to the oral health and dental care for persons with special needs are well known.[1–7] In general, the oral health of persons with special needs is reflective of, but not limited to:

Lack of oral health knowledge by caregivers and medical health professionals.[1–7]
Lack of knowledgeable and experienced dental health professionals in dental care for special needs.[1–7]
Lack of education standards in dental school and postdoctoral education in the oral health counseling and care of the special needs population.[4–8]
Lack of *effective* daily oral health supervision for individuals with special needs by caregivers and agencies.[9–16]
Lack of evidenced-based standards of oral care for community-based programs.[9–16]
Unrealistic expectations of the benefits and goals of dental care and patient management.[9–16]

As the impact of oral illness on general health is gaining attention, the importance of establishing an accountable "home oral health practice" (ie, activity by the patient to

[a] Dental Care for the Developmentally Disabled Program, Department of Children's Dentistry, Rockland Hall, Room 122, School of Dental Medicine, Stony Brook University, Stony Brook, NY 11794-8700, USA
[b] Dental Care for the Developmentally Disabled Program, Department of General Dentistry, Rockland Hall Room 148B, School of Dental Medicine, Stony Brook University, Stony Brook, NY 11794-8700, USA
* Corresponding author.
E-mail address: fferguson@notes.cc.sunysb.edu (F.S. Ferguson).

Dent Clin N Am 53 (2009) 375–387
doi:10.1016/j.cden.2008.12.009 dental.theclinics.com

achieve daily, effective oral hygiene; or that of a caregiver to provide daily effective oral health supervision for another individual who cannot accomplish this activity alone) becomes an essential protector for general health. Given the implication of developmental delays (which includes cognitive and physical growth, emotional and social maturation, speech and language development, and neuromuscular function) the lack of a knowledgeable, motivated, and properly trained support system for home oral health practice presents significant threats to health for the person with special needs.

Accountable and effective oral health for the individual with special needs requires a partnership between the caregiver (eg, parent, relative, daily health aide, agency) who is responsible for the individual with special needs and the professional dental care team appropriate to the environment of that patient. The primary responsibility of the dental health team is to provide information and training to the patient and caregiver, culminating into an individualized and evidenced-based treatment plan which will provide protection of the patient's oral health and development in the patient's place of residence. This is an evolving partnership of the oral health team (ie, dental professional, caregiver, and, if possible, the patient), each confirming their responsibility to protect the health and quality of life of the patient.

RISK ASSESSMENT DISCOVERS OBSTACLES TO ORAL HEALTH

Risk assessment is the first step in the journey of this partnership–establishing an approach to patient management that promotes learning and supports home oral health practice. This approach requires that the dental provider is knowledgeable about the epidemiology of common oral illnesses. Predictable patient management for home oral health practice is essential for successful outcomes of professional dental care. Knowledge of risk concerns directs the dental professional to identify potential problems and obstacles in the care of the patient which, in turn, points to potential options for management of patient learning and home oral health practice. Approaches to management will be different for different patients depending on the risks discovered in the assessment process. For example, a patient who cooperates with home oral health practice, accepts oral treatment without resistance, and has a dedicated caregiver with a high dental IQ will be able to receive complex treatment plans (eg, fixed prosthetics) with a high probability of success. A patient who is noncompliant, resistant to treatment, or does not have a caregiver providing effective home care would not be a candidate for complex treatment that requires effective daily home management as he or she would be at risk for treatment failure and continued oral illness.

Risk identification begins with a systematic discovery of threats to the patient's oral health including developmental concerns, health and health care history, and risks within the patient's home environment. The patient's environment includes (but is not limited to): caregiver knowledge, attitude and expectations about oral health, caregiver ability to provide the patient daily home care, patient's access to care, daily health habits (eg, home hygiene practices, dietary controls), social environment (eg, smoking controls, food reward practices), oral hypersensitivity, sensory motor limitations, and behavioral obstacles specific to self care or assisted oral hygiene. This discovery process starts with communication between the caregiver and the dental care team before the clinical examination. A clear estimation of the patient's risk factors and oral condition can be easily determined through discussion with the caregiver–including a series of very simple questions. Having an open exchange of information also serves to prepare the patient (if possible), the caregiver, and the dental provider about potential behavioral concerns before the clinical examination. This can prevent stressful outcomes and fosters informed consent for patient management. The following protocol can serve as a guide to obtain critical information in preparation for the clinical examination visit:

Step 1. Preliminary information (via phone or mailed questionnaire) including legal guardianship and medical and behavioral histories. This prepares the dental care team for possible health-related oral problems, behavioral obstacles, and informed consent barriers.

Step 2. The caregiver and patient interview ensures that the caregiver understands the requirements for oral health, and identifies the patient's social and cognitive competence and potential response to the examination. Additionally, the caregiver and dental provider have defined expected patient obstacles to the examination, potential clinical findings, and can agree on the approach to care.

Step 3. The clinical examination will confirm oral illness, treatment requirements, and the options for patient management relative to his or her cooperation and level of cognitive and social function. The identified risks are explained to the patient (if appropriate), the caregiver, and legal guardian. The consequences to both oral and general health and the methods to eradicate or reduce the risk factors are discussed. This supports patient and caregiver learning, and oral home care efforts.

In summary, effective communication with the caregiver (ie, an exchange of information) and observation of the patient before the hands-on examination provides the best opportunity to promote a partnership with the caregiver and the dental care team, begin the foundation for "informed" consent, and achieve a favorable outcome for the patient's oral health. Additionally, risk assessment provides information important to development of evidence-based care for each patient.

THE IMPORTANCE OF EFFECTIVE HOME ORAL HEALTH PRACTICE FOR ORAL HEALTH AND DENTAL CARE OF THE SPECIAL NEEDS GROUP

Self or assisted home oral health practice is critical for oral health as it controls growth of common oral pathogens responsible for the common oral infections (caries, gingivitis, bone loss, and oral malodor). Also, oral cleansing provides beneficial oral motor therapy stimulation and massage for oral tissues that is essential for circulation, cellular turnover, and reduction of oral hypersensitivity.[17] Determining this practice and the patient's oral hygiene status should be a standard of care performed at each patient visit. Specifically, an oral state free of plaque, oral debris, and accretions facilitates the successful delivery of optimal dental rehabilitation (operative, endodontics, periodontal surgery, implantology, etc) and the prognosis of therapy over time. A suggested guide in developing a treatment plan is presented in **Table 1**.

CAREGIVER'S EXPECTATION AND ROLE IN ORAL HEALTH FOR THE SPECIAL NEEDS PATIENT

Caregivers are generally aware of their effectiveness or lack of ability to provide good oral care to a child or adult who presents oppositional behaviors.[12,13] Agencies and caregivers may have expectations regarding the benefit of frequent and short appointments or "desensitization visits" as they may believe that desensitization visits will increase cooperative behavior of persons with developmental delays when receiving dental care.[11] The dental literature shows use of desensitization does not work for the patient with severe neurologic impairment who presents oppositional and avoidance

Table 1
Relationship of patient compliance and oral cleanliness to level of definitive care

Patient Status	Level of Definitive Care
A. Patient presents with clean oral tissues ■ Has effective caregiver support ■ Tolerates oral procedures	Consider all options for comprehensive care based on patient's cognitive, social needs and activity, neuromuscular and skeletal concerns, caries risk, strategic importance of tooth or teeth, isolation requirements, behavioral obstacles, habits, dietary and medication risks, etc.
B. Patient presents with clean oral tissues ■ Has effective caregiver support ■ Does not tolerate oral procedures C. Patient presents with poor oral hygiene (ie, debris and gingivitis) ■ Does not have effective caregiver support ■ Tolerates oral procedures D. Patient presents with poor oral hygiene ■ Does not have effective caregiver support ■ Does not tolerate oral procedures	Remove sources of pain and infection: ■ Pulp therapy: Pulpotomy of primary molars with carious exposures; consider endodontic therapy for selected adult teeth ■ Restoration therapy ■ Extraction of nonrestorable or pulpally-involved adult teeth ■ Periodontal therapy beyond scaling and root planing considered on a limited basis ■ Consider prosthetics in selected cases only (risk–benefit ratio for the patient) Provider must consider behavioral obstacles, medication, diet, oral hygiene risks and isolation requirements that would compromise operative, periodontal, and prosthetic therapy. The method (ie, patient management) of care must be considered in regard to future prognosis and need for medical immobilization.

To develop an appropriate treatment plan, the provider must consider the following:
- Patient safety
- Potential for recurrent infection (gingival, periodontal, caries risk, tooth surface or location).
- Isolation demands for treatment (technique)
- Patient movement or behavior (as it affects above)

behaviors. If patient cooperation cannot be accomplished by an experienced dental provider through modification techniques, physical or pharmacologic immobilization should be considered for future visits.[9–11]

In dental practice, desensitization is the systematic presentation of situations that would be regarded as low threat (ie, digital examination) and slowly increasing to higher threats (mirror and explorer) with the intention to reduce patient anxiety and gain trust and cooperation. Unfortunately, transferring skills to enable caregivers to provide oral health cleansing to individuals who present oppositional behaviors is not a routine or standard of care component of health care encounters or training to direct care staff. Studies demonstrate that caregivers and daily care staff can become skilled in providing daily oral health care for children and adults who need supervision or assistance for oral hygiene.[12–16] Home oral health practice is the most effective form of desensitization as it has the best potential to have the patient learn that oral intervention is part of their daily routine (ie, consistent and repeated regardless of their

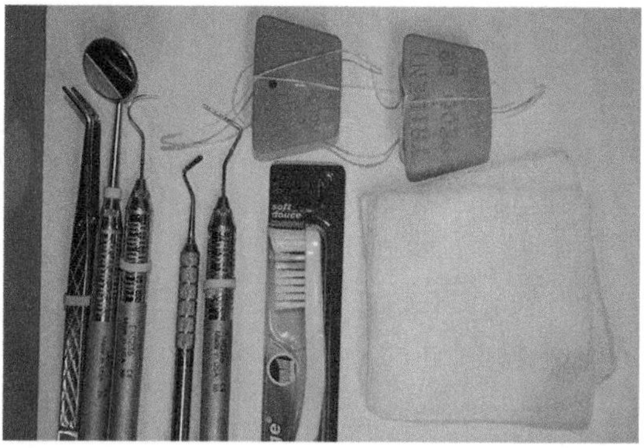

Fig. 1. Examination tray.

response). Consistent oral cleanliness over time will benefit the delivery and long-term success of dental care. Implications of cariogenic diet habits (including use of food rewards for shaping behaviors), self injurious behaviors, pouching of foods, or medication and side effects of oral medications are also significant risks for poor oral health. No matter how challenging for the oral health team, management of these threats is critical for the overall health of the patient. As daily effective oral health practice is the best means to prevent, reduce, and control oral infections, caregivers and agency daily care staff must receive proper training from capable and experienced oral health professionals, provide competent oral health cleansing to the patient as directed, and be monitored over time to assure effective outcomes.

THE INTRAORAL EXAMINATION BEGINS AND ENDS WITH ORAL CLEANLINESS

At the examination visit, the patient's oral cleanliness should be the first intraoral assessment. Depending on the clinician's impression of the patient's oral hygiene, the first intervention may be a toothbrush (**Fig. 1**). During the use of the toothbrush for oral cleansing, caregivers and daily care staff should remain silent as it is essential that the patient and dentist develop a trusting relationship through Tell-Show-Do and other behavior modification techniques (eg, voice control, contingency reinforcement, time out). During this activity, the provider describes the change in the patient's oral

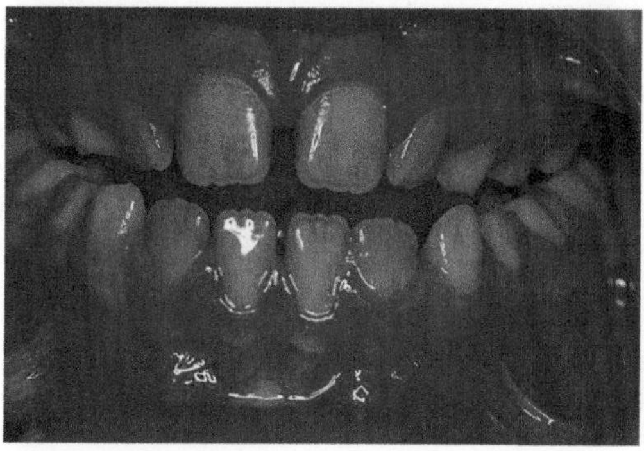

Fig. 2. Disclosing aid showing oral debris.

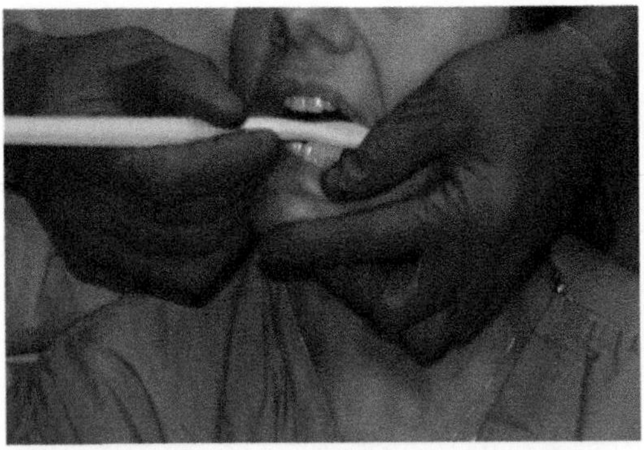

Fig. 3. Right-hand caregiver position.

cleanliness as the caregiver and patient (if possible) observes. This reflects the importance of oral cleanliness for the examination and treatment visits; which holds the caregiver, patient (if possible), and the provider accountable to this health goal that is shared by the oral health team. If possible, patients should actively participate in learning about their oral health by observing their examination with a patient mirror–independently or with caregiver support. This also serves to occupy one or both of their hands. Assertiveness and active communication by the dentist or hygienist is essential during the activity. To help the caregiver or patient appreciate the presence and implication of dental plaque, it may be helpful to have the caregiver and patient see an area of concern. To do this, wipe the tissues with moistened gauze, show the plaque-laden gauze, view the area that has been wiped clean, and the provider must discuss the cause and importance of home care and provide training. Illustrations or drawings by the dental professional may also assist caregiver and patient understanding. This exercise should be followed by reintroduction of a toothbrush to the patient, followed by the provider brushing the patient's oral tissues (ie, Tell-Show-Do). The patient's response during oral hygiene training should be noted and discussed with the patient (if possible) and caregiver. Patients who have the potential for self care but have difficulty staying on task or limitations for fine motor control may benefit from using disclosing aids **Fig. 2**. Disclosing aids enable caregivers to better view and direct the patient's self care as they and the patient can easily see where

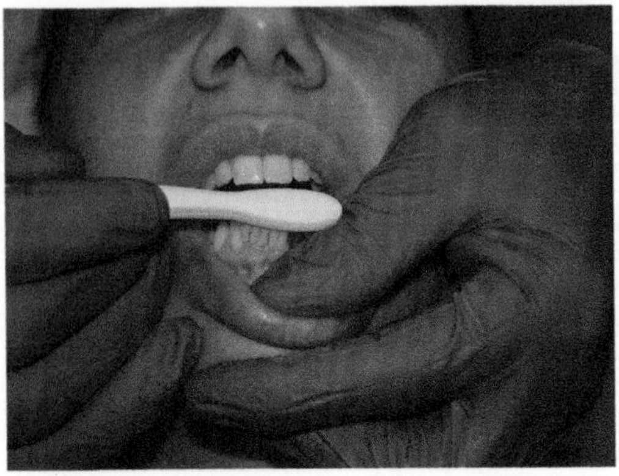

Fig. 4. Brushing lower interiors.

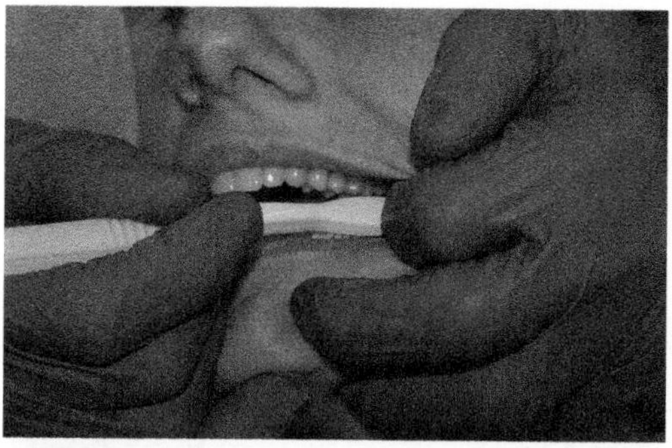

Fig. 5. Brushing lower left buccal.

staining persists. Disclosing aids are very helpful for the patient who can develop independence for self oral hygiene. Use of a timer may also facilitate patient staying on task for cleaning specific areas of concern. Rewards (eg, stickers leading to purchase of a nonedible prize) may also help to motivate patient learning.

THE PROPHYLAXIS VERSUS EFFECTIVE HOME ORAL HEALTH PRACTICE AS A STANDARD OF CARE FOR ORAL HEALTH FOR SPECIAL NEEDS

A prophylaxis is indicated when there are extrinsic accretions (ie, stain, tartar, calculus) that are not removed by the toothbrush or there is need to debride chronic gingival margin inflammation. Prophylaxis is regarded as a "standard of care" in dental care; however, its effect on oral health and dental care is temporary. As this service is commonly applied in dentistry, it has been our experience that the public has misconceptions about the long-term benefit of a dental prophylaxis, its value relative to oral health, and lack of appreciation for the need for home oral health practice. Also, caregivers do not receive sufficient and repeated demonstration and training to be able to provide daily oral health care to patients with special needs. We commonly observe that patients with poor oral hygiene who have had previous dental visits, do respond favorably to oral debridement with the toothbrush. After training, their caregivers are often able to take on the responsibility of home oral health practice. At subsequent visits, the authors observed obvious improvement in patients' gingival health and

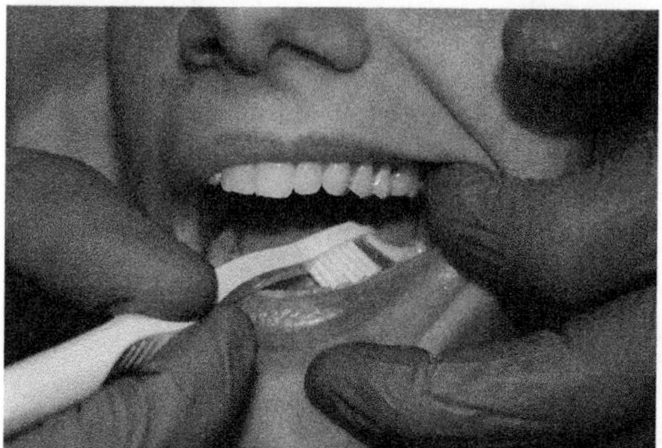

Fig. 6. Brushing lower left lingual.

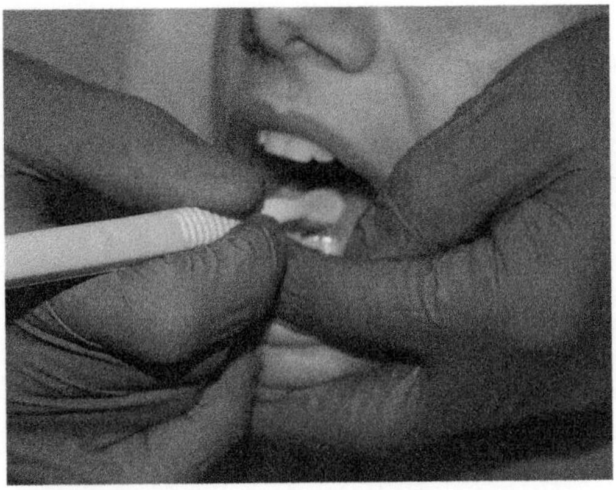

Fig. 7. Brushing lower right lingual.

reduction in oral debris. Long-term effectiveness of dental care is dependent on effective home oral health practice. Specifically, if the patient presents with oral debris:

Step 1. The oral condition should be demonstrated to the caregiver and patient (if possible), the caregiver and patient should be educated about the implication of the patient's condition, and the patient and caregiver should be trained on cleaning the patient's dentition with the toothbrush.

Step2. If extrinsic accretions are present on the patient's teeth that cannot be removed by the toothbrush, the patient should then receive a dental prophylaxis. It is important that the caregiver understands the importance of home oral health practice relative to a dental prophylaxis.

PATIENT MANAGEMENT FOR CAREGIVERS PROVIDING HOME ORAL HEALTH PRACTICE FOR SPECIAL NEEDS

Management of the patient during oral cleansing is the significant obstacle to home oral health practice. Specific obstacles to safe delivery of oral hygiene are: caregiver and patient positioning, head control, and hand positioning. As special needs patients

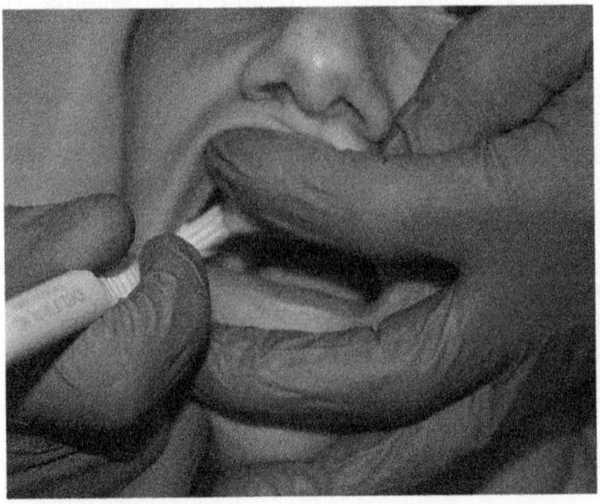

Fig. 8. Brushing upper right buccal.

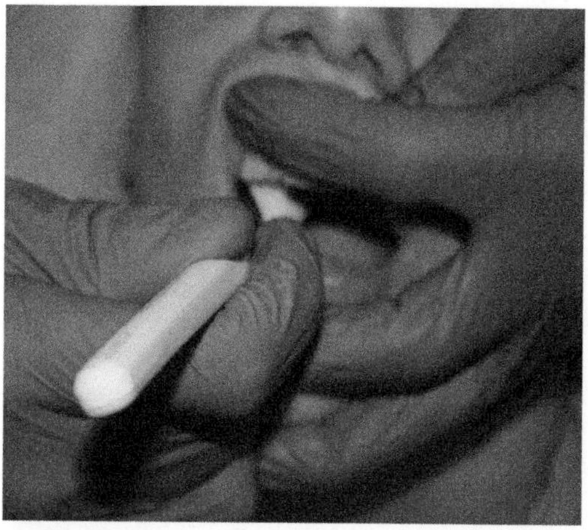

Fig. 9. Brushing upper right lingual.

(and very young children) can present an array of oppositional behaviors, health providers should personally experience the patient's reaction to oral cleansing or observe the caregiver's oral care so that they can provide suggestions to facilitate oral cleansing. Positioning of the caregiver relative to the patient is the first essential step to assure patient control and stability, and comfort and safety for the caregiver and patient. Basically, caregivers should provide patient oral cleansing in a position similar to that of the dental provider: behind the patient and to one side (11 o'clock for right-handed caregiver (**Fig. 3**); 1 o'clock for left-handed caregiver). This provides the best opportunity to control the patient's head and for the caregiver to position his or her hands to control the patient's oral musculature and gain access to the oral cavity (**Figs. 4–9**). This can be done with the patient seated and the caregiver standing behind the patient or the caregiver sitting as the patient is seated in front. A patient's wheelchair, as it may be customized, will also provide good support for patient management and caregiver positioning (**Fig. 10**). In addition to head control, a common obstacle to oral cleansing and dental care is hand interference (ie, patient grabs caregiver's or dental provider's hands). Stabilization of the patient's elbows can

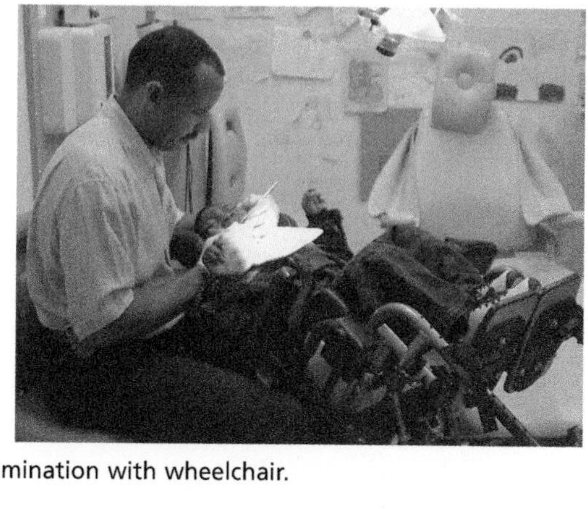

Fig. 10. Patient examination with wheelchair.

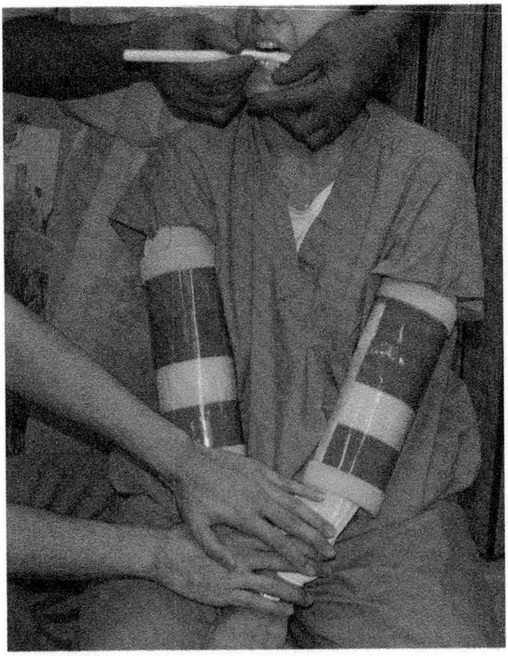

Fig. 11. Elbow stabilizers to control hand interference.

contribute to oral cleansing, provides safety for the patient and caregiver, and enables support personnel to restrict movement (**Fig. 11**). These aids (and others) which facilitate home oral health practice can be obtained through a prescription from the provider or can be developed by the oral health team (**Figs. 12, 13**).[18] It is essential that caregivers embrace home oral health practice as a necessity for health and well-being as important as any other care for special needs patients. As caregivers' attitudes and expectations begin to change, their charge will learn that home oral health practice is part of their daily routine. With time and attention, the patient's

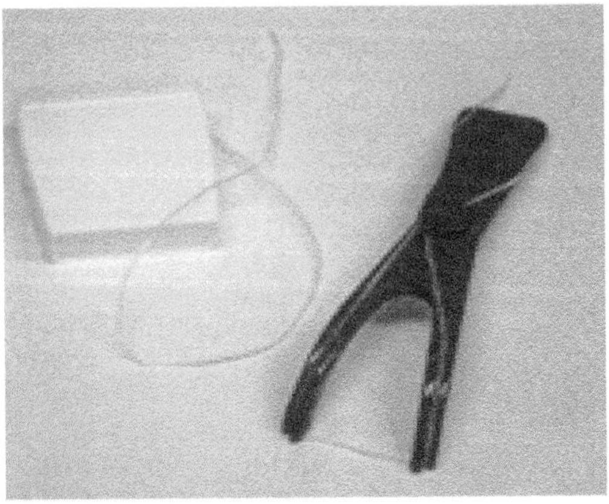

Fig. 12. Floss holder.

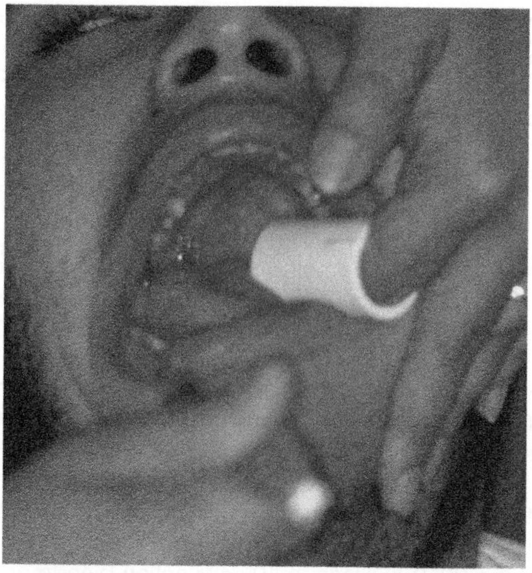

Fig. 13. PVC tubing to keep mouth open.

tolerance for home oral health practice and dental visits has the best potential to improve. Their health and dental care depends on it.

SUMMARY

Oral hygiene assessment at dental care visits provides the most reliable behavioral health indicator for the special needs population. As oral health is increasingly recognized as a foundation for general health and wellness and a primary indicator for the success of dental treatment, caregivers for special needs patients are an essential component of the oral health team and must become knowledgeable and competent in home oral health practice. Education and training for caregivers should be become a standard of care early in the first year of life for any child with developmental delay or any person, regardless of age, who experiences an illness or event that compromises their ability to provide self oral health care. Home oral health practice is a significant component in establishing healthy dental care at home. Given the implication of poor oral health to general health and health care costs, home oral health practice is a significant factor in dental care, general health, quality of life, and controlling health care costs.

ACKNOWLEDGMENTS

The authors acknowledge Forouzan Alvai and Nameeta Gupta (Health Sciences/ Pre-dental majors) at Stony Brook University for their literature search.

DENTAL PROFESSIONAL ORGANIZATIONS FOR SPECIAL NEEDS, WEB SITES

Special care in dentistry. Available at: http://www.scdonline.org/. Accessed September 1, 2008.

OMRDD Task Force on Special Dentistry. Available at: http://www.omr.state.ny.us/hp_dentistry_index.jsp. Accessed September 1, 2008.

Southern Association of Institutional Dentists. Available at: http://saiddent.org. Accessed September 1, 2008.

Healthy Kids Healthy Care. Available at: http://www.healthykids.us/. Accessed September 1, 2008.

National child care and information center. Available at: http://www.nccic.org/poptopics/itcurricula.html. Accessed September 1, 2008.

American Association of Pediatric Dentistry. Available at: http://www.aapd.org/pediatricinformation/brochurelist.asp. Accessed September 1, 2008.

Specialized care. Available at: http://www.specializedcare.com. Accessed September 1, 2008.

REFERENCES

1. Oral health in America: a report of the Surgeon General. Rockville (MD): US Department of Health and Human Services, National Institute of Dental and Craniofacial Research, National Institutes of Health; 2000.
2. McPherson M, Honberg L. Identification of children with special health care needs: a cornerstone to achieving healthy people 2010. Ambul Pediatr 2002;2:22–3.
3. Maternal and Child Health Bureau, Health Resources and Services Administration. All aboard the 2010 express: a 10-year action plan to achieve community-based service systems for children and youth with special needs and their families. Rockville (MD): MCHB, HRSA; 2001.
4. Standard 2–26, accreditation standards for dental education programs, Commission on Dental Accreditation, American Dental Association, Chicago: 2007.
5. Nowak AN, Casamassimo PS. The dental home: a primary care oral health concept. J Am Dent Assoc 2001;133:93–8.
6. Nowak AN, Casamassimo PS. Oral health in children with neurodevelopmental disorders and other CSHCN: Key research questions and implications for training. Mouradian W. Proceedings of a Conference. "Promoting Oral Health of Children with Neurodevelopmental Disabilities and Other Special Health Care Needs: Training and Research Agendas. May 4–5, 2001, University of Washington, Seattle.
7. Schwenk DM, Stoeckel DC, Rieken SE. Survey of special patient care programs at U.S. and Canadian dental schools. J Dent Educ 2007;71(9):1153–9.
8. McTigue DJ. Dental education and special-needs patients: challenges and opportunities. Pediatr Dent 2007;29(2):129–33.
9. Connick CM, Barsley RE. Dental neglect: definition and prevention in the Louisiana Developmental Centers for patients with MRDD. ASDC J Dent Child 1999;vol. 19(3):123–7.
10. Connick C, Palat M, Pugliese S, et al. The appropriate use of physical restraint: considerations. ASDC J Dent Child 2000;67(4):256–62, 231.
11. Connick C, Pugliese S, Willette J, et al. Desensitization: strengths and limitations of its use in dentistry for the patient with severe and profound mental retardation. ASDC J Dent Child 2000;67(4):250–5.
12. Isaksson R, Paulsson G, Fridlund B, et al. Evaluation of an oral health education program for nursing personnel in special housing facilities for the elderly. Part II: Clinical aspects. Spec Care Dentist 2000;20(3):109–13.
13. Glassman P. Practical protocols for the prevention of dental disease in community settings for people with special needs: preface. Spec Care Dentist 2003;23(5):157–9.
14. Glassman P, Miller CE. Effect of preventive dentistry training program for caregivers in community facilities on caregiver and client behavior and client oral hygiene. N Y State Dent J 2006;72(2):38–46.

15. Arch LM, Jenner AM, Whittle JG, et al. The views and expectations regarding dental care of the parents of children with special dental needs: a survey in the County of Cheshire, England. Int J Paediatr Dent 1994;4(2):127–32.
16. Akpabio A, Klausner CP, Inglehart MR, et al. Mothers'/guardians' knowledge about promoting children's oral health. J Dent Hyg 2008;82(1) [Epub2008 Jan 1].
17. Barks L, Lord D. Oral sensitivity, dental health and prevention. The Exceptional Parent 2002;32(12):82–3.
18. Day J, Martin MD, Chin M, et al. Efficacy of a sonic toothbrush for plaque removal by caregivers in a special needs population. Spec Care Dentist 1998;18(5): 202–6.

Index

Note: Page numbers of article titles are in **boldface** type.

Dent Clin N Am 53 (2009) 389–397
doi:10.1016/S0011-8532(09)00009-3

B

C

J

L

M

N

O

P

R

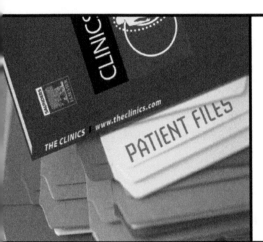